Speech Protocols in Audiology

Speech Protocols in Audiology

Edited by

Ralph R. Rupp, Ph.D.
Professor of Education and Audiology
Program in Special Education,
Speech and Hearing Sciences
School of Education
The University of Michigan
Ann Arbor, Michigan

Kenneth G. Stockdell, Sr., M.S.
Assistant Professor of Audiology
Speech and Hearing Clinic
Middle Tennessee State University
Murfreesboro, Tennessee

Grune & Stratton
A Subsidiary of Harcourt Brace Jovanovich, Publishers
New York London Toronto Sydney San Francisco

Library of Congress Cataloging in Publication Data
Main entry under title:

Speech protocols in audiology.

Includes bibliographical references and index.
1. Audiometry, Speech. I. Rupp, Ralph R.
II. Stockdell, Kenneth G.
RF294.5.S6S64 617.8′9 80-12120
ISBN 0-8089-1254-2

Grune & Stratton, Inc.
111 Fifth Avenue
New York, New York 10003

Distributed in the United Kingdom by
Academic Press, Inc. (London) Ltd.
24/28 Oval Road, London NW 1

Library of Congress Catalog Number 80-12120
International Standard Book Number 0-8089-1254-2

Printed in the United States of America

Contents

Acknowledgments

The following individuals and publishing houses are gratefully acknowledged for granting us permission to reprint material from scholarly works. We express our appreciation to those whose tables and illustrations are credited throughout the text of this book, as well as to the following whose statements are more effective quoted than paraphrased:

To Ada Z. Heavenrich for permission to quote in Chapter 1 from her unpublished master's essay, "A view from within: a consideration of how hearing loss is mediated into behavior," Wayne State University, Detroit, Michigan, 1964.

To Derek A. Sanders and Prentice-Hall, Inc., for permission to quote in Chapter 2 from *Aural Rehabilitation,* 1971, and from *Auditory Perception of Speech: An Introduction to Principles and Problems,* 1977. Reprinted by permission of Prentice-Hall, Inc., Englewood Cliffs, New Jersey.

To The American Speech-Language-Hearing Association (formerly The American Speech and Hearing Association) for permission to quote in Chapter 2 from "Hearing Impairment and the Audiologist" (Career Information Bulletin), 1973, and in Chapter 4 from "Guidelines for Determining the Threshold Level for Speech," May, 1979.

To Thomas Tillman and Academic Press for permission to quote in Chapters 2 and 4 from T. Tillman and W. Olsen's "Speech audiometry." In J. Jerger (Ed.), *Modern Developments in Audiology* (2nd ed.). New York: Academic Press, 1973.

To Norma Hopkinson and The Williams & Wilkins Company for permission to quote in Chapter 4 from "Speech reception threshold." In

J. Katz (Ed.), *Handbook of Clinical Audiology* (2nd ed.). Baltimore: Williams & Wilkins, 1978.

To Prentice-Hall, Inc., for permission to quote in Chapter 4 from Frederick N. Martins's *Introduction to Audiology,* © 1975. Reprinted by permission of Prentice-Hall, Inc., Englewood Cliffs, New Jersey.

To the *Journal of the Michigan Speech and Hearing Association* for permission to quote in Chapter 9 from Harlie R. Smith and Ralph R. Rupp's "Determination of the most comfortable loudness range (MCL-R) for normal-hearing subjects and subjects with sensori-neural hearing loss," 1973, *9,* 65–70. Reprinted with permission of both the authors and the Journal.

To Joseph Smaldino and the Academy of Rehabilitative Audiology for permission to review in Chapter 12 a membership questionnaire report on hearing and evaluation procedures, as reported to the Academy in November, 1977.

Preface

Twenty-four audiologists collaborated to create this book, *Speech Protocols in Audiology.* Fifteen major contributors compiled the first fifteen chapters, and nine associate contributors gave input to the final chapter.

The assignment given to each major contributor was a general one: compile a clinical statement on the state of the art in speech-related audiology on your special topic. The editors consider that the assignment for each contributor was carried out effectively.

Since fifteen authors may represent at least as many philosophical positions (or biases), no major attempt was made by the editors to force the contributors into a single philosophical stance. As a result, the eclectic reader may find that somewhat divergent philosophies appear in different chapters as different authors discuss related topics. Diversity of opinion may suggest to our readers that, indeed, there may be more than just one route to audiologic "heaven."

The evolution of audiology as a free-standing profession occurred in large part from efforts of enthusiastic audiologists in sharing, comparing, and synthesizing. We feel that the following discussions by our twenty-four authors contribute to this professional evolution. We acknowledge and appreciate the heavy commitments of time made by our contributors.

The editors report that the creation of this text was exciting and exhilarating as well as challenging and frustrating. In retrospect, keeping twenty-four busy audiologists moving on a voluntary labor of professional love was an interesting experience. We offer you, our readers, our collective work for your evaluation and reaction.

Finally, to our wives, Jane and Jo Ann, we wish to express our appreciation for permission to spend so much time on this project.

RALPH R. RUPP, PH.D.
KENNETH G. STOCKDELL, SR., M.S.

Contributors

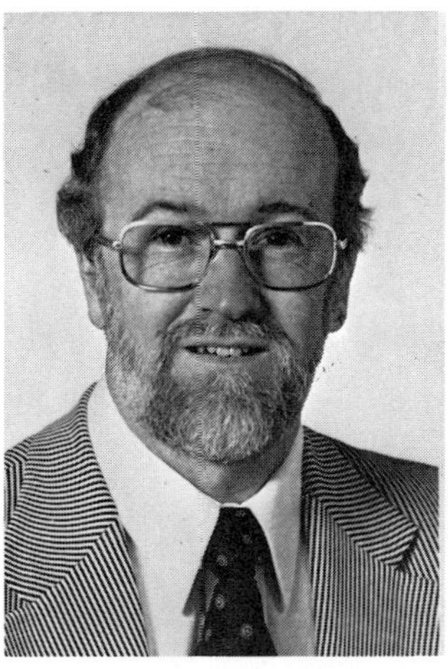

Harold L. Bate, Ph.D.
Professor of Audiology
Department of Speech Pathology and Audiology
Western Michigan University
Kalamazoo, Michigan

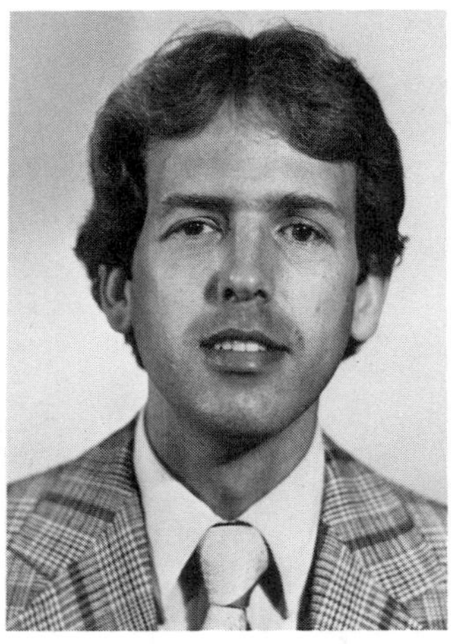

H. B. Calder, Ph.D.
Assistant Professor of Education and Audiology
Program in Special Education, Speech and Hearing Sciences
School of Education
University of Michigan
Ann Arbor, Michigan

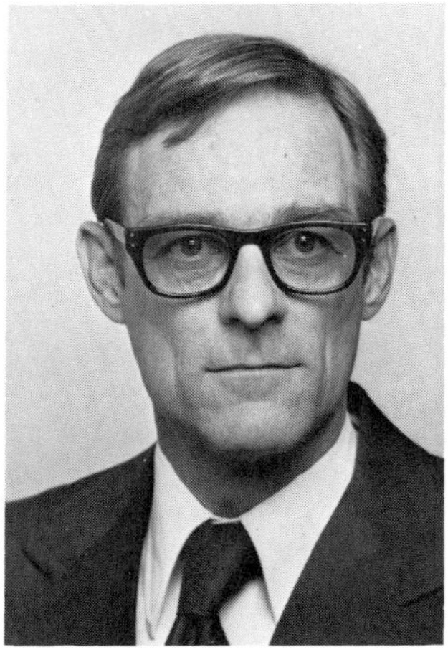

J. C. Cooper, Jr., Ph.D.
Associate Professor
Division of Otorhinolaryngology
University of Texas Health Science Center at San Antonio
San Antonio, Texas

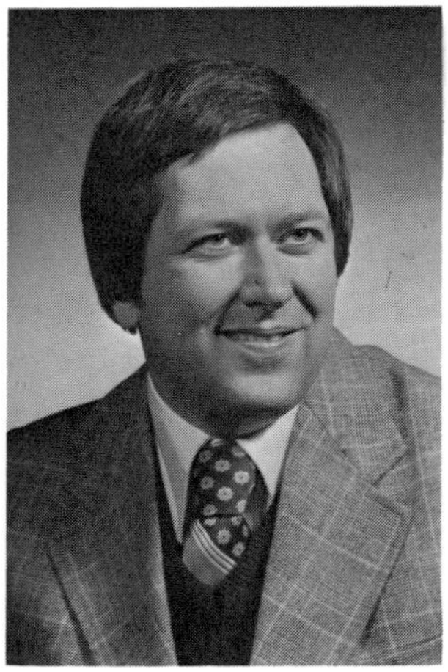

Dean C. Garstecki, Ph.D.
Associate Professor of Audiology and Hearing Impairment
Program of Audiology and Hearing
Northwestern University
Evanston, Illinois

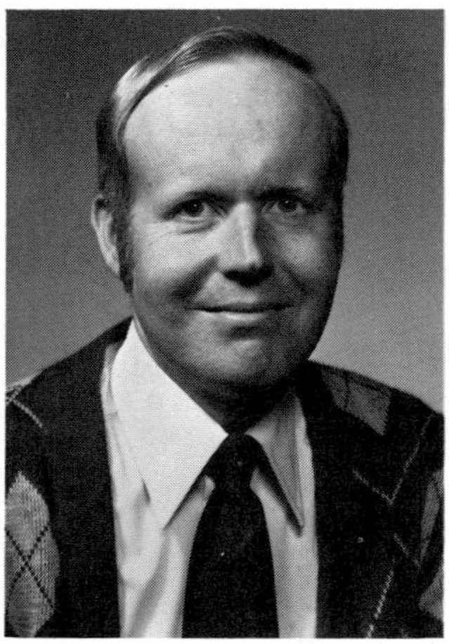

Thomas F. Hemeyer, Ph.D.
Associate Professor
Coordinator of Audiology
Department of Speech Pathology and Audiology
Ball State University
Muncie, Indiana

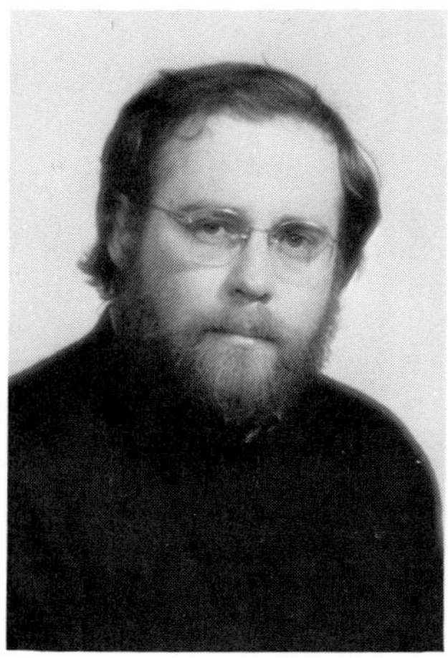

Raymond M. Hurley, Ph.D.
Assistant Professor
Department of Communication Disorders
University of Rhode Island
Kingston, Rhode Island

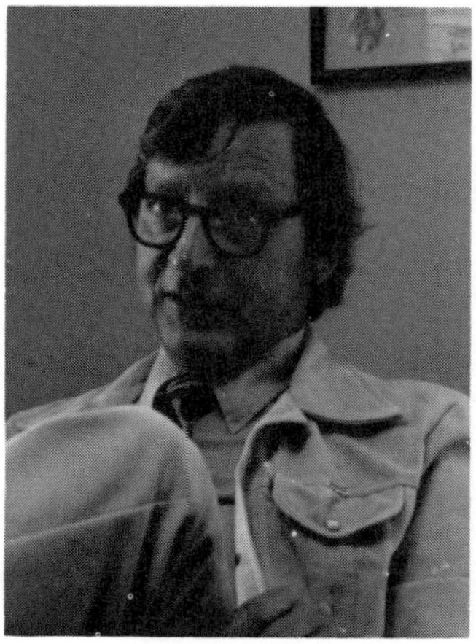

Roger N. Kasten, Ph.D.
Professor of Audiology
Department of Communicative
Disorders and Sciences
Wichita State University
Wichita, Kansas

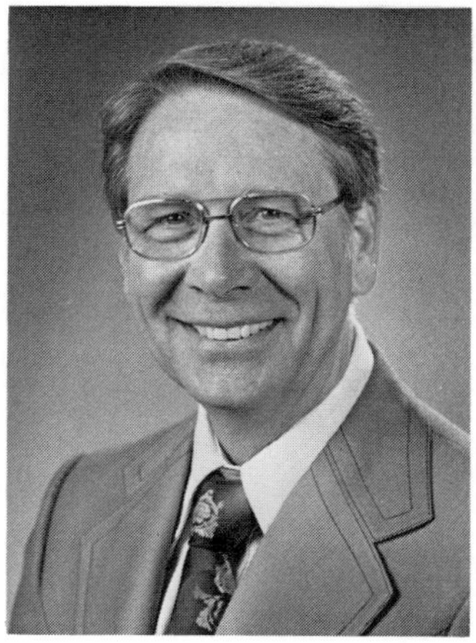

Robert L. McCroskey, Ph.D.
Professor of Logopedics
Department of Communicative
Disorders and Sciences
Wichita State University
Wichita, Kansas

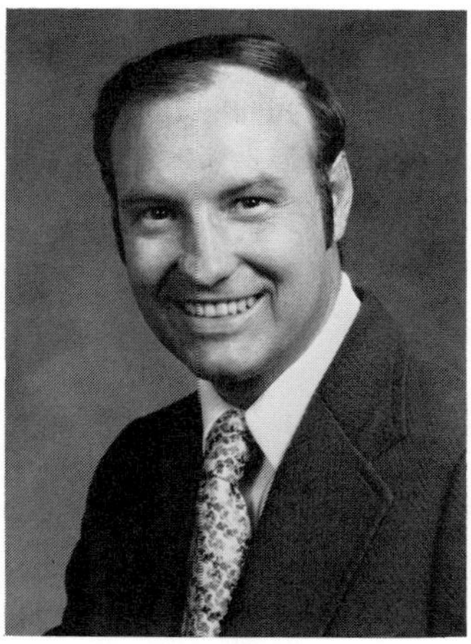

Robert M. McLauchlin, Ph.D.
Professor and Chairman
Communication Disorders
Central Michigan University
Mount Pleasant, Michigan

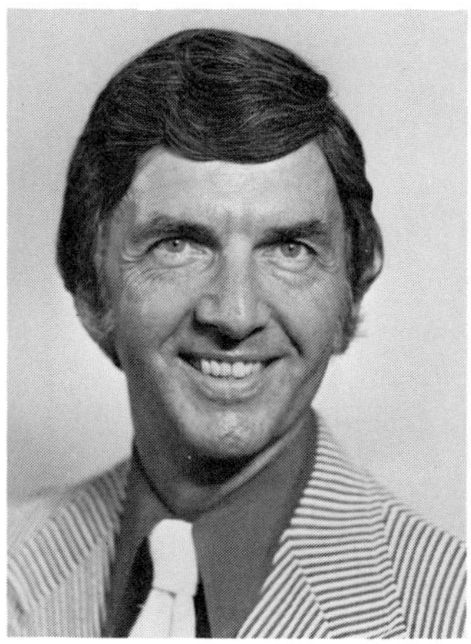

Ralph R. Rupp, Ph.D.
Professor of Education and
Audiology
Program in Special Education,
Speech and Hearing Sciences
School of Education
University of Michigan
Ann Arbor, Michigan

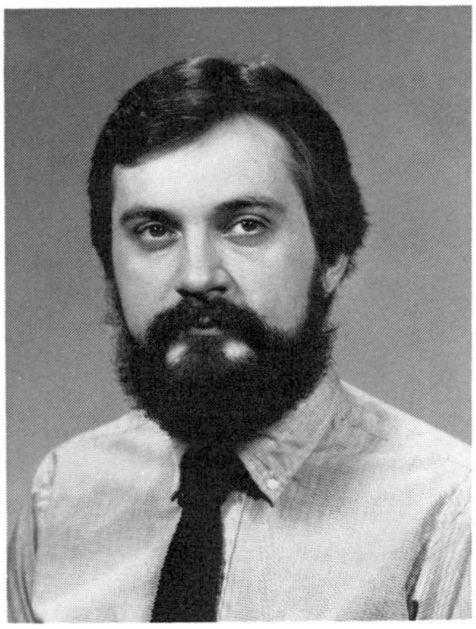

Roger A. Ruth, Ph.D.
Assistant Professor
Director of Audiology
Department of Otolaryngology and Maxillofacial Surgery
University of Virginia Medical Center
Charlottesville, Virginia

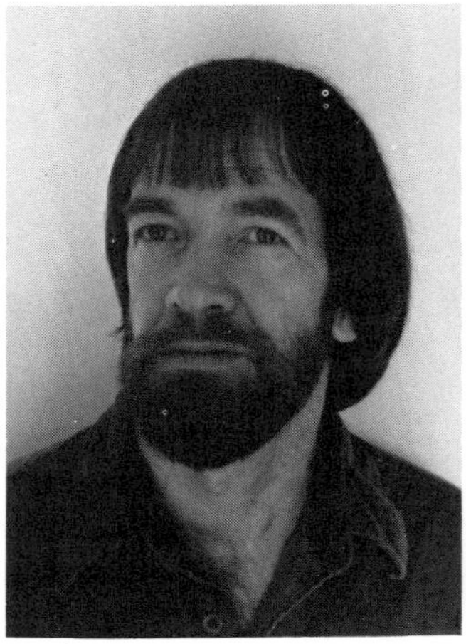

Zahrl G. Schoeny, Ph.D.
Associate Professor
Department of Speech Pathology and Audiology
University of Virginia
Charlottesville, Virginia

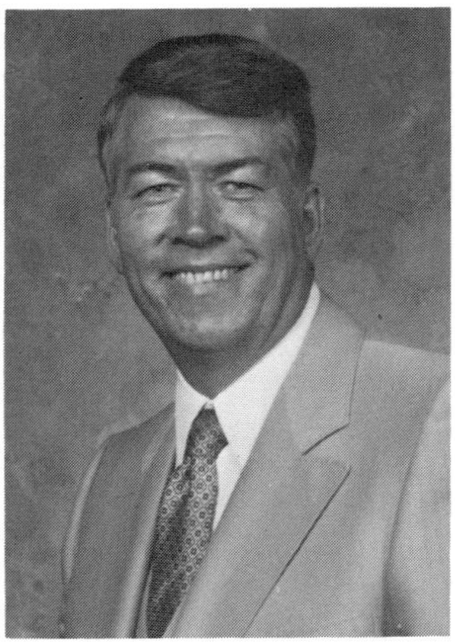

Kenneth G. Stockdell, Sr., M.S.
Assistant Professor of Audiology
Speech and Hearing Clinic
Middle Tennessee State University
Murfreesboro, Tennessee

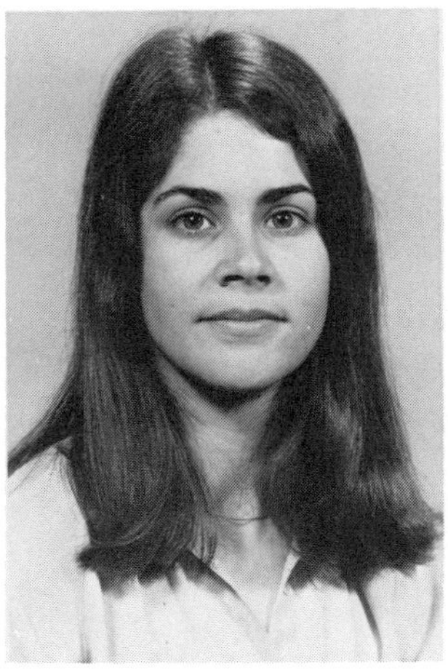

Debara L. Tucci, M.S.
Audiologist
Department of Otolaryngology and Maxillofacial Surgery
University of Virginia Medical Center
Charlottesville, Virginia

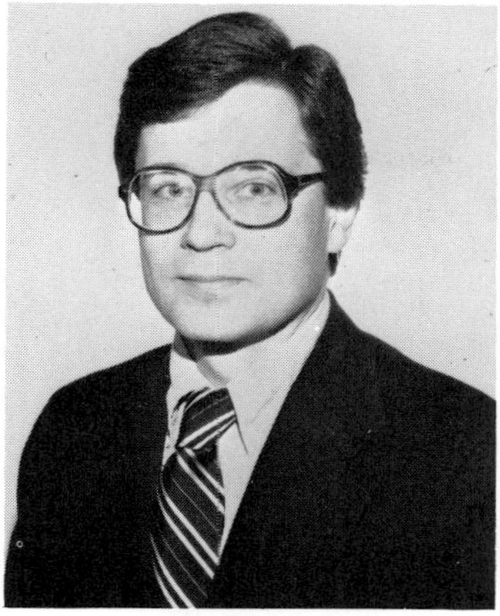

Steven C. White, Ph.D.
Assistant Professor
Department of Audiology and Speech Sciences
Michigan State University
East Lansing, Michigan

Associate Contributors

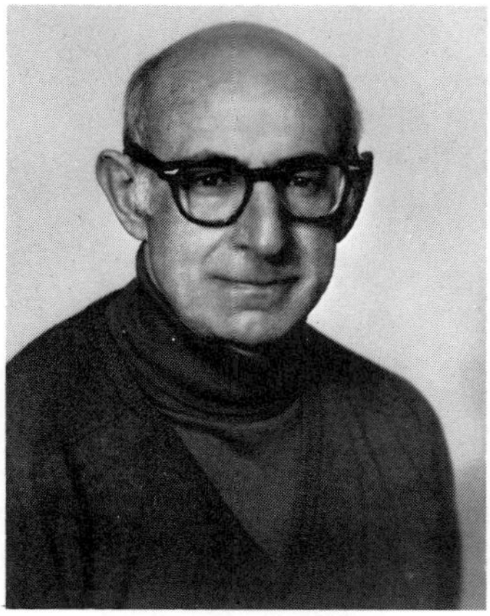

Moe Bergman, Ed.D.
Professor
School for Communication Disorders
Sackler School of Medicine
Tel-Aviv University
Tel-Aviv, Israel

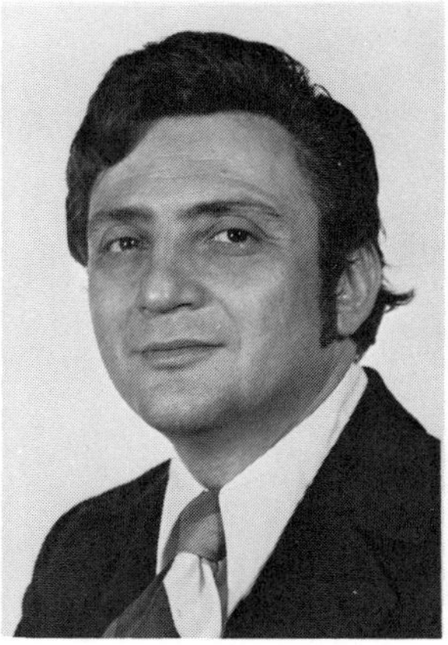

Charles I. Berlin, Ph.D.
Kresge Hearing Research Laboratory
Louisiana State University Medical Center
New Orleans, Louisiana

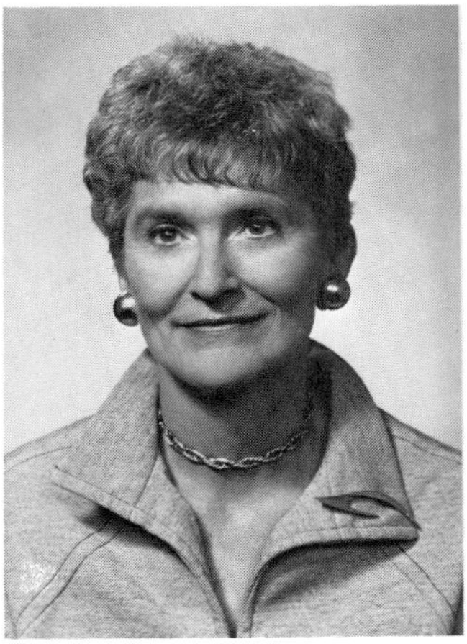

Marion P. Downs, M.A.
Associate Professor of Otolaryngology
Audiology Division
University of Colorado Medical Center
Denver, Colorado

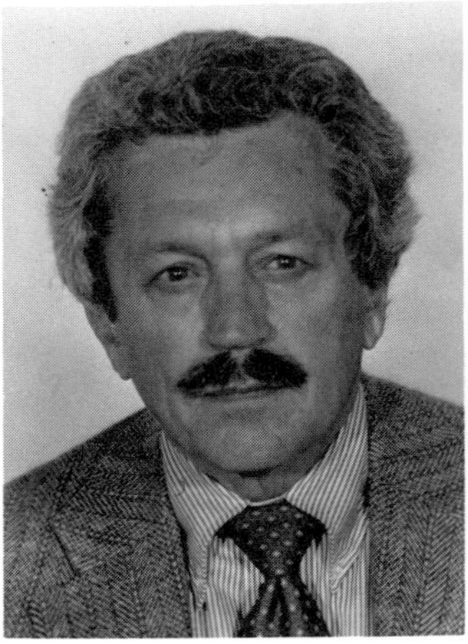

Victor P. Garwood, Ph.D.
Professor of Audiology
University of Southern California
Los Angeles, California

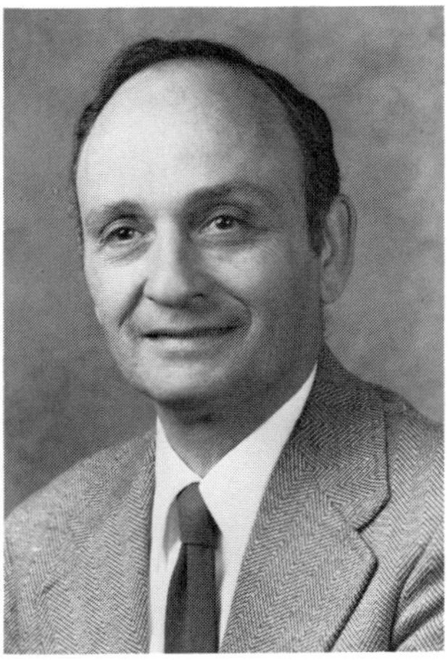

David P. Goldstein, Ph.D.
Professor of Audiology
Purdue University
Lafayette, Indiana

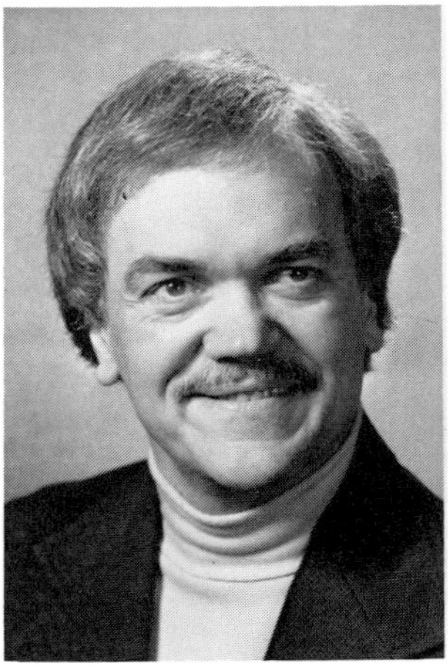

David M. Lipscomb, Ph.D.
Professor of Audiology and Speech Pathology
University of Tennessee
Knoxville, Tennessee

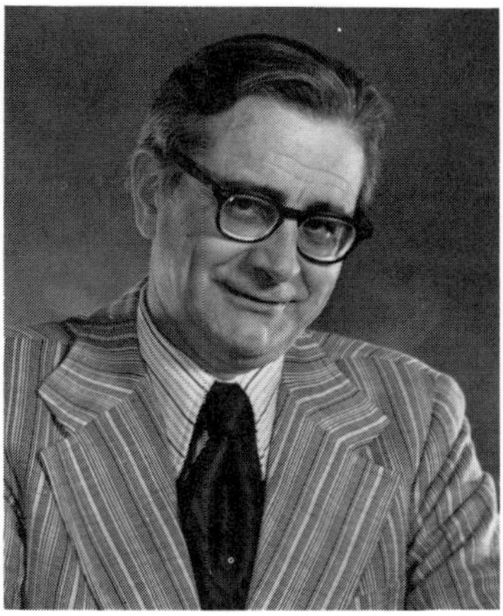

John J. O'Neill, Ph.D.
Professor of Audiology
University of Illinois at
Urbana-Champaigne
Urbana, Illinois

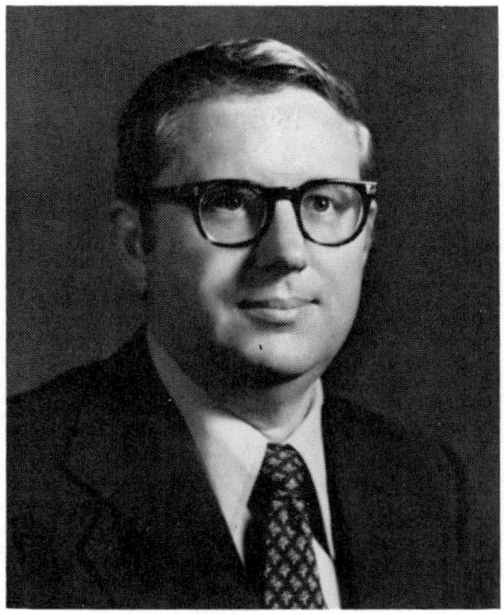

Phillip A. Yantis, Ph.D.
Professor
Department of Speech and Hearing
Sciences
University of Washington
Seattle, Washington

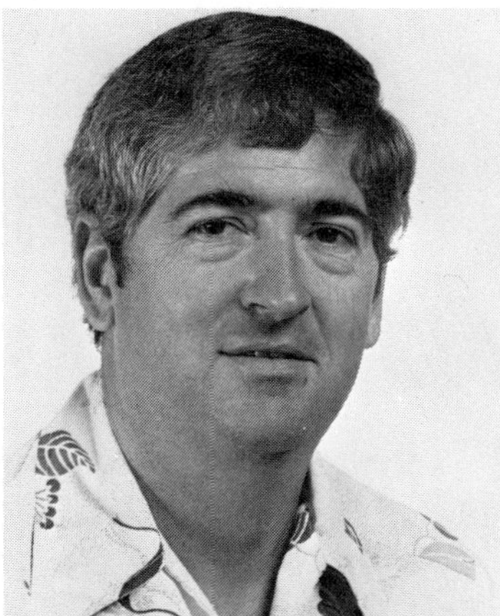

James T. Yates, Ph.D.
Professor and Chairman
Division of Speech Pathology and
Audiology
University of Hawaii at Manoa
Honolulu, Hawaii

Speech Protocols in Audiology

Ralph R. Rupp, Ph.D.

1
The Human Communicative Function

"To hear is as natural and effortless an occurrence as it is invisible. Man would as soon ask himself how breathing keeps him physically alive as how hearing keeps him psychologically alive" (Levine, 1960, p. 18). But to people who no longer hear naturally and effortlessly, the invisibility of their sensory deficits compound the frustration and anxiety created by their handicapping and disabling hearing loss. The reason for their communicative distress is confusing. They look very normal; there are no obvious visual indications of impairment; but the dehumanizing experience of unresolved hearing loss may be far more damaging than any other more obvious handicap.

"Contrary to popular opinion, hearing problems are more serious in their consequences than visual problems. Hearing is the avenue for communication, and the vast majority of what we learn throughout our lives occurs through hearing and speech" (Alexander Graham Bell Association for the Deaf, 1976).

MAN: A VERBAL CREATURE

Man is a verbally communicative being, or at least he tries to be such if he is able to speak and hear with relative ease. It is estimated that approximately 70 percent of an adult's waking activities are related to active communicative input and output by the process of speaking, listening, reading, or writing (Butler, 1975). Listening to others—on the job, out on the town, at home—constitutes the major activity of this statistical adult and involves 45 percent of his communicative time. With even a mild hearing loss, the adult will encounter deterrents to effortless listening; with a moderate to severe hearing problem, the potential for listening distress increases markedly. It is not surprising that a hearing and listening difficulty can elicit such psychological concern.

Assuming normalcy of hearing on the part of his constituent listeners, Hayakawa (1949, p. v.) wrote that "Thoughtful people in all walks of life feel, therefore, the need of systematic help in the huge task that confronts all of us today, namely, that of interpreting and evaluating the verbally received communications that pour in on us from all sides." If people who hear normally may need systematic help with this demanding task of listening effectively, how much more crucial it will be for hearing-impaired listeners to partake of a program of systematic and specific help to maintain their listening effectiveness.

SPEECH EQUALS LANGUAGE

Levine and Hayakawa agree that during the course of centuries of mutual interaction in the evolution of humankind, verbal language sporadically or systematically developed within each tribe or group into a "system of agreements" that we can call language. These symbols, used by both early and modern man, are manipulated and arranged by the speaker and received by the listener as verbal symbolic communications.

One person speaks; another listens. If these symbols have a cultural commonality, and if both speaker and listener code these pourings of symbols in sequence correctly, effective verbal communication results. If, however, either member of the communicative system falters in the interaction, the effectiveness of the verbal interaction is reduced (Carhart, 1969, p. 5; Fairbanks, 1954). In the twentieth century, the most common cause of verbal communicative failure can be attributed to hearing deficit or dysfunction on the part of the listener. Some 20 million (or more) Americans are estimated to have hearing losses severe enough to impede easy reception of speech. Verbal communication is oral speech; speech audiometry measures hearing function by employing verbal symbols common to the culture.

HEARING LOSS EQUALS WITHDRAWAL

Lest the reader be lulled into complacency regarding the debacle of unresolved or unadmitted hearing loss, consider the following observation by Gardner (1975): "There is every reason to believe that mental withdrawal from the world can be brought about by a lack of interpersonal relationships. Serious hearing impairment . . . may be one of the most important factors triggering what is commonly called senility [in older individuals]." Hearing loss is a personal disaster. The marshalling of audiologic forces to identify individuals with such handicaps and to provide them and their families with postmedical counseling and training is crucial to their continuing mental health.

The goal for each person with an irreversible hearing loss is to keep in communicative contact with important environments and the people in them.

EFFECTING AUDITORY REACH

Heavenrich (1964) labels this positive interactive contact "auditory reach." When hearing-impaired clients have built an effective listening program and when each person with whom they converse employs a cooperative approach, then improved interpersonal communication will result. As long as the background environment is relatively quiet, then the hearing-impaired older individual will be able to "reach across" auditorially and will be an effective listener. Heavenrich realistically states:

> Regardless of effort or degree of motivation the auditorially handicapped person can "hear" only within the limits of his auditory reach. . . . The point beyond which the hearing-impaired person cannot function is determined by factors in the environment, generally unpredictable, but many of which can be overcome by other persons present in a given situation. When others move in to meet the handicapped individual at the boundaries within which he is arbitrarily confined, intelligent cooperation functions to extend the limits, permit him to participate within the group, fill the gaps in his knowledge, and for the particular situation, remove the handicap.

In this environment, auditory reach is maximal, and, while the hearing loss remains, the handicap is nonexistent. It takes three factors for a hearing-impaired person to effectively reach auditorially, across a communicative interaction: (1) a well-motivated and well-trained hearing-impaired listener; (2) a cooperative and compassionate communicator; and (3) an idealized environment in which to talk and listen that is as quiet as possible. If all three factors are present, near normalcy of verbal interaction results, and effective auditory reach is achieved. When any of these factors is altered negatively, then auditory reach is reduced, and the handicap is again present.

Heavenrich reminds us that it is not hearing loss, per se, that handicaps the listener; rather, the true demoralizing facet comes from not knowing what is going on in the immediate environment. The goal is to provide a program for hearing-impaired clients to keep them tuned in, auditorially, to what is going on!

Diagnostic speech audiological techniques can help identify the magnitude of the individual's hearing deficit. Rehabilitative audiological approaches should provide the plan to enhance the individual's auditory reach.

"Because he hears, man feels himself always a part of the context of living" (Levine, 1960, p. 24). If one cannot hear, one cannot easily handle the verbal outpourings of contemporaries. If the hearing deficit remains unacknowledged or unresolved, then one's psychological alertness withers, auditory reach shortens, and psychological detachment and withdrawal may occur.

Helen Keller is reported to have said that the sound of the human voice is the most vital stimulus of all because "it brings language, sets thoughts astir, and keeps us in the intellectual company of man" (1933, p. 68). Audiologists play a crucial role in keeping their patients in the intellectual company of their peers.

REFERENCES

Alexander Graham Bell Association for the Deaf. Statement on deafness. *Hearing Alert,* 1976.

Butler, K. Auditory perceptual skills: their measurement and remediation with preschool and school-age children (an ASHA short course). *National Convention Program of the American Speech and Hearing Association.* 1975, 54.

Carhart, R. (Ed.) *Human Communication and Its Disorders—An Overview.* Bethesda, Maryland: U.S. Department of Health, Education, and Welfare, 1969.

Fairbanks, G. A theory of the speech mechanism as a servo system. *Journal of Speech and Hearing Disorders.* 1954, *19,* 133–139.

Gardner, W. Hearing loss—the route to senility? *Audecibel* 1975, *24,* pp. 74; 76.

Hayakawa, S. *Language in thought and action.* New York: Harcourt, Brace & Co., 1949.

Heavenrich, A. *A view from within: a consideration of how hearing loss is mediated into behavior.* Unpublished master's thesis, Wayne State University, Detroit, Michigan, 1964.

Keller, H. *Helen Keller in Scotland.* London: Methuen & Co., 1933.

Levine, E. *The psychology of deafness.* New York: Columbia University Press, 1960.

Ralph R. Rupp, Ph.D.
Kenneth G. Stockdell, Sr., M.S.

2
The Roles of Speech Protocols in Audiology

AUDIOLOGY: SCOPE AND DEFINITION

The more than 20 million Americans who have measurable amounts of hearing impairment are the people for whom, ultimately, this book is written. Their problems are, simply stated, hearing problems. They do not hear or understand as well as their relatives and friends. These people with hearing losses may not admit to thinking very much about their hearing problems, but the profession of audiology is concerned about them. For those five to ten percent of the 20 million who have medically resolvable hearing losses (Canfield, 1949, p. 5), the audiologist would like to measure the potential improvement and share his findings with the medical specialist who is responsible for the treatment of the reversible hearing loss. For the 90 to 95 percent of the 20 million who have irreversible hearing losses, the diagnostic findings will identify the extent of the hearing problem and suggest the magnitude of necessary postmedical rehabilitation. For the less than one percent of the 20 million who may have life-endangering hearing losses, the diagnostic procedures would enable identification of such unique losses so that lifesaving medical care may be initiated.

The diagnostician is concerned about measuring the hearing losses or dysfunctions of these people. The book is about such measurement techniques with a primary focus on speech-assessing approaches. The rehabilitative audiologist will employ similar speech-oriented techniques to determine the need for auditory remediation or rehabilitation, to assess the efficiency of personally worn amplification devices, and to evaluate the effectiveness of the intervention approach employed to improve oral-communicative reception.

Historical Beginnings

Many fields have made contributions to the audiological model. Davis and Silverman (1970, p. 5) identify the following as providing the major contributions to the field of audiology: (1) education; (2) medicine; (3) physics; (4) physiology; (5) psychology; and (6) sociology. For an exciting meander book across the centuries to the beginnings of the audiologic experience, the reader will want to review Feldmann's *History of Audiology* (1970). The first reference is to an Egyptian manuscript written about 1550 B.C. in which remedial efforts were attempted on certain hearing disorders. Feldman also carefully summarizes many of the important contributions European researchers and clinicans have made to audiology.

Earlier, in 1938, Stevens and Davis came out with their classical hearing science text entitled *Hearing—Its Psychology and Physiology.* The classical text in the U.S. was written by Bunch (1943) entitled *Clinical Audiometry.* In 1946, Polyak, McHugh, and Judd presented their work, *The Human Ear in Anatomical Transparencies.* In 1947, Davis and Silverman's *Hearing and Deafness: A Guide for Laymen* was published. Two years later, Watson and Tolan published their work, *Hearing Texts and Hearing Instruments.* In 1949, also, Canfield's *Audiology—The Science of Hearing* identified the new field with an appropriate label. In 1949, Wever's *Theory of Hearing* was published.

Definition

Since the term *audiology* came into professional use as a result of governmental action in the 1940s, it is appropriate to cite a definition from the U.S. Department of Labor's *Dictionary of Occupational Titles* (1965, p. 30).

> An audiologist is one who: specializes in diagnostic evaluation, habilitative and rehabilitative services, and research related to hearing. Determines range, nature, and degree of hearing function related to patient's auditory efficiency (communication needs), using electroacoustic instrumentation, such as pure-tone and speech audiometers, and galvanic skin response equipment. Coordinates audiometric results with other diagnostic data, such as education, medical, social, and behavioral information. Differentiates between organic and nonorganic hearing disabilities through the evaluation of total response pattern and use of such acoustic tests as Stenger and delayed speech feedback. Plans, directs, conducts, or

participates in habilitative and rehabilitative programs including counseling, guidance, auditory training, speechreading, and speech conservation. May conduct research in physiology, pathology, biophysics, and psychophysics of auditory systems. May design and develop clinical and research procedures and apparatus. . . . May act as consultant to educational, medical, and other professional groups. May teach art and science of audiology and direct scientific projects. . . . May specialize in fields, such as industrial audiology, geriatric audiology, pediatric audiology, and research audiology.

The following summarizing definition of an "audiologist" comes from a 1973 career information bulletin of the American Speech and Hearing Association:

An audiologist is a professional concerned with normal and defective hearing, prevention of hearing loss, identification of hearing loss in individuals, and rehabilitation of those who have hearing problems. The audiologist may use tests and instruments such as the audiometer to find out whether a person has a hearing loss and what kind of loss it is. The audiologist works in a variety of ways to help the person make best use of his hearing, possibly through a hearing aid or other kinds of amplification, through training in speech (lip) reading, or through many other techniques. Audiologists also perform research on the hearing problems.

Basically, audiology is concerned with assessing human hearing performance, with determining how such performance may have been altered by damage or obstruction in the auditory system, and with finding ways to improve the communicative function of individuals with irreversible hearing loss.

Normal Hearing Bases

The field of audiology did not appear instantaneously and fully mature in the educational, medical, and rehabilitative environments of the 1940s and 1950s.

Its base of normative standards is found in earlier works in physics, physiology, acoustics, and psychology. As an emerging field, in the mid 1940s, audiology played an eclectic role. The classical works of research psychologists were incorporated into a base that became the statistical standard for judging an individual's auditory performance as normal or abnormal. For all subjective responses that are elicited in any audiologic diagnostic procedure, there are normal bases of performance *against which* the individual's response is measured. It is that comparison with a normal standard that provides the power of the diagnostic instrument of any specific auditory performance. To review: the primary focus of this book is the assessment of such auditory performance as evaluated through the use of speech stimuli.

Assessing Abnormal Performance

When an individual's performance on a specific diagnostic task is different from the expected normal value, we are concerned with the extent of the abnormal response. In this regard, it becomes the evaluator's responsibility to define the responses in terms of identifying the location of the damage or malfunction in the auditory system.

The audiological search for the site of lesion does not suggest that the clinician is attempting to determine the cause of the malperformance, but rather in what section, or area, of the total auditory system the subject's performance suggests a breakdown in auditory functioning.

Obviously, the medical diagnosis, with its accompanying specified causes, is the responsibility of the physician. In cooperation with the physician who does the physical examination, the audiologist gathers performance data to support the physician's findings.

For example, if a child shows a moderate hearing loss by air conducted signals, but also shows normal threshold responses to pure tones presented by bone conduction, and the otologist finds a fluid-filled middle ear, then the audiological performance findings are in agreement with the otological physical findings. A medical diagnosis of otitis media in this case would have audiologic corroboration by the subject's performance.

In each case of abnormal auditory performance, there is concern to build a battery of performance results that are consistent with the projected location of the malfunction in the auditory tract.

Unlike the relatively uncomplicated case of middle ear fluid cited earlier, the presence of an obstruction in the eighth nerve elicits performances that are quite different. In such a case, minimal elevation of hearing level may be present, unusually poor understanding of speech may be noticed, and loudness growth may be similar to that found with individuals who hear normally. Otologically and neurologically, these signs point to a transmission problem unique to the cranial nerves that transverse the internal auditory meatus. Again, medical, physical, and auditory performance findings should be in agreement. In such a case, the physician would probably involve a number of additional medical specialists to assist in locating the precise anatomical location of the possible tumor. In this case, the concern is not merely resolution of the physical problem causing the hearing loss, but also the implementation of a life-protecting course of medical action.

To recapitulate: When auditory performance is found to be abnormal, there is an attempt to identify the location—not the cause—of the auditory malperformance. There is a relatively complete battery of diagnostic audiologic tests to help the clinician do this. These tests are designed to assess human auditory performance. When auditory malperformance is evident, the audiologist's task is to attempt to locate the site of the lesion causing the abnormal performance results.

Rehabilitative Approaches

When the otologist suggests that a subject's hearing loss is not amenable to a medical or surgical program, and when his or her review rules out the presence of any life-threatening pathology, the audiologist outlines a plan of communicative improvement with the subject. With an irreversible hearing loss that interferes with normal auditory reception, the subject will probably be in need of a long-range habilitative or rehabilitative program of audiological help. As an example, the very young child with a moderate sensori neural hearing loss as a result of maternal rubella will need several years of habilitative work under the joint guidance of the educational audiologist and the teacher of acoustically-impaired children. Similarly, the successful attorney with very gradual reduction of hearing efficiency will need the continuing support of the rehabilitational audiologist. In both cases cited, medical examination indicates irreversible hearing losses for the patients. Since both patients are expected to perform as normally as possible in terms of hearing efficiency, both patients will be referred to the audiologist for full programs in rehabilitation. Obviously, the approaches to be used with the young child will be quite different from those suggested for the practicing attorney. Both subjects, however, can be helped to a marked degree by a carefully organized program in communicative improvement. Such rehabilitative approaches usually include some of the following:

1. Counseling with the subject and/or the subject's family. What are the subject's listening problems? What can be done to meet such challenges successfully?
2. Direct observation of improvement potential with wearable amplification. Will a hearing aid be helpful?
3. Recommendations regarding wearing a hearing aid. Which aid, or aids, provide the greatest amount of improvement?
4. Hearing aid orientation. How well can the subject manipulate and adjust to the hearing aid?
5. Auditory training to strengthen listening ability. Which sounds are understood less well?
6. Speechreading training to augment diminished hearing ability. Which sounds are not heard, and which of these have high visibility?
7. Speech and language training (with children). Will the child need special help for speech and language acquisition?

8. Speech conservation (for adults). Can the subject keep the present level of speech production in the light of a reduced efficiency in self-monitoring by auditory cues?
9. Environmental modification. Are there ways to reduce the noise in the listener's environment and to "set the stage" for more optimal listening?
10. Periodic reassessment and supplemental training after the initial program of communicative improvement has been completed. What listening problems continue to concern the subject, and what can he or she and the audiologist do to overcome these problems?
11. Annual review of auditory performance and adjustment. Is the subject's hearing level remaining stable? Are there new listening problems that should be resolved? What communicative skills have proven most effective? Should a supplemental rehabilitative program be initiated?

The above list is by no means complete or applicable to all subjects with hearing deficits. The list is presented only to suggest possible audiologic approaches available to a client working through a program of rehabilitation.

Synthesis

The field of audiology deals with measuring a hearing deficit (known as *diagnostic audiology*) and helping people with hearing losses to improve their communicative skills (known as *rehabilitative audiology*). Both these functions are based on the knowledge of normal hearing performance.

In this way, audiology may be considered as a pyramid with three essential levels (see Fig. 2-1). Each higher level builds upon the one below it. The base of the audiologic pyramid is all of the information on the human function of normal hearing. Firmly interlocking with this normative base are the assessment techniques for evaluating abnormal hearing performance. At the top, and following the diagnostic regime as a logical conclusion, is rehabilitation with improvement of communicative function for individuals with hearing losses as its main goal.

In a final definition, Davis and Silverman (1970) suggest that audiology is the mobilization of professional skills to cope with the phenomenon of hearing and deficient hearing. Individuals who concentrate their training, their competence, and their experience on resolving problems of auditory communication may be considered to work in the field of audiology.

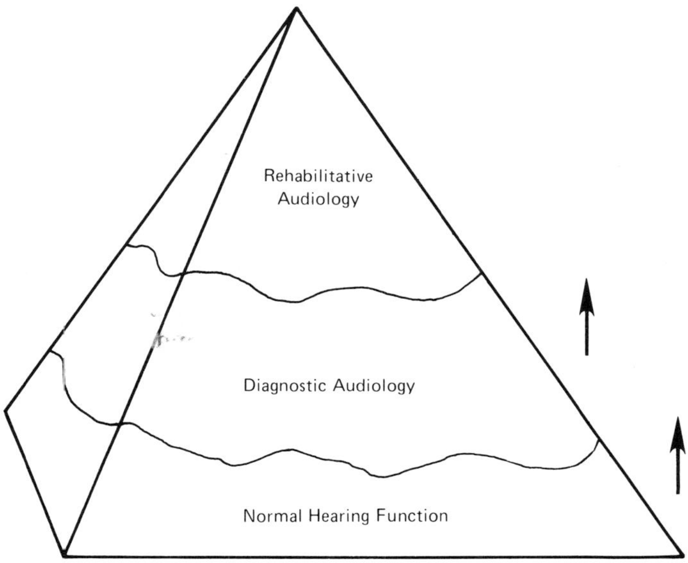

Fig. 2-1. The audiologic model.

FUNCTIONAL AUDITION

The ear, with its associated ascending and descending central and peripheral neural pathways, is a complex unit. In his review of the auditory system and the central nervous system, Davis (1970, p. 77) cautions that "Everything is very much more complicated than we can readily conceive."

The structure of this section is threefold: To outline a model of functional audition, to relate the parts of this model to respective anatomical locations in the human auditory system, and to review a classification system of audition according to levels or routes from the outer ear to the cortex.

Psychological Bases of Audition

Ramsdell (1970, p. 436) suggests that the individuals who hear normally employ hearing, or audition, at three psychological levels.

First, audition serves as the monitor system to keep the individual's background in focus. The hearer is aware of surrounding sounds, such as a ventilator fan running overhead, or the sounds of traffic outside the window. By an almost unconscious awareness of these sounds, normal-hearing listeners maintain contact with the world about them.

At the second psychological level, the listener uses this sound monitoring as an alert to changes in the background. When an unusual or different sound occurs in the background, the signal or warning level of the monitor comes into action. For example, the sudden wail of an ambulance siren causes the drive to pull to the side of the road; the sound of "shots" outside the window alerts the city-dweller to a readiness stage; the hungry cry of her baby awakens a mother who is able to sleep through other types of background noises.

Finally, the normal hearer uses audition to comprehend spoken language. Sounds arranged in specific sequences are symbols representing objects. The auditory sequence of "C-A-T" in English refers to a small, furry, domesticated animal. To a teenager deeply in love, the auditory sequence of "D-I-A-M-O-N-D" elicits an image of an engagement ring. Symbols also are used to identify activities. "S-T-R-I-K-E T-H-R-E-E" to a frustrated baseball batter carries heavy and discouraging linguistic meaning. The cry of "F-I-R-E" in a crowded room carries a frightening message. At a birthday party, the question "W-H-O W-O-U-L-D L-I-K-E M-O-R-E I-C-E C-R-E-A-M?" suggests a happy symbolic message. The statement of the boss that "Y-O-U H-A-V-E B-E-E-N P-R-O-M-O-T-E-D" leads to an equally positive symbolic message. How different the meaning would be if the boss said, "Y-O-U A-R-E F-I-R-E-D." Sounds in specific sequence are used to refer to objects, persons, places and activities by symbolic representation. Oral–aural references to important life experiences constitute the symbolic communicative level. Human beings are unique in their ability to manipulate symbols for abstract communication. Oral expression of symbols by a speaker permits a normal-hearing listener to respond to these symbol sequences when the symbols have common definitions for both speaker and listener.

Psychologically, the normal-hearing subject uses an intact auditory system to keep the auditory background of life sounds under surveillance. He or she uses hearing as a warning device when the background of sound changes markedly. Audition is employed to communicate orally and aurally through the grammatical manipulation of commonly defined linguistic symbols.

Functional Levels of Audition

There are five basic functional levels of audition in the human auditory system. Four of these are distinct levels of auditory processing, and the fifth functional aspect is the synthesization of auditory phenomena with those of the other sensory modalities. The functional levels are:

1. Conduction level

2. Reception level
3. Transmission and dissemination level
4. Perception level
5. Association level (from Hardy, 1956).

The outer ear receives air-conducted sounds and transmits these pressure waves across the middle ear to the fluid-filled inner ear. This mechanical coupling of eardrum with the ossicular chain is classed as the conduction level.

Within the fluid-filled inner ear, the analysis of the fluid movement by the cochlear sensory hair cells converts these movement patterns into electrochemical reactions. The frequency and the intensity analysis of these selected stimuli over a period of time produce neural patterns, which are then transmitted centrally to the brain. This conversion of fluid pressure motion into electrochemical stimulation patterns is considered the reception level where encoding of the "auditory" signal occurs.

Transmission of the signal toward the central nervous system occurs as the first order neurons move the neural signal through the acoustic branch of the eighth cranial nerve into the central nervous system. Such transmission and dissemination of the neural signal continues as second, third, and fourth order neurons transmit the signal up both the ipsilateral and contralateral neural routes within the brain stem and midbrain.

Perception of the neural signal occurs when neuronal activity presents the electrochemical signal to the cortex in the cortical projection areas. Here the signal is decoded, the information found in the signal is synthesized, and the essential information is projected on to other cortical centers for additional integration.

The final phase of "audition" occurs at the association level, which is not unique to audition alone, but which also serves as the master synthesizer and unifying cortical integrator of all sensory input. The association level puts all sensory patterns, including auditory patterns, into a meaningful wholeness upon which language is built. With an intact association network, the individual is able to listen naturally, to build understanding of linguistic units, and to store and recall symbolic structures. The association process permits the development of a human memory "bank" so that the individual continues to develop greater and greater recall facility. The integration of experience occurs broadly within the association area. With effective memory, symbolic references are coded and stored for future use. The language code is set. When new auditory signals are processed through the association level, recognition of these patterns is achieved because of past experience and memory of such patterns.

When a completely new and strange auditory pattern is processed for which no prior stimulation or memory exists, the integrative process of association attempts to build a meaning with which to associate this sound for future use.

For example, adults may vividly recall their first, perhaps traumatic, exposure to a sonic boom. At the psychological level, an attempt was quickly made to determine whether fight or flight was necessary as a result of the "warning" from the background monitor. After determining that no subsequent disaster had occurred, the association function processed the auditory experience to the memory bank for recall if such a boom is ever heard again.

Similarly, one can observe the way children savor and play orally with new words that they finds linguistically exciting. In using the words "ice cream," "cold," and "more," a child may combine several sensory patterns to develop the use of a linguistic code for gastric satisfaction.

The child learns that the container of ice cream is stored in a refrigerator and that a parent must scoop this stuff into a dish; the child listens eagerly as Mother describes it as "ice cream" or "cold", delighted when the repetition of the word "more, more, more" achieves the desired goal of another helping. By repeated stimulation in meaningful situations, the intact child quickly develops both input and output language skills at the appropriate readiness periods. Such acquisition of meaningful language is dependent on an intact association system; which, in turn, is dependent on intact processing for the various sensory modalities of audition, vision, touch, proprioception, taste, and olfaction. The unifying aspect of association transcends and integrates all sensory inputs into a meaningful integration of sensory experiences.

Terminology to Designate Levels of Audition

In 1966, Kirikae, Shitara, and Sata proposed a classification of deafness based on anatomical sites of the lesions. Their classification proposal was sorely needed because of the generalized confusion in the use of terminology among professionals in describing the location of possible hearing malfunction.

The following set of descriptive terms (Table 2-1) is proposed to describe levels of audition in the normal-hearing individual. While these terms are descriptive of *normal* auditory performance, their use is appropriate for describing locations of anatomical malperformance once the site, or sites, of lesion has been determined. The outline generally agrees with the classification of deafness proposed by Kirikae et al.

In the proposed outline, the use of the term "retrocochlear" would only broadly designate the entire pathway and integration centers that are central or medial to the cochlear area. If an audiologist or otorhinolaryngologist actually meant to refer specifically to the eighth nerve, then he or

Table 2-1
Outline of Levels of Audition

Anatomical Levels	Associated Function Levels
I. Conductive level: outer and middle ear	Conduction
II. Cochlear or sensory level: inner ear	Reception
III. Retrocochlear, or Neural level: all auditory pathways and centers central to the cochlea	Transmission and dissemination
A. Peripheral, or eighth nerve level: first-order neuron	↓
B. Central, or CNS level: second- third- and fourth-order neurons plus cortical level	↓
1. Brainstem level: second-, third- and fourth-order neurons	↓
2. Cortical level: auditory cortex	Perception

she would use the term that specifies a "peripheral" site within the broad retrocochlear region as "eighth nerve." In a similar manner, a professional use of the term "central" level of hearing would only broadly identify audition within the central nervous system and inclusive of all levels from the synapse at the cochlear nuclei all the way up to the auditory cortex. If the diagnostic clinician wished to refer specifically to reception of the neural signal at the level of the auditory cortex, the use of the term "cortical" hearing would be chosen as the label.

Certainly, such a classification system may still leave many gray areas where specific designation on site is not yet possible. It does, however, contribute markedly to a clearer professional agreement as to what is meant by the terms "retrocochlear" and "cortical" hearing, to mention just two of the eight possible levels of audition. The eight descriptors are as follows:

—Conductive site or sensorineural site (avoid use)
then
—Cochlear site or retrocochlear site (avoid use)
then
—Peripheral neural site or central neural site (avoid use)
and finally
—Brainstem site or cortical site

For the most precise on site labels, practicing audiologists would generally *not* use the terms "sensory neural," "retrocochlear," or "central" because of their inherent lack of specificity. The five remaining descriptors more clearly identify specific locations of function or deficit. They include: conductive, cochlear, peripheral neural, and brainstem or cortical.

SPEECH AUDIOMETRIC DATA

Classically, in the late 1970s, most audiologists routinely gathered two basic speech audiometric measures (Martin & Forbis, 1977), and these included the speech reception threshold (SRT) and word discrimination scores (WDS). These two performance tasks are markedly different in their focus. The SRT attempts to measure threshold sensitivity by the identification of an intensity level where the individual is able to correctly identify 50 percent or more of a list of bisyllabic words. Alternatively, the WDS assesses "the ability of the listener to make fine distinctions among similar speech sounds at suprathreshold intensities" (Tillman, 1973, p. 38), and these findings are reported as percentage correctly identified as a measure of speech discrimination.

The SRT, or spondee threshold (ST), as proposed as a more precise term in the ASHA "Guidelines for Determining the Threshold Level for Speech" (1977, 1979), is considered to be the speech audiometric correlate to the average of the pure-tone thresholds at the classical speech frequencies of 500, 1000, and 2000 Hz. An expanded formula proposed by the American Academy of Otolaryngology (AAO) would add the frequency 3000 Hz to the calculation (S/V News, 1978; "Guide," 1979). The scoring procedure for the ST requires a 50 percent or better recognition level, and such an intensity level is considerably greater in sound pressure than that required merely to detect the presence of a speech (or pure-tone) signal. It has been calculated (Egan, 1948) that it requires about 12 dB to move from awareness to a 50 percent understanding level of bisyllabic words.

The audiologist compares threshold findings for pure-tones and the ST, both of which are expressed in dB HTL dial levels, and then makes a decision about consistency between the two sets of data. With the mature, cooperative adult, good agreement should obtain. Variability between the two sets of information should not usually exceed ±5–6 dB.

Alternatively, WDS results are calculated at one or more suprathreshold levels and permit the audiologist to make conservative estimates of the understanding efficiency for the individual's ear(s) under study. Obviously, both ST and WDS data can be gathered monaurally under headphones or in the soundfield. Calibration bases are different for the sound pressure level (SPL) undergirdings for phones and for soundfield with audiometric "0" db HTL at approximately 20 dB SPL for headphones (ANSI S3.6-1969) and at 12.5 dB SPL for soundfield environments (Tillman, Johnson, & Olsen, 1966; Dirks, Stream, & Wilson, 1972).

Articulation/Intelligibility Functions

An eclectic set of articulation/intelligibility curves is found in Fig. 2-2. For the normal-hearing person, the threshold of detectability for speech is shown to be at 8 dB SPL, and the spondee threshold (ST) is found to be at 20 dB SPL (or 12 dB greater, as Egan proposed in 1948). The spondee curve function is a steep one (Curve C), and the intelligibility for familiar spondees moves from "0" percent understanding at 12 dB

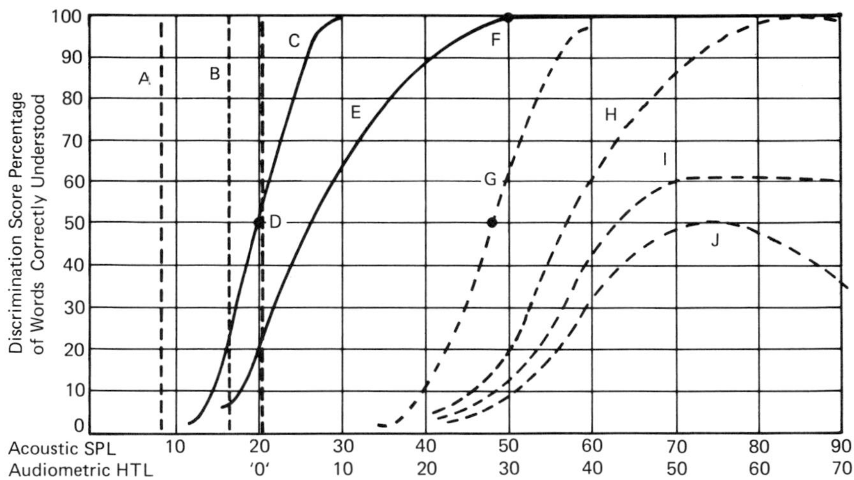

Fig. 2-2. Performance Intensity Relations, expressed as Articulation/Intelligibility Curves, for normal-hearing and abnormal-hearing subjects, determined monaurally, with TDH-39 headphones. Notes: (A) threshold of detectability (awareness of speech); (B) threshold of intelligibility (50 percent correct response for spondees); (C) spondee word list intelligibility threshold (normal curve); (D) spondee threshold (ST) or speech reception threshold (SRT), 50 percent point; (E) phonetically balanced word list intelligibility curve (normal curve), list W-22 from CID lists; (F) hundred percent understanding point for a normal-hearing listener, W-22 lists; (G) an abnormal spondee curve; (H) an abnormal phonetically balanced curve—conductive loss; (I) an abnormal phonetically balanced curve—cochlear loss; (J) an abnormal phonetically balanced curve—VIII$_n$ loss. [Adapted from Carhart, 1965; Davis, 1970, p. 212; Hochberg, 1973, p. 23; Hopkinson, 1978, p. 143; Hudgins et al., 1947; Keith, 1976, p. 17; Martin, 1975, p. 31; Rupp, 1978; Tillman, 1973, p. 52.]

SPL to 100 percent understanding at 28 dB SPL, for a function intensity spread of approximately only 18 dB in width.

The curve function for lists of phonetically balanced words (cited in the Fig. 2-2 legend as Central Institute for the Deaf [CID] W-22 lists) shows a much more gradual slope for our statistically normal subject. It requires approximately a 30 dB sensation level (SL) or greater for the subject to achieve a good word discrimination score. The intact, native English-speaking adult should achieve a score of 90 percent or better as he identifies such monosyllables at 30–40 dB SL (or at a 50–60 dB SPL level).

It is against these two basic speech audiometric measures of ST and WDS for a normal-hearing listener that the new and unknown clinical patient's hearing performances are then compared. Spondee threshold scores of 0–15 dB HTL are considered within normal. What are the dB values of the new client's STs? Similarly, what are the patient's WDSs compared with a normal function of 90–100 percent at a 3–40 dB SL re: a normal ST?

Curve G in Fig. 2-2 reflects an elevated ST at 48 dB HTL (at the 50 percent correct identification level). Additionally, Curves H, I, and J represent "examples" of WDS curves associated with the following: a conductive hearing loss (H) with good understanding at a minimal comfort level; a sensory or cochlear loss (I) with an understanding level that plateaus at approximately 60 percent; and an eighth nerve transmission deficit (J), which shows a maximum efficiency at 50 percent, its best functional level, with rollover (or reduction) in performance as signal intensity increases.

The performance–intensity relationship shows the change in speech intelligibility for any patient as the intensity of the spoken signal is changed. A low intensity for the presentation of a word list predicts low intelligibility or understanding scores for the normal-hearing subject. Higher intensity presentation levels project better performance or understanding scores for both ST and WDS values.

In Fig. 2-2, point D on curve C is the base-line normal ST point at "0" dB HTL (or 20 dB SPL); point F on curve E represents ideal understanding at a minimal comfort level of 30 dB SL re: normal "0" dB HTL.

Usually, the audiologist will not build curve C, but will search or probe for point D, which by definition is the 50 percent correct level on the abscissa, expressed in dB HTL, for spondees. When the audiologist wishes to determine a maximum percentage of understanding for monosyllabic, phonetically balanced word lists, he or she may elect to gather WDS values at two or more suprathreshold levels, i.e., at 30 dB SL, at 40 dB SL, and perhaps at 50 dB SL. If the audiologist uses a variety of intensity levels to determine the optimal WDS, then, and only then, may the findings be reviewed in terms of a "PB max score," or the maximum intelligibility for a phonetically weighted word list consistent with general English phonetic distribution.

Social Adequacy Index: A Revisit

Pure-tone audiometry identifies sensitivity for the specific frequencies under observation. From such threshold findings, it is considered appropriate to employ a formula to calculate a "percentage" of loss according to the guidelines of the AAOO's Committee on Conservation of Hearing (Davis, 1970, 265; "Guide," 1979). The limitation of such a percent loss, based on the sensitivity levels of the central speech frequencies of 500, 1000, 2000, and 3000 Hz, is that it does not give direct information about the effect upon the person's communicative input abilities. "What is needed is some measure based on the results of speech audiometry which will represent the degree of handicap so far as hearing and understanding speech is concerned" (Newby, 1972, p. 127).

The prototype for such a "measure" is the Social Adequacy Index (SAI) (Walsh & Silverman, 1946; Silverman et al., 1948; Davis, 1948; Newby, p. 127; Tillman & Olsen, 1973, p. 64). While the original research information on the SAI was gathered more than three decades ago, the basic rationale remains sound. Walsh, Silverman, and Davis developed the concept that an interacting relationship between the individual's speech reception threshold (sensitivity) and his or her word discrimination scores (understanding) should predict a potential for hearing and listening effectiveness. They gathered data on several patients for the SL and for WDS at 33 dB HTL, 48 dB HTL, and at 63 dB HTL, described by Newby (p. 128) as "the average levels of faint, average, and loud conversational speech, respectively." They then correlated their speech scores with the patients' subjective reports of the extent of their hearing handicaps in a variety of professional and/or social environments. Their rationale for the SAI was that a person with normal (low ST scores) and low discrimination loss scores could perform with good social ability for hearing. Conversely, a person with an elevated ST and high discrimination loss scores would function with poor social communicative effectiveness. Their charts provided a method for predicting the magnitude of the hearing "social adequacy" of new and unknown patients by entering their data scores into their index. In its shortened version, the WDS was obtained at only an intensity level of 40 dB HTL. An example of the SAI graph can be found in Newby's book, *Audiology* (p. 129).

Tillman and Olsen (p. 64) warn that fallaciously good scores will be found if recorded CID W-22 lists are used instead of the original Harvard PAL PB-50 lists as recorded by Rush Hughes. Since the original recordings, on disc or cassette, are still available from Technisonic Studios in St. Louis, Missouri (Berger, 1977, p. 4), the conscientious audiologist can continue to use the SAI with its original standardization lists. The shift from ASA to ISO to ANSI standards for audiometric "0" dB has reduced the basic undergirding SPL value by only 2 dB (Newby, p. 128). Close approximations of current findings for a new client can be made, therefore, with the original standardization for the SAI.

Walsh and Silverman as well as Silverman et al. established the following ranges of hearing efficiency for their SAI:

1. Within normal limits for effortless communication: SAI of 94 or better.
2. Difficulty in hearing and understanding speech: SAI of 67, and higher.
3. Threshold of social adequacy: SAI of 33.
4. Inability to follow speech by hearing alone: SAI values below 33.

As the early authors reported their procedures in the 1940s, they compared ST and WDS results with their subjects' subjective impressions of communicative adequacy. It was from these observations, with support from the speech scores, that the above four adequacy areas of the SAI were developed (see Fig. 2-3). If audiologists are willing to add two

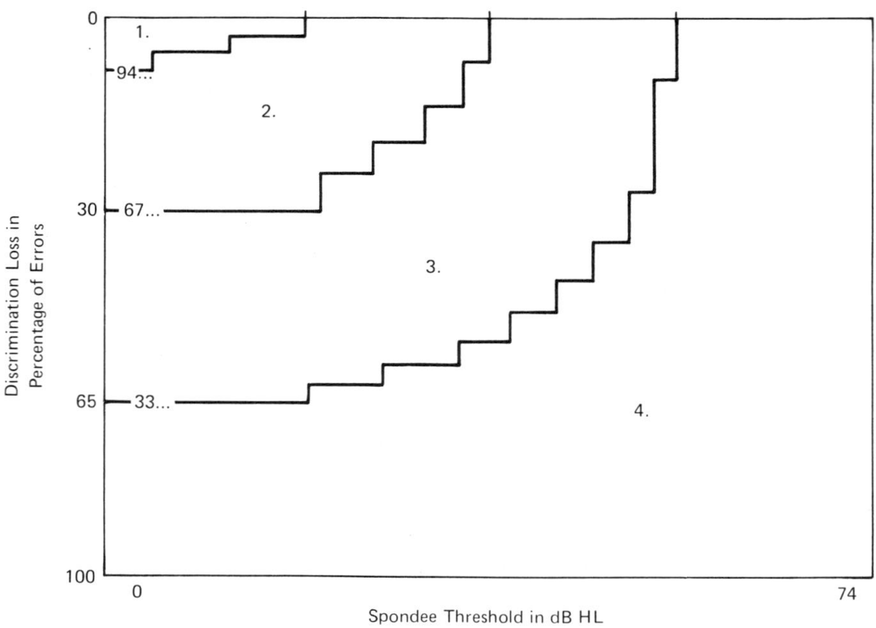

Fig. 2-3. Special Adequacy Index (SAI): four areas of communicative adequacy or inadequacy. Areas: (1) within normal and adequate; (2) some difficulty and marginally adequate; (3) major difficulty and inadequate; (4) total difficulty and noncommunicative.

additional word lists to their discrimination task in the diagnostic battery (PB-50 sets), then a strong supplemental observation of communicative adequacy can be obtained. Comparisons between the SAI findings and personal reports of communicative deficit can be made.

Other Self-assessment Scales

Since the development of the SAI (1946–1948), a number of other scales have been proposed that attempt to correlate personal evaluation of communicative deficit with the basic speech audiometric data. The classical Hearing Handicap Scale (HHS) (High, Fairbanks, & Glorig, 1964) is a questionnaire in which respondents judge the extent of their hearing difficulty for 20 different environments on a five-part continuum from "almost never" to "almost always." The authors suggest that the HHS effectively relates to sensitivity shifts, but does not predict as well on understanding ability.

Speaks, Jerger, and Tramel (1970) found similar results in a followup study and agreed that the majority of the questions were actually related to loss of hearing sensitivity.

Alternatively, the self-assessment questionnaire developed by Dirks and Carhart (1962) and studied further by Nelson (1968) suggests a closer relation "between speech discrimination scores for monosyllabic word lists and subjective impression of hearing difficulty than for thresholds" (Tillman & Olsen, p. 64).

The HHS was studied again by Berkowitz and Hochberg (1971) with an aging population; for this special population, the HHS agreed with both CID W-22 performance and CID Sentences.

In 1970, Noble and Atherley developed the Hearing Measurement Scale. Their interview questionnaire was highly effective in estimating spondee thresholds but less strongly related to precipitous high tone hearing loss or discrimination deficit.

Four years later, Shotola and Maurer (1974) introduced their 14-item interview questionnaire, which they later revised following a field study on 87 elderly females down to a six-item hearing screening task. They propose that this screening relates closely to hearing sensitivity loss. The utility of such a quick and easily administered screening approach is obvious.

The Social Hearing Handicap Index (SHI) by Ewertsen and Birk-Nielsen (1973), a 21-part forced-choice response questionnaire, was developed from a population of over 500 adults. Subjects who responded to the questionnaire felt that severe hearing loss and marked high-tone deficits were inordinate impairments to easy social conversational interaction.

Schow and Nerbonne (1976) developed two hearing handicap measures, which they designated as the (1) Self and (2) Staff Nursing Home Hearing Handicap Indices. Interestingly, and perhaps disturbingly, the Staff scores correlated better with pure-tone and speech thresholds than did the Self scores. The reader should recall that the subjects in the study were nursing/convalescent home residents.

The Denver Scale of Communicative Function (DSCF) (Alpiner, 1975, pp. 176–183; Alpiner, 1978) was designed to allow the adventitiously impaired adults to judge the effects of their hearing loss on their families, on themselves, on their social-vocational activities, and on their communicative listening abilities. Alpiner urges that individual attitudes and impressions of communicative problems are crucial to the success of any eventual auditory rehabilitative program with any subject. The scale was especially engineered to permit pre- and posttherapeutic review by the subject and, indirectly, by the educational audiologist.

In 1979, Giolas and his colleagues reported on their 158-item "Hearing Performance Inventory," which was designed to assess hearing performance in problem areas encountered in everyday listening situations. Their inventory represents probably the longest and most diverse self-assessment protocol available to the hearing-impaired individual. It includes self-appraisal of communicative ability in the six following areas: understanding speech, intensity, response to auditory failure, social, personal, and occupational. (A shortened version of this inventory has also been made available by the authors, and it contains 90 items for review.)

The essential challenge to any self-evaluated problem has to do with the capability of the self-evaluator to be truthful and honest in judging crucial areas that may depreciate the individual's own concept of self-worth or self-esteem. The psychological defense mechanisms that many employ so effectively may negate the reliability of a self-study. The client may use one or several of the following protective mechanisms to keep the self secure against the actual recognition of the effects of disabled audition: rationalization, projection, insulation, negativism, regression, repression, or fantasy. With a specific client, wide disparity between relatively objective speech audiometric findings (ST and WDS) and self-perceived deficit or disability may be encountered (Maurer & Rupp, 1979, Chapters 2 and 5).

With well-motivated clients who are capable of evaluating their listening abilities and disabilities more objectively, any of the above reviewed protocols would give corroborative findings to the basic speech audiometric findings and their application to the SAI. The ingenius audiologist could even graph results from a self-assessment scale to further heighten the patients' interest in further otological/audiological activities designed to improve listening skills. For example, consider the following

Table 2-2
Comparing Relationships Between Audiologic and Self-Assessment Findings for the Hearing-impaired Individual

University of Michigan Descriptions*	Pure-tone and Spondee Thresholds in dB HL	AAOO Descriptions of Handicap	Possible HHS Scores (Range 20–100)
Within normal	0–15*	"not significant"	20–25
Minimal hearing loss	16–25*	"not significant"	20–30
Mild hearing loss	26–40	"slight"	25–40
Moderate hearing loss	41–55	"mild"	35–55
Moderately severe hearing loss	56–70	"marked"	50–80
Severe hearing loss	71–90	"severe"	75–95
Profound hearing loss	91–110	"extreme"	95–100

*This system agrees in general with that of Goodman (1965), Green (1978), and the AAOO (Davis, 1970, p. 255). It does, however, further subdivide the most efficient classification in the Goodman and AAOO systems into two more descriptive classes. An individual with a 22 dB ST cannot be considered to be functioning in a normal manner in terms of hearing and listening abilities.

theoretical relationships between the University of Michigan Classification System for Hearing Levels and scores obtained on the HHS of High et al. (1964) as proposed in Table 2-2. As an individual's level of hearing improved, either through medical intervention or amplification, we would hopefully expect the subjective impression of hearing efficiency to improve also.

THE IDENTIFICATION OF "SPEECH" BY THE LISTENER

With its central projections to the auditory cortex and association areas of the brain, the human ear is capable of sound analysis far superior to that of any computer. Stevens and Davis (1938, p. 153) reported that an individual with an intact auditory system is able to analyze about 340,000 "different" auditory signals when the parameters of frequency and/or intensity are varied minimally. Speech signals in a general American dialect have less than 50 just noticeably different components. Sanders (1971, p. 25) suggests that such standard American speech contains 38 phonemes (16 vowels and 22 consonants). Simply speaking, as far as listening is concerned, the basic goal for a maturing child would be to master recognition of the 38 unique auditory phonetic signals, and at approximately the same time, to develop an articulatory ability to produce them effortlessly and appropriately. Davis (1972, p. 217) counters this "easy" approach to sound analysis and production by cautioning the observer "that a given phoneme does not always have the same sound spectrum, that the transitions from vowel to consonant and consonant to vowel are as characteristic and as important as the steady state of either the vowel or the consonant." Beyond these factors, the duration of the sound as well as the associated silent intervals will influence the identification of certain sound patterns. This influence of adjacent phonemes on each other has been labeled "coarticulation" and represents "a bidirectional phonomenon which involves the overlapping of articulatory movements for two or more phonetic segments" (Parnell & Amerman, 1978). This bidirectional phenomenon has an obvious auditory effect upon the listener. It has been suggested that coarticulatory cues increase the numbers of actual sound-like units in the speaker's oral expressive and aural receptive repetiore and help "lighten the perceptual load" (Ali et al., 1971).

Additional production variables may interact from speaker to speaker in terms of speech–sound production and their influence on the acoustic signal. The perceptual analyzing task for the normal-hearing or hearing-impaired listeners can be increased markedly. Consider, for example, the modification of the core speech sounds in Americanese by any or several of the following speaker's alterations: rate, duration, intonation, regional accent, precision of articulation, nasality or other modified resonance, frequency, intensity, directionality, and perhaps unique grammatical structure. When one considers that many speakers alter their speech production from an idealized one, it is not surprising that hearing-impaired subjects find the listening task a challenging one—and one in which they frequently are not successful.

Intensity/Frequency/Time Interactions

In the normal auditory system, the cochlea (or sensory end organ) functions as the encoder of the acoustical signal, either of speech or other environmental sounds. With infinite sophistication, it analyzes the signal rapidly according to the frequency and intensity composition of the signal at one point in time. Since speech components hit the ear by the thousands within each minute of input, or at the rate of 30 phonemes per second (Orr, Friedman, & Williams, 1965), this human computer analyzes remarkably well. While most younger ears can hear within a broad frequency range from 20–20,000 Hz, the frequency range considered necessary for effortless identification of speech sounds is within the range of 250–8000 Hz. (Interestingly, the Bell Telephone System employs a frequency range of approximately 300–3000 Hz in its telephone circuit, and for the ordinary listener, such a range allows both easy understanding of the speech signals as well as identification of the speaker's characteristic voice quality.) Low-frequency formants (energy concentration ranges) contribute to the identification of the various vowels (at 250–1000 Hz); recognition of the consonants is generally dependent on the contribution of additional higher-frequency components. Low-frequency vowels carry the intensity (energy) of the spoken signal while the higher-frequency consonants provide the cues for its intelligibility.

The "Signature" of the Different Sounds

The classical work of Fletcher (1953) shows such intensity–frequency relationships graphically displayed (Sanders, 1971, p. 100). For example, /*u*/ as in *cue* has its primary frequency concentration at 400 Hz and at a relative sensation level of 57 dB (GTL). In opposition, /th^{b}/ as in *think* has its energy mass at 6000 Hz with a relative sensation level at 32 dB (HTL).

Reinforcing the Fletcher data is the significant contribution of Potter, Kopp, and Green (1947, p. ix). They have shown spectrographic patterns for various speech sounds, which are seen to be highly individualistic and consistent. These "signatures" of the specific sounds are capable of creating "an automatically written phonetic alphabet" by their highly specific intensity and frequency interactions and patterns. The influence of coarticulation of adjacent phonemes can also be clearly seen in the hundreds of spectrographic patterns of visible connected discourse that enrich the pages of this classical work.

In the following years, subsequent enrichments have been reported on the analytic analysis of the acoustic characteristics of speech signals. Fujimura (1962) studied the nasal consonants; Halle, Hughes, and Radley (1957) concentrated on the stop consonants; Heinz and Stevens (1961) reported their findings on mapping the voiceless fricatives; Hughes and Halle (1956) observed fricative consonants; Lehiste and Peterson (1959) studied the effects of filtering on vowel formants; and Peterson and Barney (1952) analyzed the vowels.

The presence of conductive, sensory, or peripheral neural hearing losses upon the efficiency of the listener's analytic and encoding ability have a marked effect. Conductive losses reduce the perceived "loudness" of the acoustic signal; sensory deficit with its usual sloping audiometric configuration distorts the incoming signal by changing the crucial intensity–frequency relationship patterns; and a peripheral neural hearing disorder destroys clear transmission of the signal because of pressure on the eighth nerve.

The several sounds of the American-English language constitute the primary units of our oral language. When these sounds are linked together to make words, and when these words are strung together in a continuity to make grammatically appropriate sentences, oral communication between speaker and listener will occur. The usual cortical processing of speech by the listener includes the triad of sensation, perception, and cognition (Witkin, 1971; Semel, 1976; Wepman et al., 1960; Rupp, 1978). Whenever hearing loss or perceptual deficit interferes, the listener may be in communicative jeopardy.

Theories of Speech Perception

Speech, or its resulting acoustic stimulus, constitutes a progression of time-related interactions. A speaker speaks; a listener listens. "The acoustic signals of speech do not in themselves convey messages: They do convey information, from which messages equivalent to the speakers' are hopefully reconstructed by the listener." (Sanders, 1977, p. 98). The end result is communicative interaction.

Sanders (1977, p. 100) reviews two theoretical approaches for the way meaning is eventually derived from a speech signal. These include the passive (or nonmediated) theories and the active (or mediated) theories. The general theme of the passive theory is that the auditory perceptual process is essentially a filtering system that identifies and combines "information so as to restructure the pattern." Proposed models for this theory include: the distinctive feature theory of Jacobson, Fant, and Halle (1963), the acoustic theory of Fant (1967), and the neurological theories of Corcoran (1971), Abbs and Sussman (1971) and Uttley (1966). Their writings contribute to the passive theory of speech perception in which "the process of auditory perception involves the direct structuring of active neural patterns by the pattern information content (distinctive features) of the acoustic stimulus" (Sanders, 1977, p. 114).

Conversely, the active theory, and synonymously the motor theory of Liberman (1972), propose that speech components are "perceived by reference to the place and manner of production of the acoustic signal" (Sanders, 1977, p. 117).

In summary, Denes (1967, p. 313) creates a unifying compromise between these two theories, suggesting that "there is probably more than one method by which speech perception can be achieved and normally we may use several different methods simultaneously."

The problem for the hearing-impaired listener, with either congenitally or adventitiously acquired auditory deficit, is that he or she does not process these rich speech signals normally or easily. The individual with prelingual auditory deficit never develops such a processing base, and the older individual with gradually diminishing auditory skills can no longer perceive speech signals clearly without some special assistance. Each of these individuals may need considerable training and guidance in order to more effectively manage the oral flow of the language of the culture. For some with significant and handicapping loss, alternative forms of language routing may be more appropriate.

Linguistic Constraints

"The hearing child [and eventually the normal-hearing adult] lives in a world where a language that has taken countless centuries to evolve awaits his developmental needs and is his just for the hearing" (Levine, 1960, p. 23). Because children hear, they acquire oral language with its rich phonologic, semantic, and syntactic systems.

Within their oral language systems, certain restrictions are built into the progression of the sounds within a word and into the ordering of words within a series. Beyond that, topical boundaries will prescribe the general limits of the vocabulary, and the environments within which the communicators find themselves may also restrict the extent and types of vocabulary employed.

Sanders (1971, p. 25) categorizes these restrictions or limitors in three groupings: structural restrictions, contextual constraints, and situational controls. Orally fluent and auditorially capable adults employ these constraints, consciously or unconsciously, to reduce the listening demands upon themselves as they communicate with their peers. They develop a maturational understanding that restrictions exist. And knowing these subtle yet effective "rules" of constraint, they listen and comprehend more easily.

Structural restrictions "are those at the level of the phoneme, the form, and the construct" (Sanders, 1971, p. 25). The phonemic limitations are numerical in nature, and in standard American-English, they total the 38 regular speech sounds cited earlier. While these 38 sounds can be arranged somewhat loosely, the usual progression is in a consonant-nucleus-consonant cluster (as *cat* or *run* or *game*). In English, certain phonemic combinations do not occur; for example no word begins with a */tl/* blend. Form constraints refer to the phoneme groups that the language permits to be placed in sequence. Morphemes (or clusters of morphemes) represent forms; for example, three forms can be grouped and ordered together to form a new form: *faith* plus *ful* plus *ly* becomes *faithfully*. Finally, construction limitations prescribe the usual order in which the forms may be linked together. In English, a usual construction restriction could be "four beautiful women" (to satisfy the construction order limit of "how many," then "what kind," and finally, "what"). A German might say, *"Ich muss nach Hause gehen,"* but an English speaker would not say, "I must to my home go."

As the listener refines an understanding of structural constraints, he or she is able to follow oral communication without actively having to hear each unit or form completely. For the prelingually hearing-impaired child, the lack of an awareness of structural constraints may be the basis for stilted, error laden, and sometimes awkward language use.

A contextual constraint refers to the topic under discussion by the communicators. As long as the listener knows the discussion is about the last Superbowl football game, the vocabulary spread will be minimal. When a topic is changed and the hearing-impaired listener does not realize it, a certain confusion may exist until the new topical limit has been clarified. A friendly guide for talking with a hearing-impaired communicator in a group discussion would be to let him know when the topic has been shifted and the content of the new topic.

Finally, situational limits refer to the choice of the vocabulary to be used in the communicative interation. Sanders suggests, "Situational constraints may be considered to be a function of the people present, the relationship of the speaker to these people, and the social structure of the particular environment" (1971, p. 31). The "colorful" vocabulary used at a stag party will be quite inappropriate for use in a professor's formal lecture.

These linguistic constraints are an aid to the listener. Knowing the rules of such limitations allows him or her to listen and understand with less expenditure of effort. The same benefits can accrue to hearing-impaired listeners—if they know the rules.

Synthesis

The peripheral human ear analyzes a signal by encoding intensity and frequency interaction over a time base. The central extensions of the auditory system decode these analyzed signals and ascribe linguistic uniqueness to them. Subtle rules of linguistic restraint or constraint allow the listener to interact more readily and efficiently in the integrative process of comprehending oral speech. The hearing impaired listener may be in communicative jeopardy. A disabled conductive system reduces the magnitude of the speech signal, and a sensorily damaged system reduces the clarity of such signals. Signal processing gaps can then occur, which impair the easy flow of oral language input.

The speech audiometric techniques to be described in this book are designed for two main purposes: (1) to diagnostically assess communicative efficiency; and (2) to measure the effectiveness of aural rehabilitational intervention techniques.

SPECIFIC ROLES OF SPEECH PROTOCOLS IN AUDIOLOGY

Speech procedures in audiologic diagnostic and remediational activity constitute a majority of the time an audiologist spends when gathering volitional data with hearing-impaired subjects. While objective type techniques, such as immittance, electrocochleography, electroencephalograph-evoked response audiometry, electrodermal audiometry, and heart rate response audiometry contribute markedly to the evaluative information on acoustic signal transmission, they are limited in their measurement of speech-carrying information. To assess communicative efficiency conductively, sensorily, or neurally, speech processing approaches must be employed. The audiologist plans the measurement technique, instructs the patient in the task assignment, and records and reports the information as subjectively and volitionally supplied by the listener.

The basic purpose of this book is to review the current status of the art in speech audiologic techniques. The chapters that follow are organized, philosophically and broadly, around the various roles (or goals) assigned to speech audiometric techniques. A brief overview on such assigned roles follows.

Assessing Basic Communicative Competence for Aural Language Input

Generally, the task of assessing speech for an ear under study begins with a search for the speech threshold. Depending upon the definition of the term *threshold,* such procedures may include: speech detection threshold, speech reception threshold, spondee threshold, or speech perceptibility threshold. Such a threshold is usually defined in terms of some 50 percent performance ability.

Rupp's "Classical Approaches to the Determination of the Spondee Threshold" (Chapter 4) reviews a variety of approaches used to measure the client's functional level of hearing sensitivity to a speech-type signal.

Equally important to the general basic battery is the determination of some measure of understanding ability or efficiency when obtained at some suprathreshold comfortable level(s). The clinician wishes to obtain an estimate of aural input effectiveness. Classically, such estimates are obtained from the use of phonetically balanced word lists presented to the listener at 30–40 dB SL (or greater) using clinically established and popular lists (PAL PB-50s, CID W-22s, NU-6s). Stockdell's "Classical Approaches to Measuring Discrimination Efficiency Via Word Lists" (Chapter 5) will overview the current procedures used to assess the client's understanding by means of word discrimination scores. It will include discussions on performance findings in both quiet and noisy listening environments.

Many audiologists consider that phonetically balanced lists are an arbitrary, conservative, and perhaps unrealistic way to evaluate this understanding ability. Garstecki's "Alternative Approaches to Measuring Discrimination Efficiency" (Chapter 6) will include an in-depth discussion on the use of sentences and questions that carry more linguistic patterning, and which many regard as more appropriate for such measurements. In addition, he will review the use of nonsense syllables, closed set word lists, and synthetic sentences as tools to measure understanding or coding skills.

Corroborative Information in the Identification of Site(s) of Lesion

A basic responsibility of the diagnostician is to determine, if possible, the location of damage or deficit of auditory function. This has been repeatedly described in audiologic literature as the search for the site of lesion. The interest is obviously in the etiology of the damage, but the main diagnostic charge is to determine the general location(s) within the total auditory network in which the system may be malfunctioning. In Calder's "Overview of the Anatomy and Physiology of the Peripheral Hearing Mechanism" (Chapter 3), the stage is set for later discussions on normal and abnormal auditory function. Subsequent chapters relate speech protocol findings to broad lesion sites. Such chapters include White's "Speech Protocols in the Assessment of Sensory and/or Peripheral Neural Lesion Sites" (Chapter 7), Hurley's "Speech Protocols in the Central Auditory Nervous System Evaluation" (Chapter 8), Hemeyer's "Speech Protocols in Determining Dynamic Range" (Chapter 9), and in part, Chapter 14 by McCroskey and Kasten, "Assessment of Central Auditory Processing."

Rosenberg (1972, p. 275) suggests, somewhat whimsically, that searches for lesion(s) may be complex. "Indeed, it is not at all uncommon for two or even three or more pathological entities to coexist in a single ear. One patient who had a cerebellopontine angle tumor had a prior history of noise-induced hearing impairment, endolymphatic hydrops, clinical otosclerosis and chronic otitis media."

Identification procedures for audiological determination of lesion sites are crucially important for the patient. Conductive losses indicate the need for medical intervention for possible resolution. Sensory deficits suggest the need for full range postmedical rehabilitational programs. Neural transmission dysfunction, of either peripheral or central origin, dictate medical interaction as a lifesaving process. The audiologist's search for the loci of auditory performance disorders is a sine qua non in his or her practice.

Assessing Language Input Competence in Populations With Linguistic Limitations

Traditionally, speech audiometric materials assume a basic competency with the oral language of the American culture. Realistically, audiologists must accept the fact that not all of the patients who arrive at their facilities for evaluative or remediational interaction have such competencies. Young children, individuals with slowed mental skills, severely brain-injured persons, and individuals of foreign extraction may require different kinds of speech approaches. McLauchlin's "Speech Protocols for Assessment of Persons with Limited Language Abilities" (Chapter 11) will review specialized speech and nonspeech procedures for use with these special populations.

Measurement of the Effectiveness of Personal Amplification Devices

Basic to the predictive success of a patient's hearing aid is an indication of its contribution to improved communicative input. What is the magnitude of performance enhancement the hearing aid offers its wearer? Does the optimally performing aid found in the hearing aid evaluation process offer sufficient hearing, listening, and understanding improvement to warrant its acquisition? Kasten's "Speech Protocols for Hearing Aid Evaluations" (Chapter 12) will provide an overview on hearing aid performance as judged by speech and other corroborative procedures.

Identification of the Possibly Pseudophyoacusic Listener: Evidences of a Functional Component to the Hearing Levels

In every audiologic practice, and especially in certain kinds of practices, such as a Veterans Administration facilities, there exist patients who demonstrate exaggerated and/or inconsistent hearing levels. To assist the practicing audiologist to heighten his awareness for and ability to manage such clients, Cooper has written Chapter 10: "Speech Protocols in the Assessment of Functional Hearing Loss." The section on special speech tests should be especially practical and useful to the clinician who only occasionally encounters such unique and challenging clients.

Measurements on Central Auditory Dysfunction With Emphasis on Identification of Central Lesion Site

Hurley's "Speech Protocols in Assessment of Central Auditory Dysfunction" (Chapter 8) clearly falls within the broad philosophical role reviewed above, by virtue of its discussion of identification of lesion sites. It is highlighted here again because of the recent explosion of interest in and the development of central lesion-specific speech procedures. Traditional audiologists, out of their training programs for more than 10–12 years, may need a special boost to update their understanding of the philosophy behind central speech tests and their practical application. Probably no area of this book will become obsolete and dated more quickly than this area, but the historian will be able to look back (perhaps with subsequent intellectual amusement) at the state of this art of central assessment in the early 1980s, and know where we were in the "art" process. Such central auditory function studies have become a major force in unraveling the mysteries of central audition. The pioneers continue to push forward in their searches.

Measurements on Central Auditory Processing Abilities: Identification Systems for Locating the Individual With Auditory Perceptual Deficits

Especially challenging (and frustrating to their parents and to the classroom teachers who refer them) are the children who appear for audiologic assessment because they just don't seem to be able to hear or interact effectively in the classroom. Generally, such children do not appear to be in actual listening distress prior to the first or second grades.

Their oral language developments are not noticeably different from other children's, and at home in a relatively quiet kind of listening background, they function normally. These children, however, appear to be struggling very hard, auditorially, and only achieve marginal success in their attempt to maintain their academic skills at the level of their peers. Chapter 14, by McCroskey and Kasten, entitled "Assessment of Central Auditory Processing," is about such children and the adults which they ultimately become. These children hear with normal sensitivity and have intelligence within normal levels, but they show one or more major auditory processing deficits when assessed by an almost wholly different kind of audiologic battery. This new evaluative process represents an allied central frontier equal in its importance to that of the search for central lesions.

Evaluating the Effectiveness of Aural Therapeutic Intervention: The Quantification of the Remedial Approach

This final assigned role for special protocols represents a logical extension beyond diagnostic speech appraisal techniques. In Chapter 13, "Speech Protocols in Aural Rehabilitation With Adults," Bate focuses his discussion on measurement approaches that assess the effectiveness of the adult educational audiologic therapy programs. Bate presents the situation that occurs when medical and audiologic diagnostics have been completed, the hearing aid evaluation has been finalized, and the client is participating in a full spectrum, auditory-rehabilitational program. To what extent can the audiologist improve this client's hearing and listening effectiveness? How can such improvement be measured? What are the tools needed to quantify listening skill enhancement? In Chapter 13, Bate gives the reader a kaleidoscopic review of the effectiveness of a long-running, adult aural-rehabilitation program.

THE RECOMMENDATIONS FOR CLINICALLY APPROPRIATE SPEECH PROTOCOLS

Each chapter contributor has been given the professional independence to develop the theme of his or her chapter assignment as fully and as effectively as space limitations permit. When the assignment relates to protocols, as such, most of the authors have elected to recommend a "preferred" approach based upon their literature observations and their rich clinical experiences. If a contributor does not cite a protocol or procedure of choice, it is because the assignment was to present the information as effectively as possible, in order that the reader may make the logical decisions and choices. This book, then, becomes a logical and logistical approach for the effective use of speech protocols in both diagnostic and rehabilitative audiology.

CALIBRATION APPROACHES FOR SPEECH AUDIOMETERS

In his book *Clinical Audiometry* (1943, p. 44), Bunch reported the following disastrous case: An otologist discounted audiometric data "because he secured three entirely different audiograms in tests of the same patient by three different examiners. A report of this kind would not have been possible if the tests had been conducted under proper conditions by trained examiners, using standardized audiometers and careful technique." Bunch made a sweeping charge against a then quite immature profession. Such charges might still be made today if soundroom environments do not meet ANSI requirements for background noise attenuation, if the audiologist is unqualified and uncertified by the American Speech and Hearing Association, if the equipment is not under an effective calibration monitoring regime, and if the measurement approaches are inconsistent.

The primary purpose of this book is to propose consistent and effective speech audiometric protocols for use by the professional audiological community. In addition, the calibration monitoring procedures in many clinical programs may be in need of improvement. To this end, Chapter 15, "Calibration for Speech Audiometry" by Tucci, Ruth, and Schoeny, is herein included in order to provide the reader with a functional and practical approach to the calibration measurements appropriate for speech audiometers. The author trio begins this chapter by reporting on a 1978 questionnaire survey, which indicated that a real need continues to exist for a practical "cookbook" (step-by-step) type of guide for calibration. Detailed calibration techniques for testing under phones and in the sound field will be proposed.

Within the limits of this book, we are not planning to address Bunch's concerns over ambient noise levels in testing environments or qualifications of the audiologist. We refer the interested reader to the American National Standards Institute, 1430 Broadway, New York, New York 10018, for its specification room attenuation, entitled, ANSI S3.1-1960, "Background Noise in Audiometer Rooms." For current information on the requirements for the Certification of Clinical Competence in Audiology, the reader is referred to the Committee on Clinical Certification, the American Speech-Language-Hearing Association, 10801 Rockville Pike, Rockville, Maryland 20852.

REVIEW AND PREVIEW

By the time readers have "processed" the first 15 chapters of this book, they will have completed the review of the book. The best reading, like a fascinating dessert after a bountiful smorgasbord, may be in the pages of Chapter 16, entitled "Speech Protocols: New Frontiers and New Horizons." Within this final chapter, a small group of "Wonderful Wizards of Audiological Oz" have volunteered to look into the future from their positions of leadership in the audiological community in an attempt to predict new frontiers for the audiological profession.

REFERENCES

Abbs, J., & Sussman, H. Neurophysiological feature detectors and speech perception: a discussion of theoretical implications. *Journal of Speech and Hearing Research,* 1971, *14, 23*–36.

Ali, L., Gallagher, T., Goldstein, J., & Daniloff, R. Perception of coarticulated nasality. *Journal of the Acoustical Society of America,* 1971, *49,* 538–540.

Alpiner, J. Hearing aid selection for adults. In M. Pollack (Ed.), *Amplification for the hearing impaired.* New York: Grune & Stratton, 1975.

Alpiner, J. Evaluation of communication function. In J. Alpiner (Ed.), *Handbook of adult rehabilitational audiology.* Baltimore: Williams & Wilkins, 1978.

American National Standards Institute. Specifications for audiometers. ANSI S3.6-1969. New York: American National Standards Institute, 1970.

American Speech and Hearing Association Committee on Audiometric Evaluation Guidelines for determining the threshold level for speech. ASHA, 1977, *19,* 241–243.

American Speech and Hearing Association. *Speech pathology and audiology*—career information for students from ethnic minority groups. Washington, D.C., 1973.

Berger, K. *Speech audiometry materials.* Kent, Ohio: Herald Publishing House, 1977.

Berkowitz, A., and Hochberg, I. Self-assessment of hearing handicap in the aged. *Archives of Otolaryngology,* 1971, *93,* 25–28.

Bunch, C. C. *Clinical audiometry.* St. Louis: C. V. Mosby Co., 1943.

Butler, K. Auditory perceptual skills: their measurement and remediation with preschool and school-age children (an ASHA short course). *National Convention Program of ASHA,* 1975, 54.

Carhart, R. Considerations in the measurement of speech discrimination. *Aeromedical Reviews,* 1965, 3–65.

Carhart, R. (Ed.) *Human communication and its disorders—an overview.* Bethesda, Maryland: U. S. Department of Health, Education and Welfare, 1969.

Canfield, N. *Audiology, the science of hearing, a developing specialty.* Springfield, Illinois: Charles C. Thomas, 1949.

Corcoran, D. *Pattern recognition.* Baltimore: Penguin Books, 1971.

Davis, H. Anatomy and physiology of the auditory system. In H. Davis & S. Silverman (Eds.), *Hearing and deafness.* New York: Holt, Rinehart & Winston, 1970.

Davis H. Audiology. In H. Davis & S. Silverman (Eds.), *Hearing and deafness.* New York: Holt, Rinehart & Winston, 1970.

Davis. H. Audiometry: pure tone and simple speech tests. In H. Davis & S. Silverman (Eds.), *Hearing and deafness*. New York: Holt, Rinehart & Winston, 1970.

Davis. H. Hearing handicap, standards for hearing, and medicolegal rules. In H. Davis & S. Silverman (Eds.), *Hearing and deafness*. New York: Holt, Rinehart & Winston, 1970.

Davis, H. The articulation area and the social adequacy index for hearing. *Laryngoscope*, 1948, *58*, 761–778.

Davis, H., & Silverman S. (Eds.) *Hearing and deafness*—a guide for laymen. New York: Holt, Rinehart & Winston, 1947.

Denes, P. On the motor theory of speech perception. In W. Wathen-Dunn (Ed.), *Models for the perception of speech and visual form (proceedings of a conference)*. Cambridge: M. I. T. Press, 1967.

Dirks, D., & Carhart, R. A survey of reactions from users of binaural and monaural hearing aids. *Journal of Speech and Hearing Disorders*, 1962, *27*, 311–322.

Dirks, D., Stream R., & Wilson, R. Speech audiometry earphone and sound field. *Journal of Speech and Hearing Disorders*, 1972, *37*, 162–176.

Egan, J. Articulation testing methods. *Laryngoscope*, 1948, *58*, 955–991.

Ewertsen, H., & Birk-Nielsen, H. Social hearing handicap index: social handicap in relation to hearing impairment. *Audiology*, 1973, *12*, 180.

Fairbanks, G. A theory of the speech mechanism as a servo system. *Journal of Speech and Hearing Disorders*, 1954, *19*, 133–139.

Fant, G. Auditory patterns of speech. In W. Wathen-Dunn (Ed.), *Models for the perception of speech and visual form (proceedings of a conference)*. Cambridge: M.I.T. Press, 1967.

Feldman, H. A History of Audiology. Translations of the Beltone Institute for Hearing Research, no. 22. Chicago: Beltone Institute, 1970.

Fletcher, H. *Speech and hearing in communication*. Princeton: D. Von Nostrand Co., 1953.

Fujimura, O. Analysis of nasal consonants. *Journal of the Acoustical Society of America*, 1962, *34*, 1865–1875.

Giolas, T. G., Owens, E., Lamb, S. H., & Schubert, E. D. Hearing performance inventory. *Journal of Speech and Hearing Disorders*, 1979, *44*,0169–195.

Goodman, A. Reference zero levels for pure tone audiometers. *Asha*, 1965, *7*, *262*–263.

Green, D. Pure tone air-conduction testing. In J. Katz (Ed.), *Handbook of clinical audiology*. Baltimore: Williams & Wilkins, 1978.

Halle, M., Hughes, G., & Radley, J. Acoustic properties of stop consonants. *Journal of the Acoustical Society of America*, 1957, *29*, 107–116.

Hardy, W. Problems of audition, perception and understanding. Keynote address, summer meeting, 1956, Alexander Graham Bell Association for the Deaf. Reprint 3680, Volta Bureau, Washington, D.C.

Hayakawa, S. *Language in thought and action*. New York: Harcourt, Brace & Co., 1949.

Heavenrich, A. *A view from within: a consideration of how hearing loss is mediated into behavior*. Unpublished master's thesis, Wayne State University, Detroit, Michigan, 1964.

Heinz, J., & Stevens, K. On the properties of voiceless fricative consonants. *Journal of the Acoustical Society of America*, 1961, *33*, 589–596.

High, W., Fairbanks, G., & Glorig, A. Scale for self-assessment of hearing handicap. *Journal of Speech and Hearing Disorders*, 1964, *29*, 215–230.

Hochberg, I. *Interpretation of audiometric results*. Indianapolis: Bobbs-Merrill, 1973.

Hopkinson, N. Speech reception threshold. In J. Katz (Ed.), *Handbook of clinical audiology*. Baltimore: Williams & Wilkins, 1978.

Hudgins, C., Hawkins, J., Karlin, J., & Stevens, S. The development of recorded auditory tests for measuring hearing loss for speech. *Laryngoscope*, 1947, *57*, 57–89.

Hughes, G., & Halle, M. Spectral properties of fricative consonants. *Journal of the Acoustical Society of America,* 1956, *28,* 303–310.

Jacobsen, R., Fant, G., & Halle, M. *Preliminaries to speech analysis.* Acoustics Laboratories Massachusetts Institute of Technology Technical Report no. 13. Cambridge: M.I.T. Press, 1963.

Keith, R. The audiologic evaluation. In J. Northern (Ed.), *Hearing disorders.* Boston: Little, Brown & Co., 1976.

Keller, H. *Helen Keller in Scotland.* London: Methuen & Co., 1933.

Kirikae, L., Shitara, T., & Sata, T. Classification and differential diagnosis of deafness. *International Audiology,* 1966, *5,* 71–73.

Lederer, F., & Harcy, W. Treatment and training of the hard of hearing: a program of physical and psychosocial therapy. *Archives of Otolaryngology,* 1946, *43,* 429.

Lehiste, I., & Peterson, G. The identification of filtered vowels. *Phonetica,* 1954, *4,* 161–177.

Levine, E. *The psychology of deafness.* New York: Columbia University Press, 1960.

Lieberman, P. *Speech acoustics and perception.* Indianapolis: Bobbs-Merrill, 1972.

Martin, F. *Introduction to audiology.* Englewood Cliffs, New Jersey: Prentice-Hall, 1975.

Maurer, R., & Rupp, R. *Hearing and aging: tactics for intervention.* New York: Grune & Stratton, 1979.

Nelson, D. *An evaluation of the synthetic syntax sentence test.* Unpublished master's thesis, Vanderbilt University, Nashville, Tennessee, 1968.

Newby, H. *Audiology.* New York: Appleton-Century-Crofts, 1964.

Noble, W., & Atherley, G. The hearing measurement scale: a questionnaire for the assessment of auditory disability. *Journal of Auditory Research,* 1970, *10,* 229–250.

Orr, D., Friedman, H., & Williams, J. Trainability of listening comprehension of speeded discourse. *Journal of Educational Psychology,* 1965, *56,* 148–156.

Parnell, M., & Amerman, J. Maturational influences on perception of coarticulatory effects. *Journal of Speech and Hearing Research,* 1978, *21,* 682–701.

Peterson, G., & Barney, H. Control methods used in a study of vowels. *Journal of the Acoustical Society of America,* 1952, *24,* 175–184.

Polyak, S., McHugh, G., & Judd, D. *The human ear in anatomical transparencies.* Elmsford, New York: Sonotone Corp., 1946.

Potter, R., Kopp, G., & Green, H. *Visible speech.* New York: D. Van Nostrand Co., 1947.

Ramsdell, D. The psychology of the hard-of-hearing and the deafened adult. In H. Davis & S. Silverman (Eds.). *Hearing and deafness.* New York: Holt, Rinehart & Winston, 1970.

Rosenberg, P. The test battery approach. In J. Katz (Ed.), *Handbook of clinical audiology,* Baltimore: Williams & Wilkins, 1972.

Rupp, R. The audiologist's role in the evaluation of auditory perceptual and processing abilities in young school-aged children. *Audiology: An Audio Journal for Continuing Education,* 1978a, *3.*

Rupp, R. Course syllabus, Ed.S.461: *Hearing rehabilitation.* Ann Arbor, Michigan: The University of Michigan. 1978b.

Rupp, R., Root, K., Olsen, D., Birkhold, B., Tanner, B., & Palfey, C. A library listing of audiological reference books. *Hearing Instruments,* 1977, *28,* 10–12; 14–16.

Sanders, D. A. Auditory perception of speech. Englewood Cliffs, New Jersey: Prentice-Hall, Inc., 1977.

Sanders, D. A. Aural rehabilitation. Englewood Cliffs, New Jersey: Prentice-Hall, Inc., 1971.

Schow, R., & Nerbonne, M. Assessment of hearing handicaps by nursing home residents and staff. *Laboratory Research Reports,* Idaho State University, Pocatello, Idaho, 1976, *1,* 36–45.

Semel, E. *Semel auditory processing program.* Chicago: Follett Publishing Co., 1976.

Shotola, R., & Maurer J. The development and use of a short screening form for the detection of hearing loss in older adults. Paper at the 27th Annual Meeting of the Gerontological Society, Portland, Oregon, 1974.

Silverman, S., Thurlow, W. Walsh, T., & Davis, H. Improvement in the social adequacy index following the fenestration operation. *Laryngoscope,* 1948, *58,* 607–631.

Speaks, C., Jerger, J., & Trammel, J. Measurement of hearing handicap. *Journal of Speech and Hearing Research,* 1970, *13,* 755–767.

Stevens, K., & Halle, M. Remarks on the analysis-by-synthesis and distinctive features. In W. Wathen-Dunn (Ed.), *Models for the perception of speech and visual form (proceedings of a conference).* Cambridge: M.I.T. Press, 1967.

Stevens, S., & Davis, H. *Hearing: its psychology and physiology.* New York: John Wiley & Sons, 1938.

S/V News Hearing impairment formula. *Sound and Vibration,* 1978, *12,* i.

Tillman, T., Johnson, R., & Olsen, W. Earphone versus sound field threshold sound pressure levels for spondee words. *Journal of the Acoustical Society of America,* 1966, *39,* 125–133.

Tillman, T., & Olsen, W. Speech Audiometry. In J. Jerger (Ed.), *Modern developments in audiology* (2nd ed.). New York: Academic Press, 1973.

U.S. Department of Labor. *Dictionary of occupational titles* (vol. 1). Washington, D.C., 1965.

Uttley, A. The transmission of information and the effect of local feedback: theoretical and neural networks. *Brain Research,* 1966, *2,* 21–30.

Walsh, T., & Silverman, G. Diagnosis and evaluation of fenestration. *Laryngoscope,* 1946, *56,* 536–555.

Watson, L., & Tolan, T. *Hearing tests and hearing instruments.* Baltimore: Williams & Wilkins, 1949.

Wepman, J., Jones, E., & Bock, D. Studies in aphasis: background and theoretical formulations. *Journal of Speech and Hearing Disorders,* 1960, *25,* 323; 332.

Wever, E. *Theory of hearing.* New York: John Wiley & Sons, 1949.

Witkin, B. Auditory perception—implications for language development. *Language, Speech and Hearing Services in Schools,* 1971, *4,* 31–52.

Appendix: Commercially Available Speech Materials

The following companies have a variety for recorded speech audiometric materials available for purchase. Catalogues of such materials are available on request from the respective firms.

Audiotone
Division of Royal Industries
P.O. Box 2905
Phoenix, Arizona 85036

Auditec of St. Louis
402 Pasadena Avenue
St. Louis, Missouri 63119

Folkways/Scholastic Records
906 Sylvan Avenue
Englewood, Cliffs, New Jersey 07632

Kensinger Sound Studios
4305 Mercer
Houston, Texas 77027

MRT Recording Service
4311 Moranda Avenue
Palo Alto, California 94306

Los Angeles Foundation
of Otology
2130 West Third Street
Los Angeles, California 90057

Technisonic Studios, Inc.
1201 South Brentwood Boulevard
St. Louis, Missouri 63117

H. B. Calder, Ph.D.

3

Overview of the Anatomy and Physiology of the Peripheral Hearing Mechanism

The auditory mechanism is an extraordinary sensory system capable of performing an instantaneous analysis and recoding of rapidly changing acoustic signals, and conveying these signals to the integrative centers of the brain where appropriate meanings are attached to them. The ear and its central networks accomplish this task through four basic levels of audition: mechanical conduction, sensory reception, neural transmission, and cortical synthesis. This system is required to process a virtually continuous flood of different sounds, each of which has its own unique informational content. Yet, among this vast array of acoustic signals, none is more important for humans than the speech signal.

Generally, speech processing is immediate and obvious to normal listeners. The alacrity with which we extract and code acoustic speech signals masks the complexity of the task. Consider that speech changes rapidly, with intensity variations in the range of 30–80 dB SPL across a frequency range of 50–4000 Hz. Additionally, the speech signal may have to be scanned for periods greater than 200 msec or less than 40 msec in order to identify its phonemic segments (Liberman et al., 1967). Yet, the auditory mechanism is capable of sufficiently refined signal analysis to accommodate the discriminations necessary for speech perception. For example, the ear can differentiate changes in frequency on the order of 0.3 percent (Shower & Biddulph, 1931); and intensity changes of less than 1 dB are detectable over most of the intensity range of the ear (Riesz, 1928).

The purpose of this chapter is to review the salient anatomy of the peripheral auditory mechanism and to describe its function in relation to speech processing. We will, therefore, highlight those physiological processes that contribute to the analysis of the acoustic signal, the preservation of this information in neural transmission, and the subsequent resynthesis at the cortex. Necessarily, many topics will be omitted and others discussed only tangentially. Thus, the reader is referred elsewhere for summary (Yost & Nielsen, 1977, Durant & Lovrinic, 1977) and in-depth (Dallos, 1973; Keidel & Neff, 1974, 1975) discussions of auditory anatomy and physiology.

EXTERNAL AND MIDDLE EAR

Anatomy

The cross-sectional view of the ear is depicted in Fig. 3-1, which details the relationship of the structures of the peripheral auditory system. The external ear includes those structures peripheral to the eardrum, while the middle ear is bounded by the eardrum on the lateral surface and the bony wall of the cochlea on the medial surface. The pinna or the

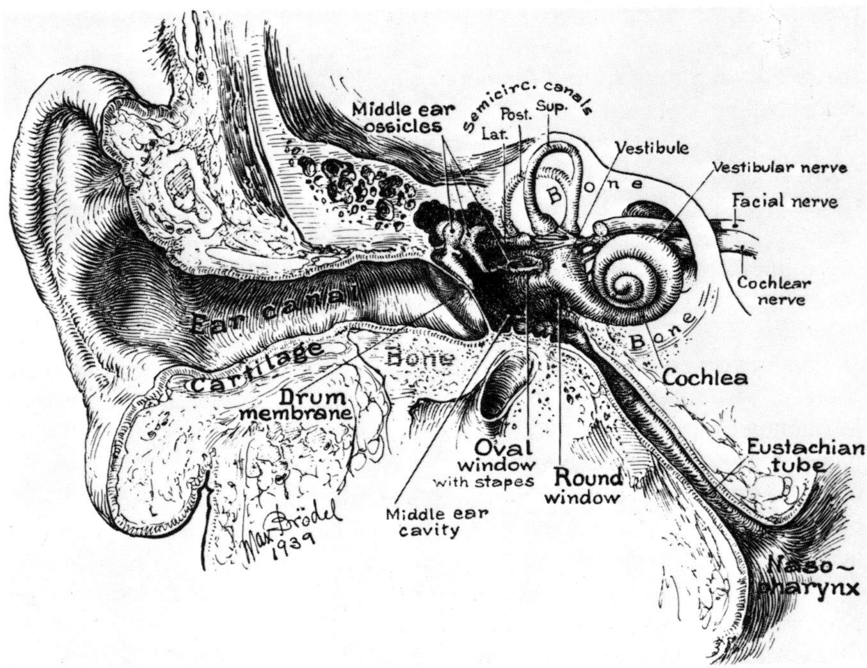

Fig. 3-1. A cross-sectional view of the human ear. [From Brödel, M. *Three unpublished drawings of the anatomy of the human ear.* Philadelphia: W. B. Saunders Company, 1946. Used with permission.]

auricle is the most visible portion of the external ear. It is the convoluted, flaplike structure that leads to the entrance of the ear canal or external auditory meatus. The pinna, as well as the lateral one-third of the external auditory meatus, is supported by a cartilaginous framework, while the medial two-thirds of the external auditory meatus is surrounded by bone. The ear canal forms a blind pouch with a length of approximately 2.5 cm, or 1 inch, and a diameter of 6–8 mm (¼ inch), the medial surface of which is formed by the tympanic membrane or eardrum. The lateral one-third of the ear canal contains cilia and cerumen glands, which serve to protect the ear canal by trapping and expelling foreign material. The external auditory meatus has an irregular course as it passes toward the middle ear, with the external portion rising gently followed by a slightly inferior-anterior direction through the remaining length.

The tympanic membrane is an important structure anatomically as well as physiologically, in as much as it marks the boundary between the external and middle ear and is the point at which the acoustic signal is converted to mechanical energy. The tympanic membrane is a taut membrane composed of three layers. Squamous epithelium comprises the lateral layer and is continuous with the covering of the external auditory meatus. A tough fibrous portion forms the middle layer and is contained in all but a small superior portion of the tympanic membrane called the pars flaccida. The medial covering is formed from mucous membrane, which is the same tissue that lines the middle ear cavity. The tympanic membrane is anchored at its perimeter by a ligamental ring called the annular ligament. The general appearance of the tympanic membrane is that of a shallow cone with an area of 55–90 mm^2, whose apex points toward the middle ear cavity. The center of the membrane, or the apex of the cone, is called the umbo and marks the tip of the manubrium (handle) of the malleus. Figure 3-2 shows a schematic representation of the tympanic membrane, the middle ear, and the ear canal.

The middle ear space is an air-filled cavity that predominately lies between the tympanic membrane and the bony labyrinthian wall. The total volume of this cavity is about 2 cc^2, with a small portion of that volume comprising the epitympanic recess; the region superior to the margin of the tympanic membrane. The middle ear cavity is ventilated to the nasopharynx via the eustachian tube, which opens into the anterior wall of the middle ear cavity. In addition to equalizing the air pressure between the middle ear and the nasopharynx, the eustachian tube functions as a drainage route for middle ear secretions.

Three small ossicles bridge the middle ear cleft between the tympanic membrane and the oval window of the cochlea (see Figs. 3-3A and B). The first of these bones, the malleus, is comprised of a bulky head, a neck, the manubrium or handle, and two short processes: the anterior

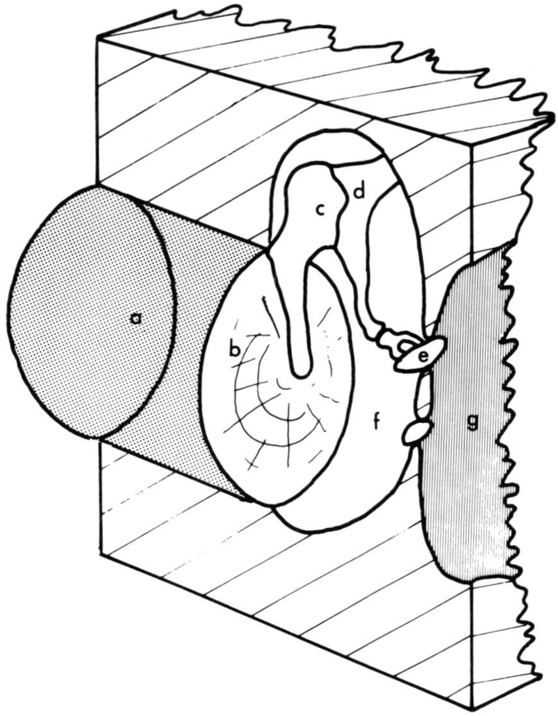

Fig. 3-2. A schematic diagram of the external and middle ear showing the (a) external auditory canal, (b) tympanic membrane, (c) malleus, (d) incus, (e) stapes, (f) middle ear cavity, and (g) lateral wall of the osseous labyrinth.

process and the lateral process. The malleus is supported by the superior ligament and the anterior ligament, which attaches to the anterior process of the malleus. Additionally, the ligament of the tensor tympani muscle inserts on the neck of the malleus opposite the lateral process. The tensor tympani muscle originates within a bony canal lying parallel to the eustachean tube. The malleus and the incus abut at their complementary articulatory facets to form the rigid malleoincudal joint. The head of the malleus and the body of the incus are situated well above the superior margin of the tympanic membrane in the epitympanic recess. From the body of the incus emerge two processes at right angles to each other. The short process extends posteriorly and is anchored to the posterior wall of the middle ear via the posterior ligament. The long process runs parallel to the manubrium of the malleus and terminates in a small bulge called the lenticular process. The articulation of the lenticular process and the head of

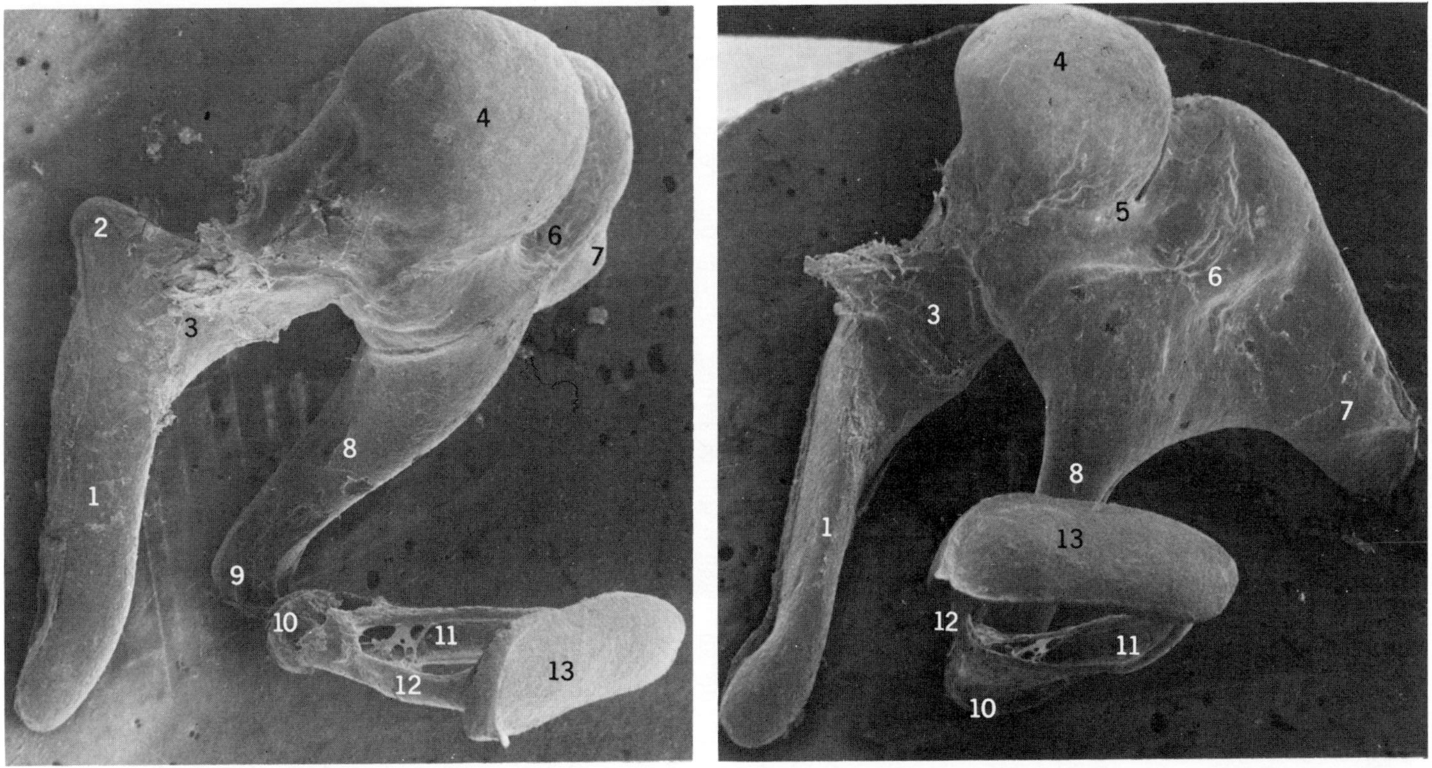

Fig. 3-3. (Left) Middle ear ossicles as seen from the front (anterior view), and (right) as seen from within the inner ear (medial view). 1–4 are parts of the malleus, 6–9 are parts of the incus, and 10–13 indicate stapes structures. (1) manubrium, (2) lateral process, (3) neck, (4) head, (5) malleoincudal joint, (6) body, (7) short process, (8) long process, (9) lenticular process, (10) head, (11) posterior crus, (12) anterior crus, (13) footplate. [Photographs by Ivan Hunter-Duvar. From Yost, W. A., & Nielsen, D. W. *Fundamentals of hearing: an introduction*. New York: Holt, Rinehart, & Winston, 1977, p. 35. Used with permission.]

the stapes forms the incudostapedial joint. The stapes consists of a flat footplate, a supporting arch formed by two delicate crura or arches, and a head. The footplate of the stapes fills the oval window and is supported around its circumference by the annular ligament. The tendon of the stapedial muscle inserts at the head of the stapes near the posterior crus. The stapedial muscle originates from a bony canal within the posterior wall of the middle ear.

Physiology

The structures of the middle and outer ear function together to transmit sound energy to the cochlea. These structures most efficiently transmit a relatively narrow band of frequencies from 500–5000 Hz.

HEAD SHADOW

The first alteration in the acoustic signal results from the placement of the ears on either side of the head. This arrangement dictates that one ear will always be closer to the sound source than the other, with the exception of sounds presented in the midsagital plane. Two significant changes occur in the acoustic signal as it proceeds to the ear most distant from the sound source. First, the additional time required for the sound to travel the extra distance will result in a time delay in the arrival of the signal at the tympanic membrane. The greatest possible interaural delay is about 660 μsec and occurs when the signal is presented directly toward one ear. This delay is a result of the time required for the sound to travel the 16.5 cm to the opposite ear (Federson et al., 1957). Psychoacoustical studies have determined that these interaural time differences are essential cues in determining the location of low frequency sound sources (Stevens & Newman, 1936; Mills 1958).

A second effect occasioned by the physical separation of the ears is an interaural difference in sound pressure. This difference is called the head shadow effect and derives from the wave phenomenon of diffraction. When a sound wave encounters a barrier such as the head, its progress is blocked, creating a sound "shadow" behind the barrier. However, the direction of propagation of some sounds, most notably low frequencies, is altered and the sound wave "fills" in behind the obstacle, thereby reducing the acoustic shadow. The magnitude of the head shadow is frequency-dependent, with the greatest sound attenuation occurring for high frequency signals which do not easily diffract.

As with interaural time differences, the magnitude of the head shadow is greatest when the sound is presented directly toward one ear (90° azimuth). Frequencies greater than 2000 Hz can produce a head shadow as great as 20 dB, but the magnitude of the head shadow decreases with frequency to near zero dB at 200 Hz (Fedderson et al., 1957). Placement of the ears on opposite sides of the head ensures maximum interaural intensity differences. This acoustic cue is extremely useful in determining the direction from which a high frequency signal originates (Stevens & Newman, 1936; Mills, 1958). On the other hand, the head shadow can prove disadvantageous in the cases of monaural hearing loss or unilateral hearing aid use. In these situations, if the signal is directed toward the poorer ear, a head shadow as great as 13 dB may occur for spondee thresholds (Olsen & Carhart, 1967; Tillman et al., 1970), significantly increasing the signal-to-noise ratio of speech and the ambient noise.

EXTERNAL EAR RESONANCE

As sound impinges upon the external ear and is funneled toward the tympanic membrane, the sound pressure of certain frequencies is enhanced due to the resonance effects of the external ear cavities. The combined resonance effects of the concha and the ear canal result in a 10–15 dB increase in sound pressure at the tympanic membrane for frequencies near 3000 Hz. This elevation in sound pressure extends over a frequency range from approximately 1500–7000 Hz. The broad frequency range of the external ear resonance results from the combination of two separate resonance systems with different resonant frequencies. The ear canal resonates with a peak sound pressure enhancement of 10 dB centered at 2500 Hz. The concha resonance has a similar magnitude, but occurs at about 5000 Hz (Shaw, 1974). Interestingly, these resonance effects correspond well with the frequency range of the low-intensity consonants of the speech signal.

ACOUSTIC REFLEX

The muscles of the middle ear, the stapedius and the tensor tympani, function together to effect a change in the transmission properties of the ear in response to intense acoustic stimuli. This feedback mechanism, called the acoustic reflex, is perhaps the most dramatic peripheral auditory control system.

For man, contraction of the stapedius muscle occurs in response to acoustic stimulation, while both the tensor tympani and the stapedius muscles contract in other mammals. The contraction of these muscles results in an increase in the stiffness of the ossicular chain, with the stapedius muscle drawing the head of the stapes in a posterior direction and causing the stapes footplate to rotate away from the oval window. The tensor tympani muscle draws the malleus inward, causing the tympanic membrane to be displaced medially. Thus, although these muscles act to draw their respective ossicles in opposing directions, they complement each other in function by adding rigidity to the ossicular chain.

Activation of the acoustic reflex feedback mechanism begins with transmission of neural activity through the auditory pathways to the superior olivary complex. The descending activity in the loop is activated from the superior olivary complex via the motor neurons of the stapedius and the tensor tympani muscles. Innervation of the stapedius muscle is through the facial nerve and the tensor tympani muscle is innervated via a branch of the trigeminal nerve. Although the acoustic reflex may be activated by acoustic stimulation of either ear, the middle ear muscles contract bilaterally. Therefore, a unilateral stimulation results in activation of the middle ear muscles of both ears.

Activation of the middle ear muscle reflex may also be initiated from nonauditory centers. It is well established that certain movements of the head and neck (Carmel & Starr, 1963; Salomon & Starr, 1963), stimulation of the eye region (Klockhoff & Anderson, 1960), tactile or electrical stimulation of the skin in the ear canal (Klockhoff, 1961; Djupesland, 1962; Klockhoff & Anderson, 1959), and vocalization (Henson, 1965) are capable of generating middle ear muscle contractions. Some people are also able to voluntarily initiate contractions of their middle ear muscles (Smith, 1943; Reger, 1960).

The acoustic reflex is elicited by pure tones approximately 80 dB above threshold, while complex signals such as noise will elicit the reflex at lower levels (Peterson & Liden, 1972). The effect of the middle ear muscle contraction is to increase the stiffness of the ossicular chain, thereby increasing the acoustic impedance of the middle ear for low frequency signals. This increased acoustic impedance presents an opposition to the transmission of sound to the cochlea, resulting in a decreased stapes velocity. However, the amount of change in transmission is not necessarily equal to the change in impedance (Møller, 1965). That is, the actual attenuation occasioned by the acoustic reflex may be less than that expected on the basis of the change in middle ear impedance. Thus, estimates of the effect of the middle ear muscle reflex upon the middle ear transmission must be based upon direct measures of cochlear input.

The most dramatic quantification of the effect of the middle ear muscle contraction has come from animal studies in which changes in the magnitude of the cochlear microphonic (CM) were measured. Since the CM is proportional to the velocity of the stapes, changes in middle ear transmission will be reflected in the magnitude of the CM. The change in middle ear transmission inferred form CM measurements amounts to 10–30 dB for frequencies below 2000 Hz. The amount of attenuation increases as the intensity of the eliciting stimulus increases, yielding a change in transmission of 0.6–0.7 dB per decibel increase above the threshold of the acoustic reflex (Wiggers, 1937; Wever & Vernon, 1955; Galambos & Rupert, 1959; Simmons, 1964; Borg, 1972).

Since the cochlear microphonic is not easily monitored in man, estimates of the attenuation effect of the middle ear muscle reflex have been derived from psychoacoustical experimentation. Smith (1943) and Reger (1960) found that the pure tone threshold increased by as much as 30 dB for a 500 Hz signal in subjects who could voluntarily contract their middle ear muscles. No threshold change occurred for stimuli above 200 Hz. Yet, it is not clear that voluntary contraction of the middle ear muscles is equivalent to acoustic reflex contractions. In fact, studies employing an acoustically elicited middle ear muscle contraction showed little change in the pure tone threshold (Loeb & Riopelle, 1960; Ward, 1961; Morgan et al., 1978). In contrast, indirect measures of the acoustic reflex attenuation indicate larger effects than do threshold measures. Loeb and Riopelle (1960) and Morgan & Dirks (1975) measured monaural loudness changes in the presence of a contralaterally elicited acoustic reflex. In general, it was found that the acoustic reflex reduced the loudness of the signal equivalent to 7–15 dB for low-frequency signals. Estimates based upon masking effectiveness of low-frequency maskers indicates an attentuation of 20 dB (Borg & Zakrisson, 1974).

ACOUSTIC REFLEX FUNCTION

Many theories have been advanced to attach functional significance to the acoustic reflex. Since the acoustic reflex attenuates low-frequency signals, it has the effect of extending the dynamic range of the ear. This amplitude compression serves to limit the input at the cochlea, thus overcoming many deleterious effects of high-intensity, low-frequency signals. For instance, it has been demonstrated that the elicitation of the acoustic reflex reduces the amount of temporary threshold shift normally caused by low-frequency stimuli (Hilding, 1960, 1961; Fletcher & Riopelle, 1960; Zakrisson & Borg, 1974).

Activation of the acoustic reflex also decreases the masking effectiveness of low-frequency stimuli (Borg, 1972) and limits the distortion products introduced by the ear for high-intensity signals. This combination of effects has the potential of enhancing the quality of the signal transduced by the cochlea by increasing the signal to noise ratio (Wang & Bilger, 1973). This reduction in masking and distortion has been thought to aid in the perception of speech signals. Investigators have demonstrated a decreased ability to discriminate speech in the presence of a competing noise for subjects without an acoustic reflex. Borg and Zakrisson (1974) and McCandless and Goering (1974) found decreased speech discrimination in noise and in quiet for subjects with normal hearing sensitivity but absent acoustic reflexes due to Bell's palsy. For subjects with interruption of the acoustic reflex due to stapedectomies, speech discrimination in noise was also reduced (Liden et al., 1963; Mahoney, 1973). Although improved speech discrimination in noise is seen when performance for normal ears is compared with performance for ears in which the acoustic reflex is absent, Rappaport (1976) found no improvement in speech discrimination in noise for normal listeners when the acoustic reflex was elicited by a contralateral stimulus.

It has been suggested that the acoustic reflex also serves to: (a) enhance ability for sound localization (Lawrence, 1965); (b) diminish middle ear resonance peaks (Simmons, 1964); (c) provide a variable auditory background, which enhances auditory attention (Tumarkin 1945, Simmons, 1964). Comprehensive reviews of the acoustic reflex can be found elsewhere (Borg, 1976; Møller, 1974; Dallos, 1973).

MIDDLE EAR TRANSFORMER

In terrestrial animals, the middle ear functions to transmit sound waves striking the tympanic membrane across the ossicular chain to the fluid system of the inner ear.

Laws of physics and acoustics describe a basic incompatibility of sound wave movement between acoustic media having different sound conduction properties (impedances). The difference in acoustic impedance between air and the fluid-filled cochlea is such that without the middle ear structures, only 0.1 percent of the signal energy would be transmitted from air to the fluid of the cochlea. Conversely, 99.9 percent of the signal energy would be reflected back (Wever & Lawrence, 1954). Such a reduction in intensity would yield a 30 dB attentuation at the cochlea. For very low-frequency signals, the estimated sound pressure loss between air and the cochlea is closer to 50 dB (Killion & Dallos, 1979).

The primary function of the middle ear is to decrease this impedance mismatch between air and the cochlea. Two mechanisms facilitate this transformer function: the effective lever raito of the malleus and the incus, and the effective area ratio between the tympanic membrane and the stapes footplate. For man, the increase in force at the cochlea due to the lever action of the ossicles is estimated to be 1.3 to 1 (Bekesy, 1960). The ratio of the affective area (that portion which actually vibrates) of the tympanic membrane to the area of the stapes footplate using the values proposed by Bekesy and Rosenblith (1951) is equal to 17 to 1. Since pressure is the product of force and area, the increase in sound pressure at the cochlea is given by the product of the ratios of force (1.3:1) and area (17:1), which is equal to approximately 22:1, or a 27 dB increase in sound pressure. This middle ear transformer has the effect of transfering to the cochlea 46 percent of the incident intensity at the tympanic membrane. (The interested reader is referred to Zwislocki, 1975, Dallos, 1973, Wever & Lawrence, 1954, and Killion & Dallos, 1979 for reviews of the impedance matching mechanism of the middle ear.)

INNER EAR

Anatomy

OSSEOUS AND MEMBRANOUS LABYRINTH

There are two inner-ear labyrinths within the temporal bone. The osseous, or bony, labyrinth is the larger cavity and contains within it the membranous labyrinth, a sac that has the same general shape as the osseous labyrinth enclosing it. The space between the osseous and membranous labyrinths is filled with a fluid called perilymph. The membranous labyrinth itself contains endolymph.

There are three distinct areas within the bony labyrinth. Medial to the oval window is the large, fluid-filled chamber called the vestibule. Posterior to the vestibule and somewhat superior are the three semicircular canals situated in their respective geometric planes. Anterior to the vestibule is the cochlea, which derives its name from its distinctive snail-like shape. In man, the cochlea spirals for 2¾ turns with the coils decreasing in diameter toward the apex.

The membranous labyrinth has three functional divisions. The membranous semicircular canals within the osseous semicircular canals contain specialized sensory structures within their ampullated endings called christae. Stimulation of the cristae due to the fluid motion within the semicircular canals allows the vestibular system to process angular acceleration. The utricle and the saccule are located within the vestibule of the bony labyrinth. Each contains a sensory receptor sensitive to linear acceleration. Finally, the cochlear duct or scala media is suspended throughout the length of the cochlear portion of the osseous labyrinth and divides it into two tubes or scala, called the scala vestibuli and the scala tympani. Within the scala media lies the organ of Corti, which is the sensory receptor for acoustic stimuli. The scala media is attached to the osseous spiral lamina on the central wall of the coiled cochlea and to the spiral ligament on the peripheral wall of the cochlea. The scala vestibuli extends from the vestibule to the apex of the cochlea, and the scala tympani extends from the round window to the apex where the two scala connect via the helicotrema. The vestibular and cochlear portions of the membranous labyrinth are connected via the ductus reuniens. The endolymph, which fills the membranous labyrinth, is thought to arise from the stria vascularis within the cochlear partition, and is reabsorbed via the endolymphatic sac.

SCALA MEDIA

The cochlea is approximately 35 mm in length; the scala media is about 31 mm long. If one were to cut the scala media perpendicular to its length, its salient structures would be visible as seen in Fig. 3-4. The common wall between the scala media and scala vestibuli is Reissner's membrane, which slopes up to about a 30° angle from the spiral limbus. The outer margin of the scala media is the spiral ligament, which attaches directly to the osseous wall. On the inferior surface is the basilar membrane on which is situated the hair cells and the supporting structures comprising the organ of Corti. A portion of the organ of Corti rests upon the rigid osseous spiral lamina; the remainder is supported by the flexible basilar membrane. The width of the basilar membrane increases from 0.16 mm at the base to 0.52 mm at the apex. The basal end of the basilar membrane is also stiffer than the apical end by a hundredfold (Bekesy, 1960).

The three outer rows of hair cells are anchored at their bases by the Deiter cells and are flanked by the Hensen cells peripherally and the rods of Corti centrally. The phalangeal processes of the Deiter cells extend to

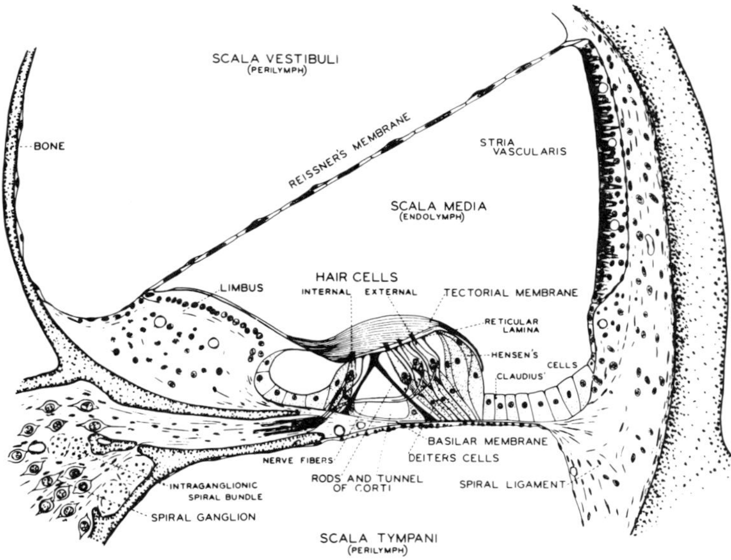

Fig. 3-4. Cross-sectional view of the scala media. [From Davis, H., Benson, R., Covell, W. P., Fernández, C., et al. Acoustic trauma in the guinea pig. *Journal of the Acoustical Society of America,* 1953, *25,* 1180–1181. Used with permission.]

the tops of the hair cells and join with the headplates of the rods of Corti to form the reticular lamina. This rigid lattice firmly holds the tops of the hair cells. The inner row of hair cells is supported by the rods of Corti and the border cells of the inner sulcus. Three rows of tiny cilia called stereocilia protrude from the top of each hair cell. The tallest row of these stereocillia is embedded in the tectorial membrane. The tectorial membrane is a soft ribbon-like flap supported on its edges by the spiral limbus and the organ of Corti. On the peripheral wall of the scala media is a rich vascular network called the stria vascularis, which serves to maintain the high potassium and low sodium ionic concentrations characteristic of endolymph.

Many of the structures of the organ of Corti can be seen in the scanning electron micrograph of a longitudinal section of the cochlea shown in Fig. 3-5.

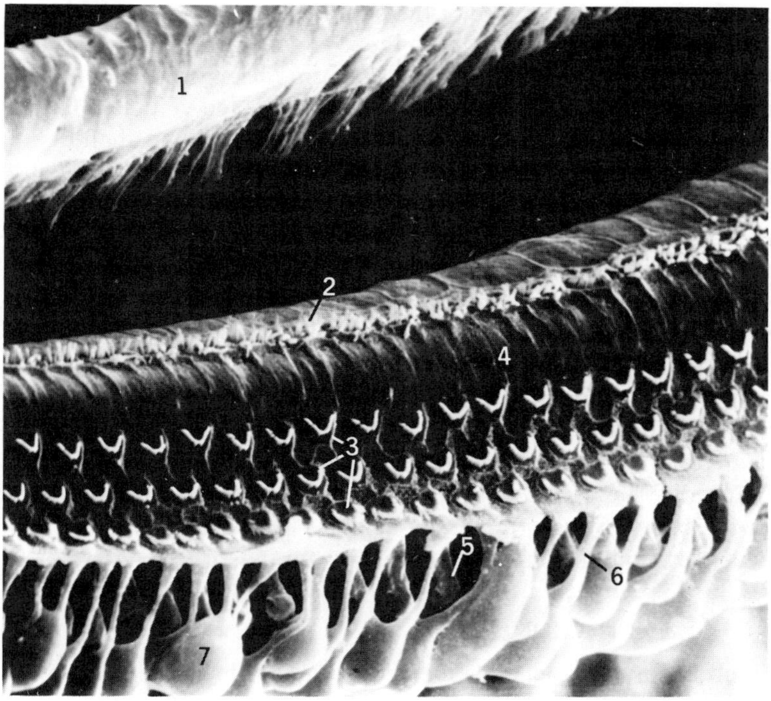

Fig. 3-5. Scanning electron micrograph of the organ of Corti showing the tectorial membrane (1) lifted back from the tops of the single row of inner hair cells (2), the three rows of outer hair cells (3), and the headplates of the inner pillar cells (4). Within the organ of Corti, the outer row of outer hair cells (5) as well as the Deiter cells (7) and their phalangeal processes (6) are visible. [Photograph courtesy of Dr. Muriel Ross, Department of Anatomy, University of Michigan.]

Physiology

TRAVELING WAVE

The cochlea is a hydromechanical system that acts to transform the piston-like motion of the stapes footplate into a wave pattern within the cochlea, which facilitates the analysis of signal amplitude, phase, and frequency.

Movement of the stapes footplate into the cochlea creates an increase in fluid pressure within the vestibule. The instantaneous increase in fluid pressure within the scala vestibuli is transfered to the scala tympani by displacement of scale media. Since fluid is a noncompressable medium, this increased pressure must be subsequently relieved by displacement of the flexible round window. The reciprocating motion of the stapes causes the scala media to be displaced alternately toward the scala tympani and the scala vestibuli, resulting in a displacement pattern proportional to the changes in the sound pressure of the acoustic stimulus. Due to the particular mechanical characteristics of the cochlea, this displacement wave induced in the scala media moves away from the base of the cochlea and travels toward the apex with changing amplitude and velocity. The amplitude of displacement increases to a maximum value and then decreases rapidly as the wave continues toward the apex while the velocity decreases to zero. Figure 3-6A is a schematic representation of the traveling wave as it would appear in one instant of time in the uncoiled basilar membrane. Figure 3-6B is a more realistic view, since it represents the traveling wave that results from the edges of the basilar membrane being anchored.

For low-frequency signals, the wave travels further toward the apex before the displacement amplitude reaches its maximum. Therefore, the peak of the traveling wave envelope is distributed along the length of the cochlear partition according to the frequency of the driving signal, with maximum displacement occuring at the apex for low-frequency signals and at the base for high-frequency signals. Different locations along the cochlear partition are tuned for different stimulus frequencies.

HAIR CELL EXCITATION

In order for electrochemical excitation of the hair cells of the organ of Corti to occur, it is necessary that the mechanical activity of the traveling wave be transfered to the receptor portion of the hair cell. The effective physiological stimulus for the hair cells of the organ of Corti is a radial shearing of the stereocilia in the direction of the stria vascularis (Bekesy, 1960). This shearing action is derived from the relative movement between the hair cell and the tectorial membrane overlying the hair cell. Some of the inner and outer hair cell stereocilia are in direct contact with

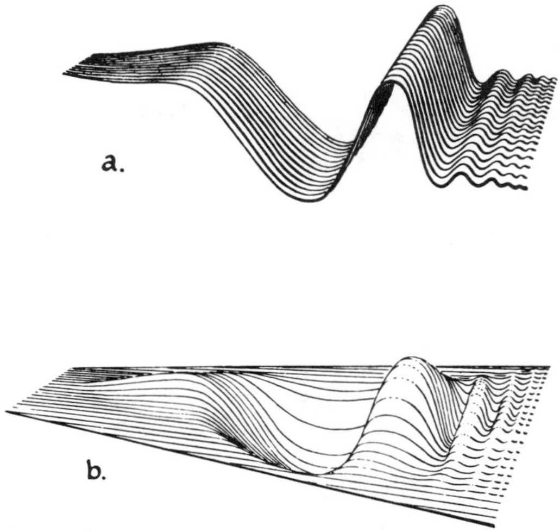

Fig. 3-6. (A) Hypothetical traveling wave pattern executed in a ribbon-like partition. (B) Hypothetical traveling wave with edges of partition anchored. [From Tonndorf, J. Shearing motion in scala media of cochlear models. *Journal of the Acoustical Society of America,* 1960. *32:* 238–244. Used with permission.]

the tectorial membrane; they either touch it or are embedded in it. The tectorial membrane itself is loosely coupled to the remainder of the organ of Corti. That is, although it is attached at the Hensen cells, this attachment is considered to be sufficiently loose to allow the tectorial membrane to slide back and forth across the tops of the hair cells. This shearing motion is accommodated by the separate pivot points of the tectorial membrane at the tip of the spiral limbus and the organ of Corti at the lip of the osseous spiral lamina as seen in Fig. 3-7. As the scala media is displaced upward, the tectorial membrane slides across the tips of the hair cells toward the stria vascularis. When the scala media is displaced downward, the stereocila are displaced in the opposite direction. Thus, the up-and-down motion of the traveling wave is translated into the back-and-forth motion of the stereocilia by virtue of the relative motion of the organ of Corti and the tectorial membrane.

The final stage of coupling between the acoustic signal and its representation as neural excitation occurs within the hair cells of the organ of Corti. The exact electrochemical basis of hair cell excitation is still unresolved, but the electrical events associated with the generation of the neural action potential suggests the general physiological mechanism.

Four electrical potentials are associated with the organ of Corti. Two of these potentials, the endocochlear potential (EP) and the hair cell potential, are resting potentials and are present at all times. The cochlear microphonic (CM) and the summating potential (SP) are stimulus-related potentials, and are only present when the cochlea is stimulated. The EP is

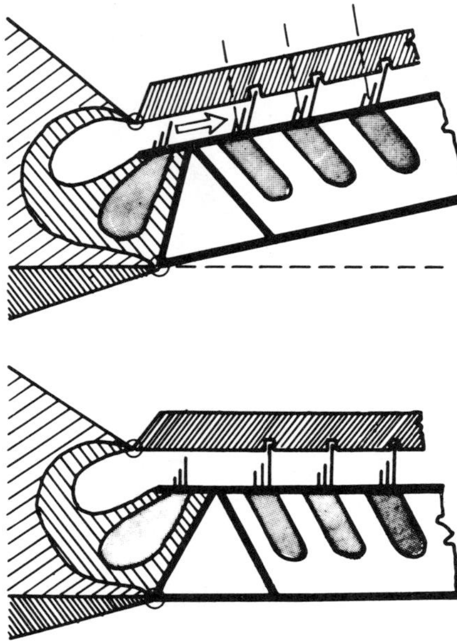

Fig. 3-7. Schematic representation of shearing action between the tectorial membrane and the organ of Corti. Bottom: organ at rest; top: during displacement toward scala vestibuli. [From Ryan, A., & Dallos, P. Physiology of the inner ear. In J. L. Northern (Ed.), *Hearing disorders*. Boston: Little, Brown & Company, 1976, pp. 89–101. Used with permission.]

a +80 mV potential maintained within the endolymph of the scala media. It is the largest positive DC potential in the body, and arises from the metabolic activity of the stria vascularis. The second resting potential is maintained within the hair cells of the organ of Corti and has a magnitude of −80 mV. Therefore, at the top of the hair cells, where they contact the endolymph of the scala media, there exists a total electrical potential gradient of about 160 mV. This difference in electrical potential is thought to aid in ion transport across the membranes of the hair cells, producing a leakage current through the hair cells (Davis, 1965). It is thought that mechanical deformation of the stereocila due to the shearing action of the tectorial membrane somehow alters the permeability of the hair cell membranes, thereby modulating the current flow through the tops of the hair cells. This alternating current appears as a variable voltage which has the same form as the amplitude waveform of the acoustic driving stimulus. This alternating voltage is reflected in the cochlear microphonic.

The CM mirrors the displacement of the cochlear partition and has virtually the same waveform as the acoustic stimulus driving the ear. Although it is not clear whether the CM is an essential link in the sensory reception of the hair cells or whether it is an epiphenomenon, measurements of the CM have been useful in studying the displacement patterns of the basilar membrane and in monitoring the physiological state of the cochlea. The fourth cochlear potential, called the summating potential, is observed as a negative DC shift in the CM. Its exact source and functional relationship to hair cell excitation have not been determined, although it may reflect nonlinearities in the sensory receptors.

EIGHTH NERVE

Anatomy

The acoustic branch of the eighth nerve is composed of the nerve fibers which innervate the organ of Corti. The most remarkable aspect of the cochlear innervation is the contrast in the pattern of innervation of the inner hair cells and the outer hair cells. Figure 3-8 shows the afferent innervation of the cochlea. The majority of the afferent neurons (95 percent) synapse with one of the 3,500 inner hair cells with a density of 16–20

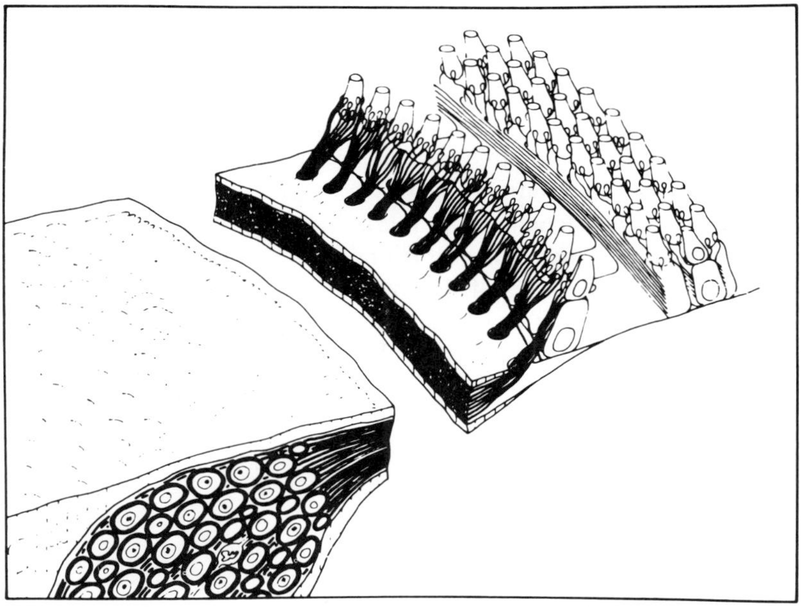

Fig. 3-8. Schematic representation of the afferent innervation of the organ of Corti. Ninety-five percent of the neurons synapse with the inner hair cells, five percent of the neurons synapse with the outer hair cells. The cell bodies of the afferent neurons are situated in the spiral ganglion. [From Spoendlin, H. Innervation densities of the cochlea. *Acta Oto-laryngologica,* 1972, *73,* 235–248. Used with permission.]

fibers per hair cell. As these fibers leave the hair cells, they accumulate in bundles called the inner radial bundles, which course into the nearest perforata habenula.

The afferent innervation of the outer hair cells is via the outer spiral bundles, so called because of the circuitous route taken by these nerve fibers as they pass toward the modiolus. Since the fibers of the outer spiral bundle comprise only 5 percent of the afferent neurons, and the number of outer hair cells is approximately three times that of the inner hair cells (12,000), the innervation density of the outer hair cells is significantly less than that of the inner hair cells. Each fiber of the outer spiral bundles synapses with approximately ten hair cells. The fibers then spiral apically between the rows of outer hair cells before crossing the tunnel of Corti and entering the nearest perforata habenula.

The afferent neurons of the eighth nerve are bipolar with their cell bodies accumulated in the spiral ganglion, which derives its name from its spiraling distribution within the center of the osseous cochlea (modiolus). The axons of these first-order neurons gather into a bundle forming the acoustic portion of the eighth nerve. The nerve fibers join this bundle as it passes through the modiolus from the apex of the cochlea. Thus, the fibers innervating the apex of the cochlea lie in the center of the bundle, and the fibers of the succeeding turns of the cochlea are added in concentric rings with the fibers from the basal turn of the cochlea lying on the outside of the nerve bundle.

Efferent innervation of the cochlea consists of 500–600 neurons arising predominately from the contralateral superior olivary complex (crossed olivocochlear bundle) or the homolateral superior olivary complex (uncrossed olivocochlear bundle). A portion of these neurons pass between the afferent neurons of the inner radial bundle, forming the inner spiral bundle. The neurons of the inner spiral bundle do not synapse directly with the inner hair cells, but rather with the afferent neurons of the inner radial bundle. The remainder of the efferent neurons cross the tunnel of Corti and synapse with the nearest group of outer hair cells.

Physiology

ACTION POTENTIAL GENERATION

In response to the receptor potentials within the hair cells, chemical excitatory substances are released at the synapse of the hair cell and the afferent neuron, producing a graded response in the unmyelinated portion of the neuron. This graded potential is transmitted to the perforata habenula where the myelin covering of the neurons begins. At this junction, the spike discharge of the action potential is initiated if the graded potential is of sufficient magnitude. Since the graded potential initiates the action potential in the neuron, it is referred to as a generator potential. Following the action potential discharge, no magnitude of generator potential will elicit a subsequent action potential until the neuron has had an opportunity to recharge. This period of time is called the absolute refractory period and lasts for about 1 msec. Therefore, given optimum excitation, the maximum rate of discharge for neurons would be about 1000 per second. Following the absolute refractory period is an interval in which the neuron may discharge if the stimulus magnitude is increased above the threshold level. As the generator potential increases, the interval between spike discharges decreases, yielding a shorter refractory period for large stimulus magnitudes than for weaker stimuli. Thus, the number of spikes per second produced by a neuron is proportional to the stimulus magnitude. For auditory neurons, increases in stimulus intensity result in increased spike rates over an intensity range of approximately 30 dB.

FREQUENCY SELECTIVITY

Of interest physiologically is the frequency range over which a neuron will respond when the ear is stimulated. This neuronal frequency selectivity is determined with the aid of tuning curves or frequency threshold curves (FTC). The FTC is obtained by presenting discrete frequency stimuli at increasing intensities until a criterion firing rate is reached. The intensity required to obtain the criterion firing rate at each frequency is the excitation threshold of the neuron. Figure 3-9 shows the frequency threshold curves for several neurons obtained from guinea pig ears. For each neuron, there is a particular stimulus frequency at which the criterion firing rate can be reached with a minimum sound pressure. This frequency is called the characteristic frequency. As the stimulus frequency is increased, the stimulus intensity must be increased greatly in order to maintain the neuronal response. For frequencies lower than the characteristic frequency, the stimulus intensity must also be increased; however, the neuron remains responsive to stimuli several octaves below the characteristic frequency. The area above the curve is termed the response area and delineates the frequency by intensity boundaries within which the neuron is responsive.

The general shape of the frequency response curve is explained in part by traveling wave mechanics. Recall that the traveling wave has a point of maximum displacement at some point along the cochlear partition. For areas toward the apex or the base, the displacement amplitude is reduced. As the stimulus frequency is increased or decreased, the point of maximum displacement is shifted apically or basally, respectively. Each of the neurons in the eighth nerve innervates only a small region of the cochlea, and the firing rate of each neuron is proportional to the basilar membrane displacement for the area that the neuron innervates. Thus, a change in stimulus frequency from the characteristic frequency will shift

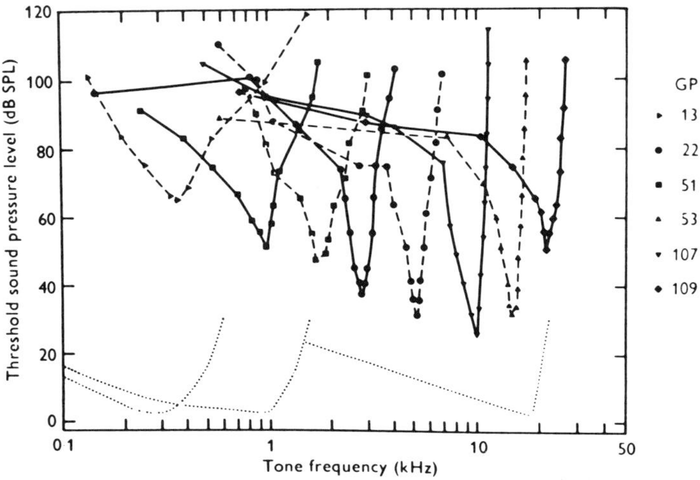

Fig. 3-9. Solid lines show frequency threshold curves for eight cochlear neurons obtained from six guinea pig ears. Ordinate is in dB SPL measured at the tympanic membrane. Dotted lines show analogous basilar membrane displacement derived from Bekesy, 1960 (curves at 0.27 and 0.9 kHz) and from Johnstone, Taylor, and Boyle, 1970 (curve at 18 kHz). SPL for displacement curves is arbitrary. [From Evans, E. F. The frequency response and other properties of single fibers in the guinea pig cochlea. *Journal of Physiology,* 1972, *226,* 263–287. Used with permission.]

the peak of the traveling wave to an adjacent region and the neural firing rate will decrease. Although this explanation accounts for the gross shape of the FTCs, it is not sufficient to explain their sharpness. In Fig. 3-8, the inverse of the basilar membrane displacement curve is shown as a function of frequency for three points along the basilar membrane. Note that the slopes of these functions are much more shallow than the frequency threshold curves. This discrepancy has led to the supposition that an additional stage of filtering occurs between the traveling wave displacement and neural activation (Evans & Harrison, 1976). This filter, called the second filter, has been hypothesized to arise from interactions between inner and outer hair cells, although no direct experimental evidence exists to support this theory.

Masking studies indicate that the sharpness of tuning demonstrated in the FTC is preserved in the auditory system. The psychoacoustical equivalent of the FTC is obtained by presenting a low-intensity signal and determining those combinations of masker intensity and frequency that will just mask the signal. The psychophysical tuning curves (PTC) determined by these masking experiments are similar in shape to FTC curves (Small, 1959; Zwicker, 1974; Houtgast, 1976; Rodenburg et al., 1974). The sharpest psychophysical tuning curves are found using paradigms in which the signal and the masker do not directly interact within the ear

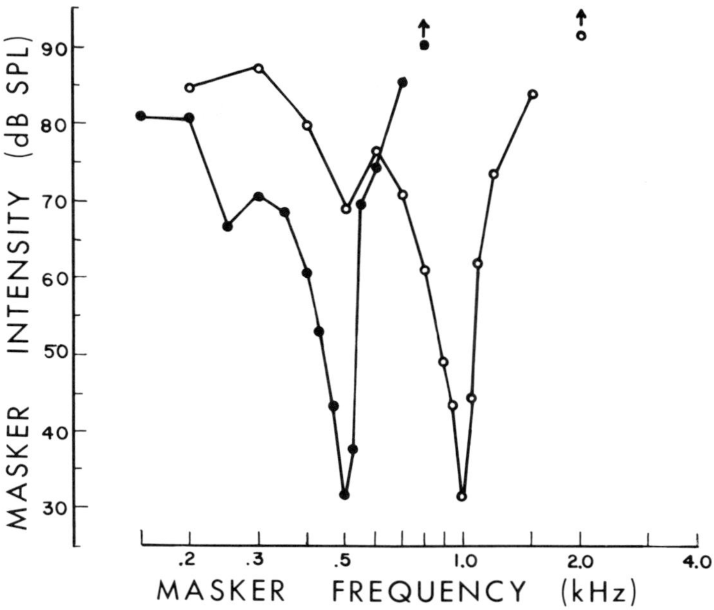

Fig. 3-10. Masker intensities required to mask a contralateral, 50 msec pure tone presented at 8 dB SL signal frequency was 0.5 or 1.0 kHz. [Adapted from Tucci, D., & Calder, H. B. Binaural frequency selectivity measured with a central masking paradigm. *Journal of the Acoustical Society of America,* 1977, *62,* 597(A).]

such as in pulsation threshold masking (Houtgast, 1974; Verschuure, 1977), forward masking (Rodenburg et al., 1974; Wightman et al., 1977), and central masking (Tucci & Calder, 1977). Figure 3-10 shows the psychophysical tuning curves obtained for two frequencies employing a central masking task. Note the similarity of the FTC curves in Fig. 3-9, which show a narrow tip portion, a steep high-frequency slope, and a more shallow low-frequency slope.

EFFECT OF COCHLEAR PATHOLOGY UPON FREQUENCY SELECTIVITY

An area of current interest in auditory neurophysiology is the effect of cochlear lesions upon the shape of the FTC. These investigations have implications for the speech-processing ability of hearing-impaired listeners, since the FTS reflects the ear's ability to selectively process the discrete frequency elements of the speech signal.

The first investigation of FTCs in lesioned ears was carried out by Kiang and his colleagues (1970), who found that for cats with lesions due to kanamycin ototoxicity or due to noise exposure, FTCs from units with characteristic frequencies within the lesion area were not obtainable. For units with characteristic frequencies lying at the border of the lesions, the

FTCs were irregular in shape, and many showed an absence of the narrowly tuned tip portion of the function. Evans (1972) measured FTCs in guinea pigs that had been treated with kanamycin. He also found that with an absence of outer hair cells, the FTCs became broadly tuned with virtually no tip section. In contrast, Dallos and Harris (1978) found that with the absence of outer hair cells in kanamycin-poisoned chinchillas, the tip portion of the FTC function retained its narrow tuning but became elevated and shortened. Two typical FTC curves are shown in Fig. 3-11.

It appears from animal studies that a complete absence of inner and outer hair cells obliterates the FTC. In regions with mixed losses of inner and outer hair cells, such as at the border of a complete hair cell-loss lesion, the shapes of the FTCs are highly variable. And, in instances of purely outer hair cell damage, the tip portion of the FTC is missing, or retains its normal width, but is elevated.

Analagous studies have investigated selectivity using psychophysical tuning curves. Dallos et al. (1977) found no changes in the shape of the

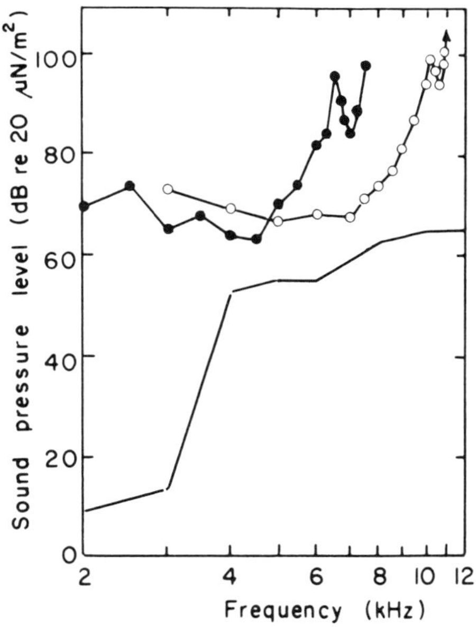

Fig. 3-11. Behavioral threshold curve for a chinchilla with a kanmycin-induced cochlear lesion, and two single unit frequency-threshold curves. [With permission from Dallos, P., Ryan, A., Harris, D., et al: Cochlear frequency selectivity in the presence of hair cell damage. In E. F. Evans & J. P. Wilson (Eds.), *Psychophysics and physiology of hearing*. London: Academic Press, 1977, pp. 249–261. Copyright by Academic Press, Inc., (London) Ltd.]

PTCs in postkanamycin-treated chinchillas. The only effect of the lesions was to elevate the entire PTC. In contrast, several investigators using human subjects have found that in the presence of moderate degrees of cochlear hearing loss, the shape of the PTC is altered, showing shallow, broad PTCs or a complete absence of the narrow tip section of the PTC (Hoekstra & Ritsma, 1977; Leshowitz & Lindstrom, 1977; Pick et al., 1977; Wightman et al., 1977; Zwicker & Schorn, 1978). Some evidence, however, indicates that in mild hearing losses where there is a high probability that only the outer hair cells are damaged, the PTC has a normal shape (McGee, 1977).

It is probable that in cases of moderate cochlear hearing loss, this breakdown in the frequency-resolving capability of the peripheral auditory mechanism may contribute to an increased difficulty in understanding speech (Hood & Poole, 1971). In order to distinguish between speech elements, it is necessary to be able to analyze both the intensity and frequency of the major energy components of the stimulus. Without the frequency-resolving ability of the normal auditory system, signal analysis fails. This would be similar to trying to measure the energy at the fundamental frequency and harmonics of a signal using a broadband filter. It would not be possible to determine what portion of the signal is contributed by each of its components.

SUMMARY

In summary, the peripheral auditory system is well designed as a sensory receptor, converting acoustic stimuli into neurophysical activity which can be processed by the central auditory system. In the process of this transformation, the intensity, phase, and frequency parameters essential for the coding of the speech signal are preserved.

[*Editors' note:* See Chapter 8, "Speech Protocols in the Central Auditory Nervous System Evaluation" for an overview of central anatomy and physiology.]

REFERENCES

Bekesy, G. von. *Experiments in hearing*. New York: McGraw-Hill, 1960.

Bekesy, G. von, & Rosenblith, W. A. The mechanical properties of the ear. In S. S. Stevens, (Ed.), *Handbook of experimental psychology* New York: Wiley & Sons, 1951, pp. 1075–1115.

Borg, E. Acoustic middle ear reflexes. A sensory control system. *Acta Otolaryngol* 1972, *Suppl*. 304.

Borg, E. Dynamic characteristics of the intra-aural muscle reflex. In A. Feldman, L. Wilber (Eds.), *Acoustic Impedance and Admittance—the Measurement of Middle Ear Function,* Baltimore: Williams and Wilkins, 1976.

Borg, E., & Zakrisson, J. E. Stapedius reflex and monaural masking. *Acta Oto-Laryngoligica,* 1974, *78,* 155–161.

Brödel, M. *Three unpublished drawings of the anatomy of the human ear.* Philadelphia: Saunders, 1946.

Carmel, P. W., & Starr, A. Acoustic and nonacoustic factors modifying middle-ear muscle activity in waking cats. *Journal of Neurophyiology,* 1963, *26,* 598–616.

Dallos, P. *The auditory periphery: biophysics and physiology.* New York: Academic Press, 1973.

Dallos, P., & Harris, D. Properties of auditory nerve responses in absence of outer hair cells. *Journal of Neurophysiology,* 1978, *41,* 365–383.

Dallos, P., Ryan, A., Harris, D., McGee, T., & Özdamer, Ö. Cochlear frequency selectivity in the presence of hair cell damage. In E. F. Evans & J. P. Wilson (Eds.), *Psychophysics and physiology of hearing.* London: Academic Press, 1977, pp. 249–258.

Davis, H., Benson, R. W., Covell, W. P., Fernández, C. et al. Acoustic trauma in the guinea pig. *Journal of the Acoustical Society of America,* 1953, *25,* 1180–1189.

Djupesland, G. Intra-aural muscular reflexes elicited by air current stimulation of the external ear. *Acta Oto-Laryngoligica,* 1962, *54,* 143–153.

Durrant, J. D., & Lovrinic, J. H. *Bases of hearing science.* Baltimore: Williams and Wilkins, 1977.

Evans, E. F. The frequency response and other properties of single fibers in the guinea pig cochlear nerve. *Journal of Physiology,* 1972, *226,* 263–287.

Evans, E. F., and Harrison, R. V. Frequency selectivity of the cochlea. In A. Møller (Ed.), *Basic mechanisms in hearing.* New York: Academic Press, 1976, pp. 519–551.

Feddersen, W. E., Sandel, T. T., Teas, D. C., & Jeffress, L. A. Localization of high-frequency tones. *Journal of the Acoustical Society of America,* 1957, *29,* 988–991.

Fletcher, J. L., and Riopelle, A. J. Protective effect of the acoustic reflex for impulsive noise. *Journal of the Acoustical Society of America,* 1960, *32,* 401–404.

Galambos, R., and Rupert, A. L. Action of the middle-ear muscles in normal cats. *Journal of the Acoustical Society of America,* 1959, *31,* 349–355.

Henson, O. W., Jr. The activity and function of the middle-ear muscles in echolocating bats. *Journal of Physiology,* 1965, *180,* 871–887.

Hilding, D. A. The intratympanic muscle reflex as a protective mechanism against loud impulsive noise. Annals of Otolaryngology, 1960, *69,* 51–60.

Hilding, D. A. The protective value of the stapedius reflex: An experimental study. *Transactions; American Academy of Ophthalmology and Otolaryngology,* 1961, *65,* 297–307.

Hoekstra, A., & Ritsma, R. J. Perceptive hearing loss and frequency selectivity. In E. F. Evans & J. P. Wilson (Eds.), *Psychophysics and physiology of hearing.* London: Academic Press, 1977, pp. 264–271.

Hood, J. D., & Poole, J. P. Speech audiometry in conductive and sensorineural hearing loss. *Sound,* 1971, *5,* 30–38.

Houtgast, T. Psychophysical evidence for lateral inhibition in hearing. *Journal of the Acoustical Society of America,* 1972, *51,* 1885–1894.

Johnstone, B. M., Taylor, K. J., & Boyle, A. J. Mechanics of the guinea pig cochlea. *Journal of the Acoustical Society of America,* 1970, *47,* 504–509.

Keidel, W. D., & Neff, W. D. *Handbook of sensory physiology,* Vol. 5, Chap. 1. New York: Sprigner-Verlag, 1974.

Keidel, W. D., & Neff, W. D. *Handbook of sensory physiology,* Vol. 5, Chap. 1. New York: Springer-Verlag, 1975.

Kiang, N. Y-S., Moxon, E. C., & Levine, R. A. Auditory nerve activity in cats with normal and abnormal cochleas. In G. E. W. Wolstenholme & J. Knight (Eds.), *Sensorineural hearing loss.* London: Churchill, 1970, pp. 241–273.

Killion, M. C., & Dallos, P. Impedance matching by the combined effects of the outer and middle ear. *Journal of the Acoustical Society of America,* 1979, *66,* 599–602.

Klockhoff, I. Middle-ear muscle reflexes in man. *Acta Oto-laryngoligica,* 1961, Suppl. 164.

Klockhoff, I., & Anderson, H. Recording of the stapedius reflex elicited by cutaneous stimulation. *Acta Oto-laryngoligica,* 1959, *50,* 451–454.

Klockhoff, I., & Anderson, H. Reflex activity in the tensor tympani muscle recorded in man. *Acta Oto-laryngoligica,* 1960, *51,* 184–188.

Lawrence, M. Middle-ear muscle influence on binaural hearing. *Archives of Otolaryngology,* 1965, *82,* 478–482.

Leshowitz, B., & Lindstrom, K. Measurement of nonlinearities in listeners with sensorineural hearing loss. In E. F. Evans & J. P. Wilson (Eds.), *Psychophysics and physiology of hearing,* London: Academic Press, 1977, pp. 283–292.

Liberman, A. M., Cooper, F. S., Shankweiler, D. P., et al. Perception of the speech code. *Psychological Review,* 1967, *4,* 431–461.

Liden, G., Nordland, B., & Hawkins, J. Significance of the stapedius reflex for the understanding of speech. *Acta Oto-laryngoligica,* 1963, Suppl. 188.

Loeb, M., & Riopelle, A. J. Influence of loud contralateral stimulation on the threshold and perceived loudness of low-frequency tones. *Journal of the Acoustical Society of America,* 1960, *32,* 602–610.

Mahoney, T. M. The effects of middle ear acoustic reflex on speech intelligibility. Unpublished doctoral dissertation. University of Oregon, 1973.

McCandless, G. A., and Goering, D. M. Changes in loudness after stapedectomy. *Arch Otolaryngoligica,* 1974, *100,* 344–350.

McGee, T. Psychophysical tuning curves from hearing impaired listeners. Unpublished doctoral dissertation. Northwestern University, 1977.

Mills, A. W. On the minimum audible angle. *Journal of the Acoustical Society of America,* 1958, *30:* 237–246.

Møller, A. G. An experimental study of the acoustic impedance of the middle ear and its transmission properties. *Acta Oto-laryngoligica,* 1965, *60,* 129–149.

Møller, A. R. The acoustic middle ear muscle reflex. In W. D. Keidel & W. D. Neff (Eds.), *Handbook of sensory physiology.* Vol. 5, Chap. 1. New York: Springer-Verlag, 1974, pp. 519–548.

Morgan, D. E., & Dirks, D. D. Influence of middle-ear muscle contraction on pure tone suprathreshold loudness judgements. *Journal of the Acoustical Society of America,* 1975, *57,* 411–420.

Morgan, D. E., Dirks, D. D., & Kamm, C. The influence of middle-ear muscle contraction on auditory threshold for selected pure tones. *Journal of the Acoustical Society of America,* 1978, *63,* 1896–1903.

Olsen, W. O., & Carhart, R. Development of test procedures for evaluation of binaural hearing aids. *Bulletin of Prosthetics Research,* 1967, *10, 7,* 22–49.

Peterson, J. L., & Liden, G. Some static characteristics of the stapedial muscle reflex. *Audiology,* 1972, *11,* 97–114.

Pick G. F., Evans, E. F., and Wilson, J. P. Frequency resolution in patients with hearing loss of cochlear origin. In E. F. Evans & J. P. Wilson (Eds.), *Psychophysics and physiology of hearing.* London: Academic Press, 1977, pp. 273–281.

Rappaport, B. Z. *The effect of the acoustic reflex on the perception of speech in noise.* Unpublished doctoral dissertation, University of Michigan, 1976.

Reger, S. N. Effect of middle-ear muscle action on certain psychophysical measurements. *Annals of Otolaryngology,* 1960, *69,* 1179–1198.

Riesz, R. R. Differential sensitivity of the ear for pure tones. *Physiological Reviews,* 1928, *31,* 867–875.

Rodenburg, M., Verschuure, J., & Brocaar, M. Comparison of two masking methods. *Acoustica,* 1974, *31,* 99–106.

Ryan, A., & Dallos, P. Physiology of the inner ear. In J. L. Northern (Ed.), *Hearing disorders.* Boston: Little, Brown, 1976, pp. 89–101.

Salomon, B., & Starr, A. Electromyogrpahy of middle-ear muscles in man during motor activities. *Acta Neurologica Scandinavica,* 1963, *39,* 161–168.

Shaw, E. A. The external ear. In W. D. Kiedel & W. D. Neff (Eds.), *Handbook of sensory physiology,* Vol. 5, Chap. 1. New York: Springer-Verlag, 1974, pp. 455–490.

Shower, E. G., & Biddulph, R. Differential pitch sensitivity of the ear. *Journal of the Acoustical Society of America,* 1931, *3,* 275–287.

Simmons, F. B. Perceptual theories of middle ear muscle function. *Annals of Ontology, Rhinology and Laryngology,* 1964, *73,* 724–740.

Small, A. M. Pure tone masking. *Journal of the Acoustical Society of America,* 1959, *31,* 1619–1625.

Smith, H. D. Audiometric effects of voluntary contraction of the tensor tympani muscles. *Archives of Otolaryngology,* 1943, *38,* 369–372.

Spoendlin, H. Innervation densities of the cochlea. *Acta Oto-laryngoligica,* 1972, *73,* 235–248.

Stevens, S. S., & Newman, E. B. The localization of actual sources of sound. *American Journal of Psychology,* 1936, *48,* 297–306.

Tillman, T. W., Carhart, R., & Olsen, W. O. Hearing aid efficiency in a competing speech situation. *Journal of Speech and Hearing Research,* 1970, *13,* 789–811.

Tonndorf, J. Shearing motion in scala media of cochlear models. *Journal of the Acoustical Society of America,* 1960, *32,* 238–244.

Tucci, D., & Calder, H. B. Binaural frequency selectivity measured with a central masking paradigm. *Journal of the Acoustical Society of America,* 1977, *62,* 598 (A).

Tumarkin, A. A contribution to the theory of the mechanism of the auditory apparatus. *Journal of Laryngology,* 1945, *60,* 337–368.

Verschuure, J. Pulsation threshold patterns and neuro-physiological tuning. In E. F. Evans & J. P. Wilson (Eds.), *Psychophysics and physiology of hearing.* London: Academic Press, 1977, pp. 237–247.

Wang, M. D., & Bilger, R. C. Consonant confusions in noise: a study of perceptual features. *Journal of the Acoustical Society of America,* 1973, *54,* 1248–1266.

Ward, W. D. Studies on the aural reflex. *Journal of the Acoustical Society of America,* 1961, *33,* 1034–1045.

Wever, E. G., & Lawrence, M. *Physiological acoustics.* Princeton: Princeton University Press, 1954.

Wever, E. G., & Vernon, J. A. The effect of the tympanic muscle reflexes upon sound transmission. *Acta Oto-laryngoligica,* 1955, *45,* 433–439.

Wiggers, H. C. The function of the intraaural muscles. *American Journal of Physiology,* 1937, *120,* 771–780.

Wightman, F., McGee, T., & Kramer, M. Factors influencing frequency selectivity in normal and hearing-impaired listeners. In E. F. Evans & J. P. Wilson (Eds.), *Psychophysics and physiology of hearing.* London: Academic Press, 1977, pp. 295–306.

Yost, W. A., & Nielsen, D. W. *Fundamentals of hearing: an introduction.* New York: Holt, Rinehart nad Winston, 1977.

Zakrisson, J. E., & Borg, E. Stapedius reflex and auditory fatigue. *Audiology,* 1974, *13,* 231–235.

Zwicker, E. On a psychophysical equivalent of tuning curves. In E. Zwicker & E. Terhardt (Eds.), *Facts and Models of Hearing.* New York: Springer-Verlag, 1974, pp. 132–139.

Zwicker, E., Schorn, K. Psychoacoustical tuning curves in audiology. *Audiology,* 1978, *17,* 120–140.

Zwislocki, J. J. The role of the external and middle ear in sound transmission. In D. Towner & E. Eagles (Eds.), *The Nervous System. Vol. 3, Human Communication and its Disorders.* New York: Raven Press, 1975. pp. 45–55.

Ralph R. Rupp, Ph. D.

4

Classical Approaches to the Determination of the Spondee Threshold

Gathering of information about a hearing-impaired client's ability to handle speech input is inherent to the classical "basic" audiologic battery. For each ear, this battery includes the four essential measures of (1) pure-tone air conduction thresholds, (2) pure-tone bone conduction thresholds, (3) spondee thresholds, and (4) an estimate of discrimination efficiency. The ASHA "Guidelines for Determining the Threshold Level for Speech" (1979). state that "Speech threshold audiometry is a procedure for measuring an individual's intelligibility threshold for speech materials. An individual's threshold for speech is defined as the (intensity) level at which he can respond correctly to 50 percent of the material presented to him."

In this book, this speech threshold will be designated as the spondee threshold (ST), since the most popular method of determining a speech threshold employs the use of such bisyllabic word lists. The ST label clearly identifies the test materials. The earlier term, speech reception threshold (SRT), usually assumed the use of such standardized spondee lists but did not clearly specify their employment. "Spondee threshold is an appropriate and precise title for reporting the hearing loss for speech" ("Guidelines", 1979).

Support for the use of the term *spondee threshold* also comes from Chaiklin, Ventry and Dixon (1971, p. 207). They state, "We recognize that 'speech reception threshold' is the more traditional usage, but chose to use the term 'spondee threshold' because it is a more accurate description of the threshold being measured." Tillman and Jerger (1959) and

Jerger, Carhart, Tillman, and Peterson (1959) also employ the term *spondee threshold* when they refer to a 50 percent correct performance for identifying such bisyllabic words.

DEFINITIONS

Audiologically speaking, the term *threshold* generally refers to a certain percentage of correct identifications as being necessary before a threshold value is affixed to the findings. Clinically, the value of 50 percent is employed for both pure-tone and speech thresholds. Through some protocol or formula, the audiologist presents tonal or speech stimuli, and the listening subject is volitionally organized to respond in a certain way whenever he or she hears the pure tone or understands the bisyllabic word. Whenever the listener's correct identifications nears the target value of 50 percent of the presentations, the intensity level of the signal that triggers these "half right" (50 percent) responses is designated as the threshold for the measure under assessment. Audilogically, such thresholds are usually designated in dB HL values. For example, Mr. X. has a threshold for a 500 Hz tone at 45 dB HL for his right ear. His spondee threshold is 46 dB HL for the same ear. At 45 dB, he can just identify the presence of the 500 Hz tone 50 percent of the time; at 46 dB HL, he can just correctly repeat the spondees 50 percent of the time.

Within the arena of speech audiometry there are three (or four) thresholds that need defining. The speech detection threshold (SDT) "is simply the level at which the listener is able to detect the presence of a speech signal about one-half of the time" (Hopkinson, 1978). On the speech-intensity-intelligibility grid, reviewed in Chapter 2, the SDT appears at a −12 dB HL (or 8 dB SPL) intensity level. Egan (1948) proposes the term speech perception threshold (SPT) as a definition for an intensity level where the listener is just able to follow the meaning of a continuing linguistically-correct speech sample (connected discourse). He reports that to move from an SDT to an SPT requires approximately 8 dB of additional intensity. Finally, we observe the speech reception threshold (SRT) now designated as the spondee threshold (ST). As suggested earlier, the task is to correctly identify half of the presented spondees, and it requires an additional 4 dB of intensity. As reviewed earlier in Chapter 2 and discussed again in Chapter 15, the statistically normal audiometric "zero" dB HL is derived from a 20 dB SPL base when Telephonics TDH-39 earphones are used (ANSI S3.6-1969, p. 21). A comparison of intensity values for a "normal-hearing" individual's various speech threshold shows the following relationships:

SDT—audiologically at −12 dB HL, acoustically at 8 dB SPL,
SPT—audiologically at −4 dB HL, acoustically at 16 dB SPL, and
ST (or SRT)—audiologically at "0" dB HL, acoustically at 20 dB SPL.

Clearly, the most popular measure of the three cited is the ST, and, as Martin states, it "is the preferred speech threshold test" among audiologists (1975, p. 128).

PURPOSES FOR ASSESSMENT OF SPONDEE THRESHOLDS

The client's speech thresholds, measured monaurally or in the sound field, and hereafter identified as spondee thresholds (ST), provide the audiologist with information that is useful in several different ways.

Hearing Level for Speech

First, the ST score establishes a hearing level for speech stimuli, both in the sound field and also independently for each ear. Relating these findings to the hearing loss classification system employed in the audiologist's facility gives a first estimate of the listener's communicative listening abilities. It establishes a basic hearing level (or "loss") for speech.

A Base Intensity Level in Calculating Word Discrimination Scores

Second, the ST serves to establish the intensity level above which the audiologist will gather speech discrimination information. Martin and Forbis (1978) report that in their survey, almost 38 percent of their audiologist responders employed a sensation level of 40 dB in relationship to the ST for checking suprathreshold understanding ability through the use of monosyllabic phonetically balanced word lists. Other cited SL values varied from 25 to 45 dB, but the reporting clinicians all used the ST as the base intensity level to determine the subsequent intensity dial level in administering monosyllabic word lists. (See the articulation-intelligibility curves presented in Fig. 2-2.)

Consistency Check with the Pure-tone Average

Third, the ST is used to check listener consistency for hearing levels by comparing the pure-tone thresholds with the ST for the ear under observation. Especially crucial are the "speech" carrying frequencies of 500, 1000, 2000, and 3000 Hz. Most audiologic writers consider a consistency factor of ±5 dB as clinically acceptable (Berger, 1971). Hopkinson (1978, p.143) warns the clinician that "To some extent the configuration of the hearing pattern and the specific spondees will also influence the SRT." She proposes a formula that makes such a consistency probe easy: "the SRT [now labeled ST] should correspond to the best of the three pure tone speech frequencies by minus 8 to plus 6 dB." (The literature abounds with citations of the unique relationships between the flat or atypical pure tone thresholds and the ST. A limited number of these findings will be reviewed later in the chapter.)

Diagnostic/Prognostic Information

Fourth, the ST provides the audiologist with both evaluative and predictive information. If bone conduction ST values are gathered along with air conduction STs, and if both ST data are in close agreement with the respective pure-tone findings, reinforcement as to possible conductive or sensory (or neural) sites can be made. Further, if ST, tonal tests, and corroborative battery findings determine that the hearing deficit is cochleo-sensory, these data provide the audiologist with quantifiable information that can be used to support recommendations for audiological rehabilitational intervention.

Assessing Amplification Assistance

Fifth, the ST serves a useful function in the assessment of possible amplification benefit through its measurement in the traditional hearing aid evaluation. Such a study assesses clients' hearing abilities as they are assisted by appropriately chosen representative hearing aids. The ST shift toward normal (audiometric "0" dB HL) represents one of the "aided" measures the audiologist may employ to help evaluate the individual's performance as enhanced by a specific hearing aid under observation. In a similar way, the effectiveness of an intensive auditory training program may be measured in part by the possible movement of the ST score toward the normal base line. While it has been established that beyond a familiarization benefit, normal-hearing individuals do not usually improve their ST scores with training, conversely, the goal for hearing-impaired listeners in an analytic/synthetic listening skills training program will be to hear the components of the aural language more effectively. One improvement may be in the movement toward normal of the ST dB HL. Obviously, the linguistic constraints for spondees are considerably larger than for monosyllabic words. With specific listening training, improvement in the understanding for both ST and WDS may occur.

Assessing Hearing Enhancement from Medical/Surgical Programs

Sixth, the use of the ST score serves as a good indicator of possible shifts in communicative efficiency for an ear that has undergone medical and/or surgical intervention, either to improve the health of the ear or to improve the hearing levels. In conjunction with the other components in the basic audiologic battery, these serial observations of the dB HL of the ST for the ear under medical treatment become effective monitor scores for hearing sensitivity for speech. People use the codes of the language for communicative interchange. Measuring this code-interpreting function by means of the ST gives important information about the ear's general capability to handle speech.

Research

Seventh, and crossing all six of the cited purposes above, the audiologist and the otologist are interested in quantifying and qualifying their activities on behalf of their patients with research-oriented studies. The audiologist wishes to classify ST hearing levels in terms of communicative ease or jeopardy. The otologist wishes to obtain hearing enhancement data for certain kinds of surgical procedures. The audiologist endeavors to assess compatibility of residual hearing with performance potential of selected hearing aids. The otologist observes resolution of middle-ear effusion, and associated improvement of the ST, as a result of his medical program. Basically, the ST measure is a primary factor in monitoring the listener's hearing sensitivity for speech. Gathering research data and acceptable clinical data requires that appropriate, consistent, and defensible methods be used by the audiologist in measuring the ST.

HISTORICAL OBSERVATIONS ON SPEECH THRESHOLD ASSESSMENTS

1800–1940

Berger's review of the development of speech audiometry (1977, p. 7–30) is fascinating reading for the audiologist interested in the historical background of the field. His detective-like devotion to detail and his zeal for uncovering many exciting audiologic clues is evident in this review of the audiologic world from the early nineteenth century.

Audiologists well versed in the history of the field agree that the first widely used recorded speech test in the United States was developed at the Bell Telephone Laboratories specifically for assessing human hearing sensitivity (Fletcher, 1929; Fletcher & Steinberg, 1929). Officially the test was labeled the "Western Electric 4-A Test" but it was dubbed the "fading numbers test" by its administrators because it employed a disc recording of groups of two (or three) digits with an intensity decreasing range of 33 dB. Run from a "spring-wound phonograph with up to 40 earphones" (Berger, 1977, p. 12), the record contained segments with both male and female voices. A revised version had only two-digit stimuli, which the listeners wrote down on their answer sheets for as long as the fading intensity permitted. In addition to the fact that 40–50 children were able to take the test at one time, calibration control was a major problem. MacFarlan (1940) also cautioned that the test missed many high-frequency hearing losses because the children could recognize most digits from their vowel formants. But it was the beginning of something big in the audiologic world!

1940–1950

Hudgins and coworkers (1947) were the pioneers in the development of spondees for measuring hearing sensitivity for speech. They built their lists around the following three prerequisites: adequacy of testing materials, appropriate equipment, and established norms for the normal-hearing population. They chose their spondees to satisfy the following requirements: familar vocabulary, dissimilarity in phonetic composition, a spread in the typical representation of English sounds, and intensity homogeneity.

The use of spondees became popular with the publication of the Harvard Psycho-Acoustic Laboratory (PAL) tests (Hudgins et al., 1947) and the commercial availability of the PAL auditory tests no. 9 and no. 12 on disc recordings. Both recorded versions contain the same two lists of 42 spondees (total 84) appearing in six scramblings. Test no. 9 is a decreasing intensity recording of 4 dB for every six words, for a total attenuation in each scrambling of 24 dB. Test no. 14 follows the same sequency, but without internal attenuation. All lists are at a constant level.

1950–1960

Further refinements in the clinical application of spondee lists came from the research of Hirsh et al. (1952) at the Central Institute for the Deaf. They reduced the total number of PAL words from 84 to 36. In doing so, they attempted to achieve greater familiarity with the vocabulary, more representative phonemic distribution, and tighter control on equality of audibility. The CID W-2 disc record had a 3 dB attenuation factor for each three-word group; the CID W-1 recording was at a constant intensity level. Six scramblings of the word list appear on each recorded version.

The reader is asked to review the intensity-intelligibility curve function for spondees (see Fig. 2–2). Tillman and Olsen (1973, p. 42) report that "The articulation score for these [spondee] materials rose from 0 to 100 percent within a range of 20 dB. An increase of 20 to 80 percent occurred within a range of 8 dB, yielding a slope of approximately 8 percent per decibel in this range." Because of their sharp change in performance with each decibel intensity change, such CID spondee lists serve well in assessing speech thresholds.

1960–1970

While both Hudgins et al. (1947) and Hirsh, et al. (1952) attempted to control the relative intensity across their recorded versions, subsequent intensity observations on the CID W-1 recordings show an intensity range of 10 dB between the easy and hard-to-understand words (Bowling & Elpern, 1961). These observers proposed an "edited" version, which employed only 22 of the original 36 words and achieved a small 3.5 dB range for intelligibility. Five years later, Curry and Cox (1966) suggested a similar editing of the W-1 recording, whereby 25 words could be retained for a 4 dB spread in intelligibility.

1970–1980

Nine years later, Beattie et al. (1975) studied the intelligibility of the W-1 word lists via a monitored live voice, and by even more stringent editing, this group proposed a list of 17 spondees with an intelligibility variability of only 1.5 dB. All such "edited" lists are found in Berger's *Speech Audiometry Materials* (1977, p. 40).

In 1976, the Committee on Audiometric Evaluation of the American Speech and Hearing Association proposed "Guidelines for Determining the Threshold Level for Speech" (1977). The committee formalized the "Guidelines" in 1978. In the documents, and with a supporting explanation by Byers (1978), a suggested "pool" of 36 spondees was proposed. These words were divided into two lists of 18 words each with six scramblings of each list. The committee recommended a minimum number of 18 words for a test list. These proposed lists appear as Table 4-1 below and are in alphabetical order.

Byers (1978) reports that the majority of the words in these lists come from the CID lists, and were selected "emphasizing the criteria of phonetic dissimilarity and homogeneity of audibility." The following six spondees were taken from the earlier PAL lists: blackboard, backbone, cookbook, earthquake, eyebrow, and nutmeg. While a commercially available recorded version of these new lists is not yet available, the

Table 4-1
Test Lists

List A	List B
Airplane	Armchair
Baseball	Backbone
Blackboard	Birthday
Cowboy	Cookbook
Drawbridge	Doormat
Duckpond	Earthquake
Eardrum	Eyebrow
Horseshoe	Greyhound
Hot Dog	Hardware
Ice Cream	Headlight
Mousetrap	Inkwell
Northwest	Mushroom
Oatmeal	Nutmeg
Pancake	Outside
Playground	Padlock
Railroad	Stairway
Sunset	Toothbrush
Whitewash	Woodwork

From the Committee on Audiometric Evaluation of the American Speech and Hearing Association. Guidelines for determining the threshold level for speech. *ASHA*, 1979, *21*, 353–356.

adroit electronics technician in a speech and hearing facility could dub a new, informally edited, taped version by carefully piecing spondee segments from both "parent" PAL and CID lists (with appropriate approval, of course). The Committee on Audometric Evaluation did not take a firm position on the desirability of recorded versus live voice presentation of such words. It stated that "Recorded presentation of the test material is the preferred procedure . . . [but] clinical situations may arise which favor the use of a monitored live voice presentation" ("Guidelines," 1977, p. 242).

The ASHA "Guidelines" were proposed by the Subcommittee on Speech Audiometry of the Committee on Audiometric Evaluation in 1976, with publication "for discussion purposes only" in 1977. In 1978, at its annual session, the ASHA Legislative Council approved the proposed "Guidelines for Determining the Threshold Level for Speech" with subsequent publication in the *ASHA* Journal in May 1979. The introduction to the document states, "The intention is to suggest a standard procedure that will improve interclinician and interclinic comparison of data that, in the final analysis, will benefit the people we serve" (1979, p. 353).

CLINICAL CONSTRAINTS INVOLVED IN THE DETERMINATION OF THE SPONDEE THRESHOLD

A review of the literature on speech thresholds suggests that a sizable number of potential variables (or influences) must be considered by the audiologist as decisions are made about creating a clinical method to determine the client's spondee threshold. This section considers only the variable themselves. The discussions on methods follows in subsequent sections. These variables, or factors, group into two major areas: those relating to speech audiometric procedures in general, and those related uniquely and specifically to the ST search. They are reviewed in a general-to-specific progression.

The Acoustic Environment

Ambient noise is a contaminant to acceptable audiologic data whenever the noise is not a part of the task design. Therefore, the American National Standards Institute (Melnick, 1973)—in cooperation with the Acoustical Society of America and almost 400 other "different private organizations"—has recently updated its requirements for restricting sound room environmental background noise levels in its revised standard, ANSI S3.1-1977. "Criteria for Permissible Ambient Noise During Audiometric Testing" (American National Standards Institute,1977).

Table 4-2
Requirements for "Quieted" Environments

Conditions:	Maximum Allowable Sound-pressure Levels for Octave Bands, Centered Hz						
	125	250	500	1000	2000	4000	8000
Ears not covered (bone-sound field)	28.0	18.5	14.5	14.0	8.5	9.0	20.5
Ears covered (earphones)	34.5	23.0	21.5	29.5	34.5	42.0	45.0

Briefly, the requirements for "quieted" environments are presented in Table 4-2.

Manufacturers and/or installers of new sound rooms should assure purchasers that the rooms meet the new ambient noise restriction, both by specifications and by postinstallation measurement. Rooms that have been in use for several years should undergo calibration review to insure that the rooms meet current suggested restrictions. Accurate audiologic data collected from a mature, intelligent, and cooperative adult first requires a sound-treated room with acceptable low levels of background noise.

Articulation Function for Spondee Threshold

As reviewed in Chapter 2, the normal-hearing individual should obtain a spondee threshold at 0–15 dB HL for both earphone and soundfield listening conditions. The SPL reference level for audiometric "zero" for speech, under phones, is 20 dB SPL when using Telephonics TDH-39 earphones (ANSI S.3.1-1969). "The TDH-39 earphone is that most often supplied by manufacturers of speech audiometers in the United States" (Hopkinson, 1978, p.142). Alternatively, soundfield norms indicate that the SPL reference level for audiometric "zero" should be at 12.5 dB SPL with the speakers carefully calibrated to a usual head placement for both distance from the speakers and the height of the receiver's ears (Tillman, Johnson, & Olsen, 1966; Dirks, Stream, & Wilson, 1972).

While the audiologist does not usually develop full articulation curves with each patient, it should be recalled that in the middle of this theoretical curve, each *one decibel* of intensity increment yields an *8 percent increase* in performance efficiency. Careful attention to intensity levels and the increments employed in the search for the ST becomes crucial.

Appropriate "Speech" Materials

Berger (1977, pp. 31–41) suggests that either spondees or cold running may be used in establishing speech thresholds. He describes cold running speech as "informative but nonemotional connected discourse." In this alternative stimulus, the threshold is established at an intensity level where "the listener, with concentration, can just barely hear and repeat key words or phrases." Falconer (1948) and Martin (1975) concur that spondee thresholds and such cold running speech thresholds will give approximately equivalent dB scores. Coversely—and depending upon the definition—Egan (1948) reports a difference of approximately 4 dB between these two stimuli, with the advantage to the discourse.

According to Tillman and Olsen (1973, p. 39), the earliest investigators to measure the "speech reception threshold" and to define the relationship between speech and pure tones in persons with impaired hearing were Hughson and Thompson (1942). Bell Telephone Laboratories Sentence Intelligibility Tests (in Berger, 1977, pp. 45–47) were employed to obtain a minimal intensity level where the individual could "just understand the sentences." A direct relationship was seen between the hearing levels for the central speech frequencies (500/1000/2000 Hz) and the hearing levels where subjects could understand 66 percent of the sentences. Hughson and Thompson's observation would agree with Egan's.

At the present time, the use of spondee lists to determine speech thresholds is the most popular approach. Tillman and Olsen (1973, p. 40) state that "spondee words now represent the standard materials for the clinical measurement of speech reception threshold." The ASHA "Guidelines" (1977, p. 241) state simply that "spondee words are specified as the standard test materials" for speech threshold audiometry.

Use of the Carrier Phrase

The question of using a carrier phrase preceeding the target spondee involves a choice available only with monitored live voice presentation of the word lists. Recorded forms of the PAL auditory tests no. 9 and no. 14 and the CID W-1 and W-2 tests all employ carrier phrases. Students in audiology will easily recall Ira Hirsh's instruction on the recorded CID lists to "say the word ____ " prior to the presentation of each word.

Martin (1975, p.129) urges that "when monitores live-voice testing is used, the carrier phrase should be omitted, since . . . the phrase [is] partially inaudible at the threshold. No real advantage to using a carrier phrase with spondee words has been proven." Hopkinson (1978, p. 143) does not push for or against the use of the carrier phrase, although she does report that "at one time it was thought that the carrier phrase prepared the patient for listening," and attributes this position to Egan (1945). The ASHA "Guidelines" (1979) do not review this issue. In their frequently cited report on the relative merits of 2–dB versus 5–dB intensity increments for determining spondee thresholds, Chaiklin and Ventry (1964, p. 1971) employed recorded versions of the CD auditory test W-1. They stated "at no time was live-voice testing used in the measurement on spondee thresholds." Carrier phrases were integral to the measurement approach. From their national survey in 1977, Martin and Forbis (1978, p. 533) found that with live-voice spondee testing, "over 49 percent of the respondents reported that they do not use a carrier phrase."

In conclusion, in clinical practice by a skilled clinician where monitored live-voice presentations are employed, the use of the carrier phrase is optional. With certain populations, as with the elderly, with young children, with mentally slowed clients, with brain injured populations, or with those with unusual loss patterns, the use of the carrier phrase may, indeed, alert the listener to attend. For this reason, its clinical use is recommended. For the novice student clinician, its use is generally mandatory, for it helps achieve the desired intensity level of the audiologist's voice on the VU meter of the audiometer, and it prohibits the clinician from presenting the spondees too quickly while the patient's own physiology is still settling down from his own voiced response.

Monitored Live-Voice Versus Recorded Presentations

"Most audiologists use monitored live voice (MLV) when presenting spondees for obtaining the SRT" (Martin & Forbis, 1978, p. 533). The ASHA "Guidelines" (1979) suggest that "recorded presentation of the test material is the preferred procedure . . . . Either a recorded or a monitored live-voice technique can be used to obtain the ST." A recorded version has the obvious advantages of standardized composition of words, standardized presentation, intensity consistency within the list, and the same testing materials and presentation for each subject.

The practicing audiologist can also identify advantages for MLV presentations: more flexible pacing to the subject's speed of response, flexibility in choice of words necessary because of severe discrimination problems, age, maturational levels, normal use of a language other than English, and elimination of concern over possible wear on the discs or tapes that might introduce "distortion in the signal and noise into the test system" ("Guidelines," 1979, p. 354).

With the use of the pause switch on tape decks, the concern over too rapid a presentation of recorded words can be managed. Flexibility in clinician–client interaction, however, may be the prime reason to use monitored live-voice spondee testing in order "to fit the test to the patient's needs" (Hopkinson, 1978, p.144). A footnote to the "Guidelines" (1979) states: "There will not be a clinically significant difference in the level of the ST between the use of recorded or live-voice presentation [employing a 5-dB step increment]". Support for this agreement has been made by O'Neill and Oyer (1966), Beattie, Svihovec, and Edgerton (1975) and Beattie, Forrester, and Ruby (1977).

Monitored live-voice routing of spondees in the search for the speech threshold appears both flexible and defensible.

The Size of the Decibel Increment—2 dB or 5 dB?

There is no unanimity on the intensity increment size for searching for the ST. Audiologists fall, philosophically, into two somewhat militant camps on this issue.

The ASHA "Guidelines" (1977, p. 243) does not discuss the relative logic for either intensity level, but states, "The basic procedure involves an ascending technique with sets of four different spondees presented at 5-dB step increments." Hopkinson (1978, p. 145) reports that "on the basis of available research there is no clinically significant difference in SRT obtained in using either . . . 2- or 5-dB increments." In her procedure outline, she suggests that "the audiologist speaks one spondee for each 2-dB or 5-dB decrease" (p. 146). In the earlier edition of this chapter, Hopkinson (1972, p. 151) interestingly suggested that "the audiologist speaks one spondee for each 2 dB decrease."

Martin (1957, p. 130) places himself strongly in the 5-dB camp with this statement: "Use of 5-dB steps makes the procedure go more rapidly and makes decision making about threshold easier, without any sacrifice in the quality of test results."

The research project that opened this audiologic Pandora's box was reported by Chaiklin and Ventry (1964, 1971). They compared spondee threshold values via 2-dB and 5-dB intensity incremental use. They state in their summary, "It is recommended that spondee thresholds be measured in 5-dB steps rather than in 2-dB steps" because it is faster "and provides more than adequate accuracy for clinical needs." Interestingly, they reported that the difference between the means was 1.83 dB (in favor of the 2-dB increment) and significant (Chaiklin & Ventry, 1971 revision, p. 244).

Support for the 2-dB increment comes from Newby (1972, p. 122) and Tillman and Olsen (1973, p. 45). Wilson, Morgan, and Dirks (1973, p. 190) did a follow-up study using 2-dB and 5-dB increments in the ST search, and also found a significant 1.2 dB difference between approaches; again, they favored the 2-dB step. Based upon their findings, which were less dramatic than those of Chaiklin and Ventry, they proposed a strict adherence to the use of standardized procedures using "only the 2-dB step method clinically."

From their survey, Martin and Forbis (1978, p. 533) report that 57 percent of their responders used a 5-dB increment step while 33.1 percent used a 2-dB step.

When one recalls that it requires only a 20 dB range of intensity to move from 0–100 percent in the identification of spondees by a normal-hearing individual, and that a single decibel intensity contribution equals an 8 percent change in understanding in the center of this range (Tillman & Olsen, 1973, p. 42), then conservative audiologists are almost mandated to employ 2-dB increments in order to most effectively identify the ST for a specific hearing assessment.

Relationship Between the ST and the Pure-tone Average

The interaction between the threshold sensitivity of the central pure-tone frequencies of 500/1000/2000 Hz and the threshold of linguistic speech units has intrigued audiologic researchers for decades (Hughson & Thompson, 1942). While the early equivalency comparisons were made by comparing tonal averages against Bell Telephone Sentences, Carhart's observations (1946) led him to the conclusion that "words and sentences are essentially equivalent in their value as materials for measuring speech reception threshold" (1946, p. 346).

In order to quantify the constancy between speech and pure-tonal sensitivity, Hudgins, Hawkins, Karlin, and Stevens (1947) identified four essentials for the speech materials: words in common usage, dissimilarity among the words, words with approximate representation in percentage of occurrance in the language, and intensity homogeneity.

As an uncomplicated quick check on compatibility of findings, Carhart's (1946) three frequency average of 512/1024/2048 cps, now 500/1000/2000 Hz, has held up well. Berger (1971) suggests that the ST should fall at an intensity level +5 dB of this pure-tone average for each ear. The use of Fletcher's (1950) proposal for averaging the better two of the three speech frequencies is an easily added modification when marked slopes appear in the pure-tone findings. Carhart (1971) and Carhart and Porter (1971) elaborate on this comparison by suggesting that a general rule for the quick calculation of an approximate ST can be achieved by averaging the 500 and 1000 Hz pure-tone thresholds. The most rapid compatability check is offered by Hopkinson (1978, p. 146), who suggests that "the SRT should correspond to the best of the pure tone speech frequencies by minus 8 to plus 6 dB."

A series of factors contribute to the efficiency of the ST: frequency formants in the sounds, intensity levels of different sounds, distortion created by hearing loss and associated frequency deficits of the listener, subjective perceptual factors, preciseness of articulation of the speaker, regional idiosyncracies of the speaker, and speed of the spoken utterance. Unlike pure-tonal thresholds, which "are obtained by a comparatively slow series of long constant tones of 1 to 2 sec." (Hopkinson, 1978, p. 143), the speech signal is a highly variable stimulus.

Why Assess the ST if Good Theoretical Compatability Exists Between it and the Pure Tones?

It is true that in a statistically large population, appropriate approaches are available to predict the ST from pure-tone thresholds. This has led Davis (1970, p. 208) to propose elimination of the ST as a routine audiologic procedure. "The correlation between these two measures of sensitivity . . . is so good that the measure of the speech-reception threshold is redundant and therefore unnecessary in most cases." The logistical problem is to determine which "cases" do not fit the statistical correlation. Carhart (1950, 1960) and Chaiklin and Ventry (1963) counter Davis's proposal by reporting that when such discrepencies do show up, they are strong indications of data incompatibility and must be investigated further. Siegenthaler (1964) and Feldman (1976) concur that "in routine testing, the best validation feature is usually the correspondence between pure-tone thresholds and speech reception thresholds." Even when good decibel agreement is present, "it serves indirectly to establish the reliability of the pure-tone test results" (Tillman & Olsen, 1973, p. 47).

In 1977, "the majority of audiologists obtain both SRTs and word discrimination scores (WDS) for their patients" (Martin & Forbis, 1978, p. 533). Conservative audiologists feel more comfortable when their clinical findings support each other; and most clinicians remain positive in their approach to maintain the ST in their audiologic armamentarium.

Which Threshold Search Should Lead: Pure Tones or Speech?

The majority of writers in the 1970s did not discuss this question. Martin (1972) suggests that the ST should be found before gathering pure-tone thresholds so that the clinician is not biased by the pure-tone data. The audiology staff in some Veterans Administration Hospitals routinely gather ST observations for this reason. Since the interaction between the ST and PTA is so strong in a mature and cooperative adult, one might argue that the preparatory set (or bias) in expected thresholds of the second threshold search will be influenced by the findings of the first search, or vice versa.

Most references propose that the beginning intensity levels in the ST method be set at some comfortable level above the estimated speech threshold based on pure-tone observations (Tillman & Olsen, 1973, p. 45; Wilson, Morgan & Dirks, 1973, p. 184; Hopkinson, 1978, p. 146). We expect these "estimated" thresholds to be based upon the pure-tone thresholds already completed for the ear under observation. Chaiklin and Ventry (1964, 1971, p. 247) propose that the clinician begin the initial [intensity] descent 25 dB above the two-frequency PTA." They offer alternative methods "if pure-tone thresholds have not been measured prior to the measurement of the spondee threshold."

Which Ear Should Be Measured First?

There is a general clinical agreement that the better ear should receive the spondee study first, either by observation of pure tones or by subjective reporting by the client in the absence of tonal information.

As the second ear is assessed for the ST, the need for masking becomes apparent as the disparity between ears reaches or exceeds the interaural attenuation factor of 35–40 dB. The well-organized clinician will employ wide band noise masking for the speech observations if masking has already been employed with some or all of the pure-tone threshold determinations for the second, more poorly functioning ear.

In cases of suspected collapsed canals, as induced by the weight of the earphones on pinnas with little cartilaginous tonicity and resultant compression of the cartilaginous external auditory canal, a soundfield ST is recommended. Hildyard and Valentine (1971, p. 448) suggest that the incidence of such audiometrically induced pseudoconductive hearing loss is about 4 percent in a routine adult population. They propose that "the average error introduced by collapse of the canal appears to be of the order of 10–15 dB, and it is greatest (14.6 dB) at 2000 Hz." Slightly larger pseudoconductive loss findings were reported by Rupp and Gruber (1970) when the average induced "collapsed" conditions gave threshold elevations of 15–30 dB in the speech frequencies.

Whenever the soundfield ST is better that the ST under earphone conditions (with the other ear under headphone masking conditions) by the order of 10 dB or more, a possible audiometric collapsed state for that ear may be suspected. Rupp and Gruber (1970) proposed nine clinical approaches for evaluating possible collapsed canal conditions.

The Need for Intensity Homogeneity

Early researchers (Hudgins et al., 1947) were concerned with the need for intensity homogeneity with respect to audibility for the sentences that comprised their speech threshold materials. The PAL and CID spondee lists also attempted to meet this requirement. Tillman and Olsen (1973, p. 40) review its importance: "First, it increases the probability that the articulation function . . . will rise from 0–100 percent within a narrow range of intensity levels . . . . Second, it is desirable to determine the threshold for speech with as small a number of items as possible."

Several additional studies stressing the need for tighter surveillance of homogeneity of audibility have been reported. Bowling and Elpern (1961), Curry and Cox (1966), Beattie, et al. (1975), the ASHA "Guidelines" (1977), and Byers (1978) have all reinforced the real need for a manageable list of spondees with essentially equal audibility.

Few audiologists will dispute the wisdom and contributions of these various reporters.

Bone Conduction Routing for Determining the ST

Martin and Forbis (1977, p.533) reported in their 1977 survey that about 33 percent of their responders "use the bond-conduction oscillator as the receiver when establishing the SRT." Martin (1975), Stockdell (1974), Goetzinger and Proud (1955), and Williams and Rupp (1975) agree that STs obtained via bone conduction speech stimuli may have their greatest value working with small children who are able to participate in "word" games (such as identifying spondees by pointing to pictures), but who will not or cannot respond to pure tone signals. Williams and Rupp (1975) proposed "that bone conduction speech reception threshold (BCSRT) should be included . . . in the pediatric audiologist's test battery . . . with the difficult to test young populations."

For audiometers that were not originally designed for bone conducted speech audiometry, biological bone conduction correction factors of approximately 38–40 dB (Stockdell, 1974; Williams & Rupp, 1975) are required to offset the attenuation effects of the skull mass. Newer diagnostic audiometers do have calibrated bone conduction speech stimulus potential. As Martin (1975, p.138) reminds the reader, unless masking is employed, "there is no way to be certain which ear is being tested . . . However, even the limited information derived from this procedure . . . often justifies the use of bone-conducted speech audiometry."

Masking Requirements and Procedures

An in-depth discussion of the rationale and procedures for masking when determining the ST is beyond the primary focus of this chapter. But "masking must be used to eliminate the nontest ear and ascertain the true threshold of the test ear in precisely the same way as for pure-tone air conduction audiometry" (Martin, 1975, p. 134).

Wide band, or white noise, is the preferred masking source because of its broad spectrum of energy across frequencies. Sanders' discussion (1978, p. 124–140) on masking serves as an excellent review for practicing audiologists. The discussion includes an identification of the problem, when to mask, variable masking noises, relative masking efficiency, how much masking is necessary, and masking in speech audiometry.

The interaural attenuation for speech is approximately 50 dB, according to Liden (1954). Conservatively, the practicing audiologist should begin to question data when disparity is at 35–50 dB between ears. The audiologist who follows the plateau search method (Hood, 1960; Studebaker, 1962, 1964, 1967), or who has developed an effective masking table (Sanders, 1978, 130–136), and who understands the special challenges of combining masking rituals with speech stimuli will be able to determine valid and reliable masked spondee thresholds.

Visual Contact Between Clinician and Client

In most diagnostic facilities, the patient is separated from the audiologists by a wall and a shared viewing window. A strong case is made here for mutual observation by both clinician and client. The adroit clinician knows how to manipulate the necessary dials and switches on the audiometer without giving clues; and a hand spread flat in front of the microphone will hide any visual clues during live-voice presentations of spondees. The advantages of mutual visual monitoring during a spondee threshold search and during most other audiologic diagnostic procedures far outweigh any constraints that may be imposed upon the audiologist by the client's observations. If a full-face observer peering back at the clinician appears too disconcerting, a 45° angle to the patient's chair in relationship to the windowed wall may be more manageable. If the audiologist is concerned about visual clues during the spondee presentation, the patient can be instructed to look toward the door during the procedure. If a 45° angle is still unnerving to the clinician, then a 90° angle with the patient in profile will still give many important clues to the clinician. The disadvantage of this arrangement is that the patient must obviously turn his or her head toward the clinician to achieve visual interaction.

Why is a mutual observation appropriate? For the same reason that patient signal buttons are not routinely used in the facilities association with the graduate audiology training programs at the University of Michigan, for the goal is to make our student clinicians "people oriented" and not light response oriented. Thus, the goal is to become astute observers of the client's behavior during the administration of any audiologic task. The best indication of patient reaction is his or her face. By gentle and continuing surveillance of the patient, the audiologist obtains a clear indication of the patient's motivation, understanding of instructions, ability to respond appropriately, and need for auditory or visual reinforcement for the task. In addition, the audiologist will be able to sense the need to reassure when performance falters, and on very rare occasions, will be ready to help if the patient develops actual distress.

As with Green's discussion (1972, pp. 81–85) on the six categories of "Useful Finger Observations in Pure-Tone Threshold Audiometry," the manner in which patients ready themselves and the speed with which they perform the volitionally assigned tasks may be almost as important as the final data derived. The two-way window provides benefits to patients that can be high, too. By observing the audiologist, the patient can know the task is being performed as instructed, that the process is moving along well, and, indeed, that segments have been completed. All of this information can be shared by verbal or visual signals from the clinician. Especially with young children, the elderly, and potential problem patients, the close eye contact between clinician and client is important to the successful gathering of required data.

Ascending Versus Descending Techniques

Hopkinson (1978, p. 144) reports that "on the basis of available research there is no clinically significant difference in SRT obtained . . . in ascending or descending technique." It becomes important, however, for the audiologist to differentiate between the orienting segment of the search and the actual probing for the intensity level that will give 50 percent success in identifying the spondees. If one begins at a 20–30 dB level above the projected ST and then moves rapidly down to bracket the ST in 5-dB steps, this process should appropriately be considered as an orienting or attending process whereby the listener is gently coaxed or encouraged to listen to less and less intense speech signals. The actual ST probe comes as the clinician moves up and down in established intensity increments within a bracketed intensity range, the top of which give too much success (80–100 percent) and the bottom of which gives little success (1–20 percent).

The ASHA "Guidelines" (1977, p. 243) propose only an ascending series: "Threshold for the hearing level for speech is defined arbitrarily as the lowest level in which half or more of the spondaic words are repeated correctly with the minimum requirement of two ascending sampling series." Martin (1975, p. 129), Chaiklin and Ventry (1964; 1971), Tillman and Olsen (1973), and Wilson, Morgan, and Dirks (1973) propose a suprathreshold beginning point at an intensity level 25–50 dB above the estimated threshold followed by a descending orientation approach and finally a descending threshold probe searching for the 50 percent success level. Jerger, Carhart, Tillman, and Petersen (1959) proposed jumping around "from level to level in 2-dB steps" without specifying an ascending or descending series of intensity progressions.

Familiarization Approaches for Spondees

The audiologic literature is unanimous in recommending that a familiarization process be used to prepare the listener for the ST task. Tillman and Jerger (1959) reported that "normal-hearing subjects given prior knowledge of the test vocabulary yield spondee threshold SPLs which are 4–5 dB lower than those yielded by subjects not given such knowledge [employing 2-dB increments in an 'up and down method']."

Tillman and Olsen (1973, p. 44) suggest that familiarization "can be accomplished simply by reading the test words in alphabetical order at a comfortable listening level and asking the patient to repeat each word." If the patient cannot repeat some of these words "even at comfortable listening levels . . . these words should be eliminated from the test vocabulary." Chaiklin and Ventry (1964, 1971) and the ASHA "Guidelines" (1977) suggest almost identical processes. Martin (1975) encourages the audiologist "to provide the patient with a list of the words before the test." Hopkinson (1978) supports this approach but warns that "the list should not be kept by the patient during the test." Burke and Nerbonne (1978) report that in their study, "each subject was familiarized with the test items by having the individual read each of the 35 spondee words."

In spite of the fact that essentially all writers urge some kind of familiarization approach, Martin and Forbis (1978, p. 534) report that "only a slim majority of clinicians familiarize their patients with the words."

Instructions to the Patient

In organizing the patient to the listening task, the ASHA "Guidelines" (1979) identify the following components in an instructional set:

1. Orient the client to the nature of the task.
2. Specify the client's mode of response.
3. Indicate that the test material is speech material.

4. Stress the need . . . to respond at faint listening levels and encourage the client to guess.

Hopkinson's specific instructions to her hearing-impaired subjects follows (1978, p. 145): "I am going to say some words to you that have two parts; words like airplane, baseball, mushroom, eardrum. My voice will get softer and softer. Just repeat the words after me. If you are not sure of a word, do not be afraid to guess." She cautions the overzealous clinician that excessive directions may confuse the listener.

The exhortation to guess appears in most sets of directions. "You may have to guess, but repeat each word if you have any idea what it is" (Martin, 1975, p. 131). "It's important that you guess if you are uncertain of a word" (Chaiklin & Ventry, 1971).

This encouragement for guessing so interested Burke and Nerbonne (1978) that they completed "an investigation to determine the extent to which guessing on the part of the listener may influence the speech reception threshold." They were intrigued with the possible differences in ST value between "aggressive" guessers and "those who choose not to engage in any guessing." As anticipated, a mean difference of 4.2 dB was observed between the two preparatory sets (employing 2-dB increments) for their 30 subjects. They found, further, that there was better agreement between the PTAs and the ST when the subjects responded in the set where the listener repeated the spondee *only* when he was sure he had heard it correctly. The alternative instruction was to "respond on every test item even if it is a guess." They proposed the elimination of the guessing factor.

Response Approaches by the Patient

How shall the audiologist evaluate the responses of his adult listener to these spondees? The majority of audiologists, in keeping with the usual instructions, judge the oral utterances repeated by the subject for correctness. Since most lists are limited in number, such an approach for bisyllabic words is generally acceptable. When the respondent is unable to repeat the word appropriately, alternate methods for assessing the efficiency of the ST must be employed.

The Need for a "Clinical Approach" to the ST

Hopkinson (1978, p. 146) states: "Since SRT is an estimate at best, . . . the most efficient method would seem to offer the greatest return for the least time investment." Conversely, almost every other writer cited in this chapter cautions for the need for a carefully developed and consistent procedure. Tillman and Olsen (1973, p. 44) proposed a clinical approach that can be a "standard method for measurement of the spondee threshold" as well as "one which confines all clinicians to the same set of operation in the definition of threshold."

The remaining major sections of this chapter review suggested methods from the literature and propose such a standard method.

SPONDEE THRESHOLD PROTOCOLS IN THE LITERATURE

Recommended approaches for determining the ST have appeared in the professional literature since the mid-1940s. The following review considers only those approaches which have appeared, or reappeared, since 1970.

Chaiklin and Ventry: 1971; Martin: 1972, 1973

A secondary goal of the Chaiklin-Ventry study, which compared the influence of 2-dB and 5-dB increments on the ST, was to provide "detailed descriptions of [the] measurement methods employed" (1971, p. 243). While they philosophically supported the use of the 5-dB step, they offered procedures for use with both intensity increments. Descending approaches were used with both protocols, and recorded CID W-1 lists were employed. In the search for the ST, threshold was defined as the lowest hearing level at which three words were repeated correctly out of a theoretical maximum of six stimulus presentations.

In both approaches, following instructions and familiarizaton, and beginning at a suprathreshold comfort level (25 dB SL re: PTA estimate of ST), single spondess were presented at 5-dB decrements until the listener could no longer respond. Then in the 2-dB method, the signal intensity was raised 5–6 dB to "an even number on the hearing level dial." The threshold probe then followed by decreasing the intensity in 2-dB steps with a minimum of three or a maximum of six stimuli presented at each step. Threshold was established by the definition cited above. In order to avoid "premature" STs, they continued testing until either four words were missed at three incremental levels, or four words were missed at two such incremental levels with no correct responses.

The 5-dB variant shows modification only after the first orientation incorrect response, as above. When the subject missed the word on the 5-dB increment descending step, the intensity was increased to 5 dB above the level of the last correct response. From this level, and descending in 5-dB steps, three to six spondees were presented at each level. The prematurity prohibition in this approach was "four incorrect responses at two consecutive levels" (1971, p. 243).

These authors shared a "Spondee Response Data Sheet " (1971, p. 248), which allows the clinician to record all responses by the listener and subsequently provide a recorded data base for the patient's file.

Martin (1972; 1975) found the Chaiklin-Ventry method acceptable for the 5-dB increment step, and he proposed a flow chart to describe the procedure graphically. He did not, however, insist that recorded spondees be used.

Tillman and Olsen: 1973
Wilson, Morgan, and Dirks: 1973

Tillman and Olsen proposed the following "standard method." Familiarization and instruction are provided. Constant level recordings of CID W-1 lists serve as the stimuli and the 2-dB step serves as the threshold probe increment. Beginning at a 30–40 dB SL "above the estimated threshold," single spondees are presented in 10-dB attenuated steps until an incorrect response (or no response) is found. At this same level, a second spondee is presented. If both words are missed, the intensity level is increased 10 dB and the "threshold seeking" begins. If the second word was correctly identified, another 10-dB decrement is made, and two more words are presented. The clinician is searching for a level where both words are missed. At stated above, the test is begun at a 10 dB SL over this failure level.

The intensity level is dropped in 2-dB steps with two spondees presented at each level. This decreasing intensity search continues until the client misses "at least five of the last six words." The assumption is also made that the listener achieved correctness on five of the six words given at the beginning of the threshold probe. "The clinician then merely counts the number of correct reponses, decreases this total by one, and subtracts the result from the hearing level setting at which the test began." The ST then corresponds to the crucial 50 percent efficiency point on the spondee articulation curve (see Fig. 2–2).

Wilson, Morgan, and Dirks (1973) reported on a statistical study using the above protocol and shared their "Spondee-threshold Worksheet," which provides documentation of actual findings. For the audiologist who prefers a 5-dB incremental step, the worksheet also permits this kind of observation.

ASHA "Guidelines": 1977 and 1979

In opposition to the above protocols, these guidelines proposed an ascending approach in the ST search. While its definition is compatible with the others, the task begins with the audiometer intensity dial set "to its lowest setting." Using one spondee at each 10-dB step, presentation continues until a correct reponse is obtained.

The intensity level is then reduced 15 dB from that success level, and "the first ascending sampling series is begun" with four spondees given at each 5-dB step. The goal is to reach a level where the listener correctly identifies three or more spondees. A second ascent is then begun at a level 10 dB below this obtained level of three correct responses. A third ascent is completed beginning 10 dB below the level of success found in the second ascent. Threshold is established at the intensity level where "half of the spondaic words are repeated correctly with a minimum requirement of two ascending sampling series" (1977, p. 243).

Hopkinson: 1978

Employing a live-voice approach, the audiologist begins testing the better ear at a level 20 dB above the 1000 Hz pure-tone threshold. Using either 2-dB or 5-dB decreasing steps, one spondee is presented. "As the patient begins to show signs of having trouble, more words are spoken at each decrease" (1978, p. 146). The ST is considered to be 2 dB above the intensity level where "the patient cannot repeat any more words correctly." Hopkinson also proposes that a derived ST can be made by adding 2–8 dB to an obtained speech detection threshold intensity value "without the laborious exercise of finding the 50 percent point."

A PROPOSED CLINICAL APPROACH FOR DETERMINING THE SPONDEE THRESHOLD

The following protocol for the cliical determination of the spondee threshold is a procedure that has been in use in the audiology area of the Section of Speech and Hearing Sciences since the mid-1970s. It employs a monitored live-voice presentation of the stimuli, an ascending 2-db intensity step series in the threshold probe phase, and a reinforcement-closure procedure as its completion exercise. It also presumes a mature, cooperative, and motivated adult. The process includes the following components:

1. Familiarization to the word list

2. Instructions to the listener
3. Orientation-attending phase
4. Threshold probe phase
5. Reinforcement and closure phase

Familiarization

The spondee list is read at a suprathreshold comfort level (35–40 dB SL) to the patient seated in the sound room facing the audiologist at an approximate 45° angle. The subject is encouraged to watch the clinician during the reading of the list through the speaker system of the audiometer. Since the publication of the ASHA "Guidelines," their proposed 18-word lists serve as the stimulus spondess. (The Curry & Cox [1966] lists were previously used.) The patient is then asked if all of the words were understood. If an affirmative response is obtained, the audiologist moves to the second level in the process. If, however, the patient reports that some words were unintelligible, the clinician then rereads the list with the subject repeating the words. Any words that are missed are removed from the word list.

Instructions

In agreement with Hopkinson (1978) that excessive instructions may confuse rather than clarify the task requirements, a short set of instructions is then given. It is approximately as follows:

> Now I am going to read these words again, but one at a time. I want you to repeat each word after me. The words will be getting softer and softer. This is deliberate, for I want to find the level where you can just understand the word as you listen carefully. It is all right to guess if you are not sure. Please listen carefully. Repeat each word if you can. Please guess if necessary. Do you have any questions?

Since many clients tend to become uncomfortable about their inability to hear all of the test words near their threshold correctly, we have found that including our goal—finding that 50 percent intensity level—in the instructions reduces this concern. The instructions inform the listener, review the goal, encourage the patient to listen attentively, and reassures the listener that guessing is acceptable behavior.

Orientation-Attending Phase

Based upon the estimate of the ST from the previously gathered pure tone data, two spondees are presented at 25–30 dB SL. The intensity level is then decreased in 5-dB steps, with two words presented at each level.

This decreasing intensity phase is designed to encourage the client to listen with more and more selective attention as the intensity levels drop. The orientation phase ends either at "zero" dB on the attenuator dial of the audiometer, or when the listener misses one or both words at some dial level above this normal baseline level. If the latter event occurs, a final 5-dB decrement is programmed with the presentation of two additional spondees, and the expectation is that both will be missed.

Threshold Probe

The orienting and bracketing procedure has identified an intensity range within which the potential 50 percent correct response should occur. At this last orientation presentation level, and with the patient now experiencing poor performance, the audiologist now adds four more spondees. It is anticipated that the client will continue to perform poorly. The intensity level is now increased by a 2-dB step, and three to six spondees are presented at this level. If four words are missed, the clinician increases the intensity another 2 dB and begins a new presentation series. Even if the first three words are correctly coded by the listener at this new level, the entire set of six words is presented, for the listener may miss the last three words. Three right and three wrong responses, however, equals 50 percent. Another 2-dB step is added, and the audiologist gives another set of up to six spondees. If the patient responds to the first four correctly or repeats four of the six correctly, the threshold probe phase is terminated, and the ST is assigned to the dB level where the listener achieved his 50 percent correct performance.

Reinforcement and Closure Phase

Following the final threshold probe presentation, the audiologist immediately increases the intensity level an additional 5 dB and presents three last words to the listerner, who should respond well to this final task (unless there is a severe discrimination loss, and if so, the audiologist will have already modified the basic approach). This final action by the clinician makes two contributions: it reaffirms the sharpness of the articulation curve for spondees, and it leaves the patient with a final impression of personal success for the task. Since the audiologist may be asking the listener to perform a number of demanding listening tasks in the course of the basic and supplementary batteries, it is important that the client receive sufficient personal reward and encouragement to help him or her work through a possibly demanding listening battery. This reinforcer and closure phase proposes to give this small psychological boost in the ST search for either ear or in the soundfield.

Figure 4-1 shows the Flow Chart Worksheet for recording the listener's responses. Figure 4-2 gives an example of a completed search for an ST of 21 dB HL for a left-ear response under headphones. The estimated ST is entered in the first column in the "orientation" phase and labeled "E"; the dial levels are then noted in the second column (at 25–30 dB SL re: the estimate); and the descending orienting phase is begun. As failure at two adjacent decreasing levels occurs, a lateral shift into the threshold-probe phase is made. An ascending intensity run in 2-dB steps is made. This probe phase ends when a 50 percent or better response pattern is observed. The final reinforcement phase is run at an intensity level 5 dB above that of the level now designated as the ST. The patient is expected to perform well at this final rewarding intensity level.

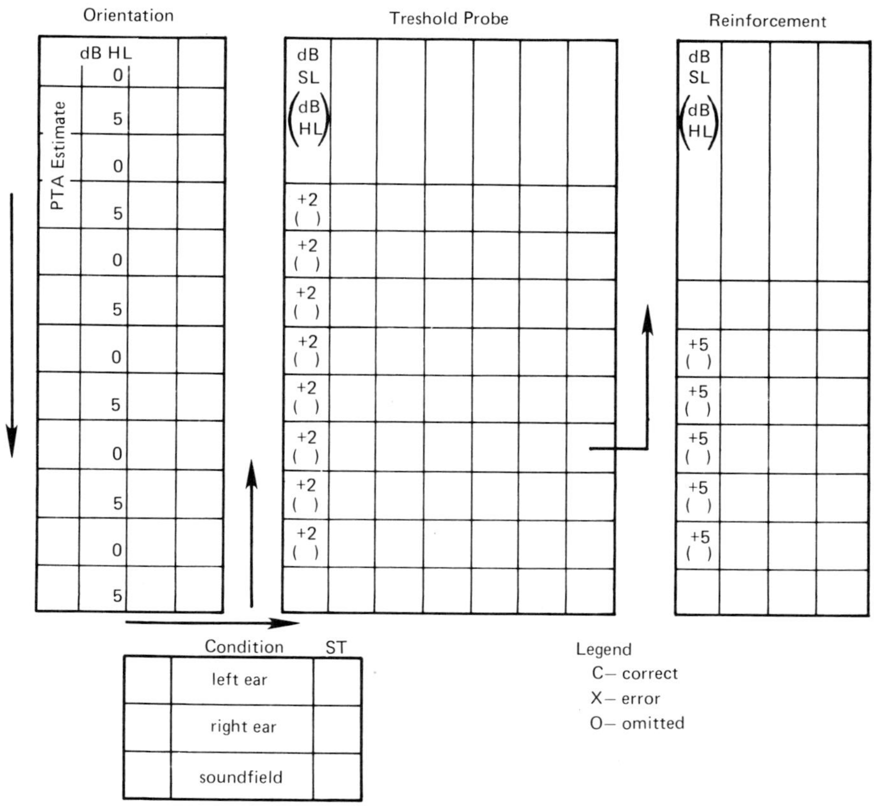

Fig. 4-1. Flow chart for the determination of the spondee threshold.

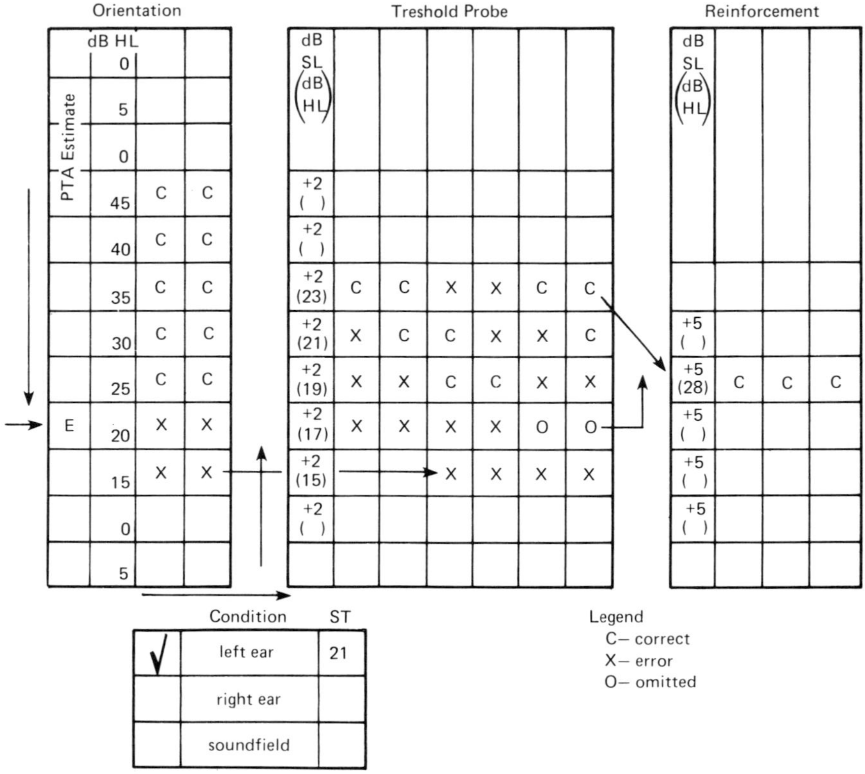

Fig. 4-2. Flow chart for the determination of the spondee threshold. Example: left ear ST at 21 dB HL.

NEW DIRECTIONS IN THE 1980s AND BEYOND WITH SPONDEE THRESHOLD MEASUREMENTS

Despite an occasional note of nonconformity by dissident or tired audiologists, the determination of a speech threshold by the use of spondees appears well entrenched in the basic assessment. As cited earlier in this chapter, the ST gives basic and practical information about the hearing sensitivity of the patient for a specific kind of speech stimulus.

A conservative prediction on the ST and its role in evaluative and rehabilitative audiology is that its measurement will continue. In the final chapter of this book, where several audiologic leaders look to the future of speech protocols in audiology, none predict the demise of the ST measure. While the ST may not have the glamour and charisma associated with some newer and more exotic audiometry, it does yet have a comfortableness and practicality that may be reassuring in an era when long-held audiologic beliefs are being subjected to much pressure.

Tillman and Olsen (1973) effectively projected the future direction in the maturational thrust of ST activity when they proposed that efforts be directed to establishing a "standard method" for determining the spondee threshold.

The ST serves as one of the essential pillars of the basic audiologic battery. As such, its role will continue even as newer procedures and protocols are developed to further refine our diagnostic and rehabilitative skills on behalf of our hearing-impaired clients.

REFERENCES

American National Standards Institute. Criteria for permissible ambient noise during audiometric testing. ANSI S 3.1-1977. New York: American National Standards Institute, 1977.

American National Standards Institute. Specifications for audiometers. ANSI S 3.6-1969. New York: American National Standards Institute, 1970.

American Speech and Hearing Association. Guidelines for Determining the Threshold Level for Speech. ASHA, 1977, *19,* 241–243.

American Speech and Hearing Association. Guidelines for Determining the Threshold Level for Speech. ASHA, 1979, *21.* 353–356.

Beattie, R., Forrester, P., & Ruby, B. Reliability of the Tillman-Olsen procedure for determination of spondee thresholds using recorded or live voice presentations. *Journal of the American Audiological Socity,* 1977, *2,* 159–162.

Beattie, R., Svihovec, D., & Edgerton, B. Relative intelligibility of the CID spondess as presented via monitored live voice. *Journal of Speech and Hearing Disorders,* 1975, *40,* 84–91.

Berger, K. Speech audiometry. In D. Rose (Ed.), *Audiological assessment.* New York: Holt, Rinehart & Winston, 1971.

Berger, K. *Speech audiometry materials.* Kent, Ohio: Herald Publishing House, 1977.

Bowling, L., & Elpern, B. Relative intelligibility of items on CID auditory test W–1. *Journal of Auditory Research,* 1961, *1,* 152–157.

Burke, L., & Nerbonne, M. The influence of the guess factor on the speech reception threshold. *Journal of the American Auditory Socity,* 1978, *4,* 87–90.

Byers, V. Revision of the spondaic word list. ASHA, 1978, *20,* 487–488.

Carhart, R. Monitored live voice as a test of auditory acuity. *Journal of the Acoustical Society of America,* 1946, *17,* 339–359.

Chaiklin, J., & Ventry, I. Spondee threshold measurement: a comparison of 2- and 5-dB methods. *Journal of Speech and Hearing Disorders,* 1964, *29,*, 47–59.

Chaiklin, J., Ventry, I., & Dixon, W. (Eds.) *Hearing measurement.* New York: Appleton-Century-Crofts, 1971.

Curry, E., & Cox, B. The relative intelligibility of spondees. *Journal of Auditory Research,* 1966, *6,* 419–424.

Davis, H. Audiometry: pure tone and simple speech tests. In H. Davis & S. Silverman (Eds.), *Hearing and deafness.* New York: Holt, Rinehart & Winston, 1970.

Dirks, D., Stream, R., & Wilson, R. Speech audiometry: earphone and sound field. *Journal of Speech and Hearing Disorders,* 1972, *37,* 162–176.

Egan, J. Articulation test methods. *Laryngoscope,* 1948, *58,* 955–991,

Falconer, G. The reliability and validity of monitored connected discourse as a test of the threshold of intelligibility. *Journal of Speech and Hearing Disorders,* 1948, *13,* 369–371.

Feldman, A. Diagnostic Audiology. In J. Northern (Ed.), *Hearing Disorders.* Boston: Little, Brown & Co., 1976.

Fletcher, H. A method for calculating hearing loss for speech from the audiogram. *Acta Otolaryngologica,* 1950, *90,* 26–37.

Fletcher, H. *Speech and hearing.* (Rev., 1953, *Speech and hearing in communication*). New York: Van Nostrand Co., 1929.

Fletcher, H. & Steinberg, J. Articulation testing methods. *Bell Systems Technical Journal,* 1929, *8,* 806–854.

Goetzinger, C. & Proud, G. Speech audiometry by bone conduction. *Archives of Otolaryngology,* 1955, *62,* 632–635.

Hildyard, V., & Valentine, M. Collapse of the ear canal during audiometry. *Archives of Otolaryngology,* 1962, *75,* 422–423.

Hirsh, I., Davis, H., Silverman, S., Reynolds, E., et al. Development of materials for speech audiometry. *Journal of Speech and Hearing Disorders,* 1952, *17,* 3211–337.

Hood, J. Principles and practics of bone conduction audiometry. *Laryngoscope,* 1960, *70,* 1211–1228.

Hopkinson, N. Speech reception threshold. In J. Katz (Ed.), *Handbook of Clinical Audiology.* Baltimore: Williams & Wilkins, 1972.

Hopkinson, N. Speech reception threshold. In J. Katz (Ed.), *Handbook of Clinical Audiology* (2nd ed.). Baltimore: Williams & Wilkins, 1978.

Hudgins, C., Hawkins, J., Karlin, J., & Stevens, S. The development of recorded auditory tests for measuring hearing loss for speech. *Laryngoscope,* 1947, *57,* 57–89.

Hughson, W., & Thompson, E. Correlation of hearing acuity for speech with discrete frequency audiograms. *Archives of Otolaryngology,* 1942, *36,* 526–540.

Jerger, J., Carhart, R., Tillman, T., & Peterson, J. Some relationships between normal hearing for pure tones and speech. *Journal of Speech and Hearing Research,* 1959, *2,* 126–140.

Liden, G. Speech audiometry. *Acta Otolarygologica,* 1954, Suppl. 114, 72–76.

MacFarlan, D. Speech hearing and speech interpretation testing. *Archives of Otolaryngology,* 1940, *31,* 517–528.

Martin, F. *Introduction to audiology.* Englewood Cliffs, New Jersey: Prentice-Hall, 1975.

Martin, F. *Clinical audiometry and masking.* New York: Bobbs-Merrill, 1972.

Martin, F., & Forbis, N. The present status of audiometric practice: a follow-up study. *ASHA,* 1978, *20,* 531–541.

Melnick, W. What is the American National Standards Institute? *ASHA.* 1973, *8,* 418–421.

Newby, H. *Audiology* (3rd ed.). New York: Appleton-Century-Crofts, 1972.

O'Neill, J., & Oyer, H. *Applied audiology.* New York: Dodd, Mead & Co., 1966.

Rupp, R., Gruber, L. The identification and resolution of audiometrically-induced hearing loss due to collapsed canals. *MSHA, Journal of the Michigan Speech and Hearing Association,* 1970, *6,* 26–32.

Sanders, J. Masking. In J. Katz (Ed.), *Handbook of clinical audiology* (2nd Ed.). Baltimore: Williams & Wilkins, 1978.

Siegenthaler, B., & Strand, R. Audiogram average methods and SRT scores. *Journal of the Acoustical Society of America,* 1964, *36,* 583–589.

Stockdell, K. Speech by bone conduction in diagnostic audiometry. *Audecibel,* Summer, 1974, 100–106, 109–110.

Studebaker, G. Clinical masking of air- and bone-conducted stiumli. *Journal of Speech and Hearing Disorders,* 1964, *29,* 23–35.

Studebaker, G. Clinical masking of the nontest ear. *Journal of Speech and Hearing Disorders,* 1967, *32,* 360–371.

Studebaker, G. On masking in bone-conduction testing. *Journal of Speech and Hearing Research,* 1962, *5,* 215–227.

Tillman, T., & Jerger, J. Some factors affecting the spondee threshold in normal-hearing subjects. *Journal of Speech and Hearing Research,* 1959, *2,* 141–146.

Tillman, T., Johnson, R., & Olsen, W. Earphone versus soundfield threshold sound pressure levels for spondee words. *Journal of the Acoustical Society of America,* 1966, *39,* 125–133.

Tillman, T.,& Olsen, W. Speech audiometry. In J. Jerger (Ed.), *Modern developments in audiology.* New York: Academic Press, 1973.

Williams, R., & Rupp, R. Comparison between speech reception threshold by air conduction and bone conduction with averaged warble-tone threshold in young children. *MSHA, Journal of the Michigan Speech and Hearing Association,* 1975, *11,* 185–195,

Wilson, R., Morgan, D., & Dirks, D. A proposed SRT procedure and its statistical precedent. *Journal of Speech and Hearing Disorders,* 1973, *38,* 184–191.

Kenneth G. Stockdell, Sr., M.S.

5

Classical Approaches to Measuring Discrimination Efficiency Via Word Lists

HISTORICAL BACKGROUND

The evolution of speech development has necessitated the understanding of speech as a result of speech reception. Early in the establishment of the universe, man was spoken to and he understood without any prior knowledge of a vocabulary or an interrelationship with others (Gen. 2:16).

In biblical history, we see that many languages developed when God said he would confound the primal language so that one person would not understand another's speech (Gen. 11:7). It is interesting to note that in these instances, there was immediate understanding of the spoken word. When a group later gathered together, the Bible tells us that all understood one another in their own language (Acts 2:6).

When one talks of speech discrimination and the process of understanding, we find that speech is that faculty of expressing thoughts by the spoken word through articulation utterance. The discrimination of speech indicates the discerning of differences or distinguishing things by their characteristics. The process by which we can discriminate speech is the fundamental act or faculty of intellect in noting differences and resemblances. This ability to recognize differences prepares material for the more highly complex forms of perception, conception, and classification of information.

It is important to note that speech is at the very core of communication, and consists of a very complex and delicate set of variables that must function as a unit to reveal man's thoughts verbally.

When one considers our development of speech materials and the protocols we use to determine speech intelligibility, we forget the ancient order and presume that this was developed in the 1940s following World War II. World War II created many problems of communication due to the injuries suffered. It was discovered from these injuries that the most debilitating problem was the injured person's inability to communicate effectively.

Although we like to consider audiology to have had its beginning in the 1940s while World War II was being fought and persons receiving noise-induced hearing losses were being treated, actual work had begun as early as 1800. G. W. Pfingsten in 1804, followed by Itard in 1821, used various methods to show and reveal improvements in hearing speech (Feldman, 1970). Through these efforts, speech discrimination was identified as a separate concern as early as 1821.

Due to the lack of sophisticated instrumentation, development of measuring techniques for speech intelligibility was not available until the early 1940s when it was developed by Hughson and Thompson (1942).

Prior to the Hughson-Thompson development, phongraphs were used in Germany that utilized cylinders to present material to the listerner. Poor reception through these instruments led to use of whispered and live-voice techniques in which the distance from subject to test administrator was varied.

Various machines, including the phonometer, micro-phonautograph, and modifications of these were used in the late 1800s, but results that enabled satisfactory diagnostic significance were minimal.

During the time of the development of instrumentation, materials for testing were also being developed. Since live voice was the primary mode of conveying the message, general speech was used to determine understanding. To enable a more critical measure, nonsense syllables were developed in the early twentieth century as a result of early telephone research, and later, certain vowel lists were prepared (Fletcher & Steinberg, 1929).

Fletcher (1929) became specifically concerned with developing a test of intelligibility to determine human hearing sensitivity. The outcome of his early work was the fading numbers test using group audiometry. There were many problems inherent to this method, but it did demonstrate the need for more critical methods that would approach the determination of speech discrimination. In addition, it pointed out the critical nature of calibration for obtaining accuracy in measurements.

TRADITIONAL TESTS OF SPEECH INTELLIGIBILITY VIA WORD LISTS

The first list of monosyllabic words was developed by W. H. Bristol in 1926 for use with children. In 1927, Fletcher produced an intelligibility test at Bell Labs that was used mainly for hearing aid testing. The use of monosyllables appeared to be successful, and most tests have used this system since the late 1930s.

Present-day methods that use monosyllabic word lists were developed through trial-and-error methods. Even today, many questions are raised concerning the difficulty of the task in determining the discrimination of the subject. The effectiveness of the word lists that are used to critically diagnose the hearing sensitivity of the subject have also been questioned.

Paired word lists were developed along with monosyllabic words in the late 1930s for hearing aid consideration and usage. In *Auditory Outlook,* West (1938) described the word lists he prepared and used to test various speech parameters in diagnosing hearing handicaps. These tests appeared to inspire others to consider the development of tests that would determine how subjects would respond to various frequency areas of the spectrum of sound in hearing.

During World War II, research in speech communications was conducted at Harvard University Psychoacoustic Laboratory (PAL). Since communication in wartime was of extreme importance, three areas were considered necessary. The Harvard studies looked at test materials, speakers, and systems of transmitting messages. Fourteen PAL tests were developed, using specific testing criteria. Each test was sufficiently different to enable the examiner to consider the effects of various stimuli upon the listener's response. The PAL tests that are more widely known include PAL no. 2, a written word test in the presence of noise; PAL no.4, which tests sentences in noise; and PAL no. 8, modified from no. 5, a multiple-choice test with 100 recorded sentences.

PAL no. 12 was a sentence test composed of 21 sentences in one test and 28 sentences in seven other lists. These tests are made up of questions that elicit short answers. They were recorded to allow a 6 dB attenuation for every three response words, This test was not designed for use with young children.

The PAL research was very thorough at the time, and it stimulated the development of articulation testing. This research brought about a large number of word lists that were used from time to time. From the initial groups, the Revised Monosyllabic Lists of 1200 word as reported by Egan (1948) were prepared in 24 lists of 50 words each. These lists consisted of words assigned according to phonetic composition of the initial portion of the monosyllable. The lists ultimately became known as the PB Word Lists.

In the original study eleven listeners were used to establish the orginal PB-50s. At the time of this early work, it was hoped a shorter version could be developed, but it was thought that phonetic balance was lost with a 24-word list test. Since this early work, Grubb (1963) and Schultz et al. (1964) prepared shorter lists, which meet current needs.

Egan (1948) clearly points out, "All articulation scores are relative scores. The scores or any of the tests are contingent upon the use of specific announcers, microphones, amplifiers, earphones, noises, listeners, and test lists."

As the curves in Fig. 5-1 show, normal listeners attain maximum scores with the PB-50s at 40 dB SL or slightly higher. For determination of the highest possible score in obtaining discrimination scores, the term ***PB max*** has been coined.

The PAL word lists for testing systems were used to test human hearing losses, and it was quickly determined that these lists were inadequate for such testing. (Eldert & Davis, 1951).

From these early questions of the tests' validity and inadequacies, Hirsh developed the W-22 lists (1952, 1954). In preparing these materials, he included a calibration of the recording and a carrier phrase. The sound pressure level (SPL) for presentation was also of concern. Many studies

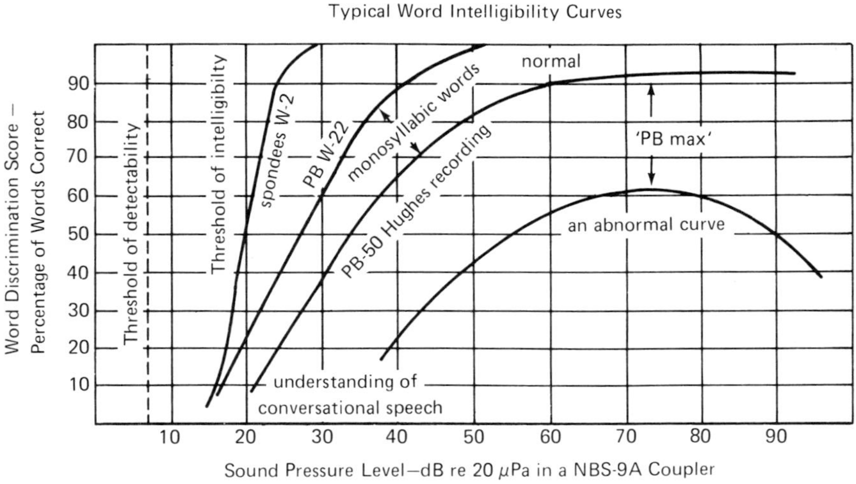

Fig. 5-1. Articulation curves for spondee words and PB words, realtive to .0002 dyne/cm² for the calibration tone (1000 cps) usually recorded on each disc. [From H. Davis & S. R. Silverman, *Hearing and deafness.* Holt, Rinehart and Winston, Inc., New York, 1970.]

have been completed to determine the reliability of the W-22 lists (Brandy, 1966; Campbell, 1965; Carhart, 1965; Creston et al., 1966; Elpern, 1960; Engelberg, 1968; Epstein et al., 1968; Huntington & Ross, 1962; LeZak, 1963; Lovrinic et al., 1968; Schultz, 1964). Several studies were made between 1961 and 1964 that questioned the reliability of the full lists and suggested the use of abbreviated lists (Elpern, 1961; Grubb, 1963; Lynn, 1962; Resnick, 1962; Tobias, 1964).

Although a number of questions have arisen about these early lists, they have remained in the armamentarium of the clinician since their development. In 1959, a large number of lists of CNC words were developed by LeHiste and Peterson. Even though these lists included 1263 words and ten lists, their popularity did not approach that of the W-22 lists of earlier years.

In creating the NU Auditory Test no. 4, Tillman et al. (1963) developed from these words a list of 95 words, plus some additional words. A total of 16 test lists were developed from this original work; included among them is the NU Auditory Test no. 6 (Tillman & Carhart, 1966).

Two of the more widely used discrimination tests are the Rhyme Test developed by Fairbanks (1958) and the Modified Rhyme Test developed by House et al. (1965). The Rhyme Test uses a semiclosed set and the listener writes down the initial consonant to a provided word stem. The modified test is a closed response format. The frequency of the word in conversational use and the phonetic balance of the words were not considered in the test's development.

Specialized test lists for different frequency regions were prepared by Glaser (1974) to assist in hearing aid selection. An abbreviated list for screening purposes was prepared by Rose (1974). In addition to these, there are specific types of sentence tests, multiple choice lists, pediatric tests, kindergarten lists, nonorganic speech lists, and foreign language lists (Berger, 1977). The different foreign languages in which these lists are available include Finnish, Japanese, Spanish, Dutch, Arabic, Norwegian, Italian, Philippines (Tagalog), German, Russian, and French.

METHODS IN DETERMINING SPEECH DISCRIMINATION

Presentation

The early developments of tests for speech intelligibility were presented via live voice prior to the 1940s because of a lack of sophisticated recording equipment. The classical works were done on recordings

(Egan, 1944, and Hirsh et al., 1952), but it has become practice to present by live voice "standardized" lists of words.

A number of problems have been pointed out in the use of speech to test hearing. The variables inherent in speech related to the uncomplicated pure-tone tests are sometimes very difficult to control. The variables include intensity, pitch, duration, consonant–vowel ratio, articulation, and voice quality (Hirsh et al., 1947; Egan, 1948; Hirsh et al., 1952).

Early studies have indicated that the acoustic wave forms of two or more talkers are sufficiently different to cause variability in listener performance. Brandy (1966) compared the presentation of speech discrimination materials by live voice and recorded presentations. The results of the study showed that recorded presentations, which are equivalent in acoustic output, provide more reliable listener performance than do live presentations, which are unequivalent in acoustic output.

List Length

The standardization of all materials included a 50-word list that was presented totally for the determination of intelligibility. To assist in reducing the time required to evaluate the hearing of patients in audiological clinics, research has been done on a number of methods.

It seems a little strange that it took fifteen years before Grubbs (1963) pointed out the reliability in the use of half-lists of 25 words to determine the discrimination ability of the patient. It was considered, however, that if a 25-word list could be derived that correlated highly with the original phonetically balanced list, and assuming it was sufficiently reliable, there should be no objection to its use since it would be producing an accurate estimate of the results that would have been obtained from the original full lists (Deutsch & Kruger, 1971).

Since this method has been established, its use has been expanded to shorten the test for the elderly, the young child, and the difficult-to-test patient. The test procedure has also been shortened further to provide a screening test for determining speech discrimination (Rose, 1974).

Word Familiarity

The difficulty and familiarity of the words used in the original PAL lists, the CID lists, and the Northwestern lists have been continually questioned. Owens (1961) studied the intelligibility of words varying in familiarity. His study matched lists of words phonetically and varied systematically with respect to familiarity. The lists characterized by greater familiarity, even to a slight degree, were significantly more intelligible.

When the CID W-22 words were first introduced as a test series, a preliminary study was undertaken to detect differences in difficulty among four main word lists. The initial study indicated the word lists were essentially equal in difficulty. Elpern (1960) designed a larger study to verify or to provide a broader evidence for or against the prevailing indiscriminate intercomparison of scores obtained by means of these lists. Differences were found among the four W-22 lists with respect to both level and range of difficulty. Numerically, the differences were small from a nonstatistical standpoint. For clinical purposes, the assumption of equal difficulty was considered tenable.

Fulton (1967) also used the CID W-22 lists to test retarded children since the word familiarity enabled good performance by most listeners. It was found that list 3A appeared to be more difficult and the subjects' response was significantly poorer than to lists 1 and 4.

Another study by Epstein (1968), utilizing low-pass filtering, as did Owens, demonstrated the effect of word familiarity when normal-hearing subjects listen to distorted speech. Errors increased as distortion increased for the lists falling in the "unfamiliar" category, while intelligibility remained undisturbed by the continuous discourse in the "familiar" lists as long as frequencies below 1560 Hz were left intact.

Additional studies have presented a higher percentage of familiar words to the listener than the original lists (Campbell et al., 1973). Giolas and Duffy (1973) have suggested using sentences once again, since they offer a more natural listening task than a list of monosyllabic words.

Questions about the effectiveness of the materials used to determine discrimination abiilty continue to arise for the clinician and the researcher. These questions deal with familiarity of word lists, mode of presentation, age grouping, dialect of presenter and, in certain materials, the familiarity of the task questions.

Hearing Aid Determination

The use of discrimination scores in hearing aid selection has been a questionable activity since its inception in the early 1950s. The major factor in this testing procedure has been how to accurately test the discrimination ability of subjects with hearing aids. The question that is generally raised is whether or not the conditions for testing give an accurate picture of the normal wearing conditions. How can we test all different types of aids and determine if improvement is available? There are those who claim that aids create greatly improved discrimination, but the person does not respond as the tests indicate from the results observed in a quiet listening situation.

The early work of Carhart (1965) in hearing aid selection was concerned with the effect of noise as it affected the wearability of hearing aids. In his early testing, he found a number of items that affected the results of the tests administered. Nielson (1976), inspired by Carhart's previous work, studied discrimination in noise more thoroughly. Nielson's research centered upon more up-to-date hearing aids and their benefit to people with marginal sensorineural hearing losses. The results indicated that no real improvement in discrimination was found for these subjects. Likewise, there was no reduction in speech intelligibility scores. The studies confirmed studies by Carhart (1970) and Olsen (1971) that a wide frequency range is of importance in obtaining good discrimination in noise.

McClellan (1967), utilizing mold venting versus unvented molds with hearing aids, found improved discrimination in high-frequency hearing loss subjects with vented molds. Subjects showed a mean gain in discrimination scores in noise of 16 percent. The gain in discrimination effected by the vented earmold was explained as an improvement in signal-to-noise ratio (S/N) at the aided ear primarily as a result of changed in acoustic impedance. With a small sample being used, generalization of these findings would suggest caution.

Cohen and Schliefer (1969) found that discrimination scores of hearing aid users changed significantly over time, with a decrease being shown in older patients for the evaluation and fitting of the aid.

In a more recent study in a Veterans Administration Center, Dennison and Kelly (1978), utilizing high-frequency consonant tests in hearing aid fittings, obtained results that supported the selection of the aids previously shown by using the NU Auditory Test no. 6.

The literature has many different studies that suggest the need for more critical measurements of discrimination ability and hearing aid use. Although different materials have been used, the methods of determining speech intelligibility and hearing aid use have not been researched extensively. It would appear that this area could use some creative thinking to spark discovery of newer and more critical determinations of speech understanding with hearing aids.

METHODS IN DETERMINING SPEECH DISCRIMINATION IN NOISE

The measurement of speech discrimination in the presence of noise has been studied considerably in recent years. The failure of the traditional intelligibility tests in quiet to yield important diagnostic information has precipitated these investigations. The use of noise and its effect upon discrimination was studied by several researchers between 1970 and 1975

(Olsen et al., 1975; Morales-Garcia & Poole, 1972; Katinsky et al., 1972; Cooper & Cutts, 1971; Young & Harbert, 1970; and Keith & Talis, 1970).

While the early studies varied as to the different concerns being tested, specific problems were viewed, such as the assessment of selective auditory attention (Heilman et al., 1973) and auditory perceptual problems in learning-disabled children (Willeford & Billger, 1978).

In 1978, Rupp provided normative data for the CID W-22 lists in the presence of noise under three conditions (ratio 1:1; 50 dB HL):

1. Sound field, speech and noise combined: 70–80 percent correct
2. Sound field, speech and noise separated: 80–90 percent correct
3. Monaural, combined findings: 70–80 percent correct

Rupp's findings supported previous researchers' discoveries that discrimination efficiency decreases in the presence of noise. Other findings showed that white noise is less interfering than speech spectrum noise; spatial separation between speech and noise in the sound field is a superior environment for listening with both types of noise; monaural headphone is comparable to sound field listening with speech and noise from the same speaker; and a high individual variability exists.

Some very interesting individual items have been observed in the studies with noise and its effect upon discrimination. The effect of noise on sensorineural-impaired listeners was poorer than normal, but the articulation functions were not appreciably different (Cooper & Cutts, 1971). Variability in response by listeners increased between the sensorineural impaired and the normal as the signal-to-noise ratio decreased (Keith & Talis, 1970).

After reviewing the evidence of these studies, Olsen et al. (1975) concluded that an abnormal speech performance in noise should exist if there is a 40 percent reduction between the quiet and noise conditions.

In using this criterion, all of the groups one would expect to have difficulty with understanding in the presence of noise did have a problem. The difference between noise and quiet response of 40 percent occurred in the following types as seen in Table 5-1 below.

In addition to the study by Olsen et al., Katinsky et al. (1972), Morales-Garcia and Poole (1972), and Heilman et al. (1973) found similar evidence in cases they studied.

Additionally, Heilman et al., and Morales-Garcia and Poole reported results that show significantly poorer speech in noise test scores in the ear contralateral to temporal lobe lesion when compared to the ipsilateral ear. Likewise, Olsen et al. found that a considerable portion (42 percent) of the contralateral ears had abnormal scores, but failed to find the between-ear difference. Heilman (1973) contends that these patients display a dis-

Table 5-1
Occurrence of Noise and Quiet Response of 40 Percent

Population	Incidence Showing Disparity
Noise trauma	8%
Meniere's	48%
Eighth nerve tumors (confirmed)	62%
Temporal lobe (contra-to lesion)	42%
Multiple sclerosis	14%

ruption of selective auditory attention that is unrelated to language mechanisms, because when patients who had dysfunctions in their dominant hemisphere were compared with patients who had dysfunction in their nondominant hemisphere, no significant differences were found.

Willeford and Billger (1978), in attempting to identify children with auditory learning disabilities, observed that measurement of speech reception in the presence of noise is the most effective procedure. The use of the Goldman-Fristoe-Woodcock test of auditory discrimination has been used routinely in this setting.

Since all of the tests mentioned have pointed out the problem the clinician faces in testing discrimination in the presence of noise, there are those who would advise against this procedure (Willeford & Billger, 1978, and Keith & Talis, 1970). Even though this has been suggested, Olsen et al. (1975) state, "Results from speech-in-white-noise tests may have some clinical usefulness in revealing abnormalities in auditory function but not in suggesting a particular site of involvement as being reponsible for the dysfunction."

A study by Rupp et al. (1977) found that by utilizing different noise environments, several conclusions could be noted for normal-hearing subjects:

1. Noise interferes with understanding efficiency.
2. White noise is less troublesome than speech spectrum noise.
3. The ratio of 1:1 signal/noise does not change performance with intensity change.
4. Speechlike noise is more interfering than white or traffic noise.
5. The noise, if separated spatially, is less disabling than presentation of speech and noise from the same sound source.
6. The greater the intensity of the noise, the more disabling are its effects.

In addition, various studies have been performed on different materials with comparisons of the difficulty of lists and comparison with the original CID lists and other earlier lists. It is interesting to note that under noise conditions, the CID W-22 lists showed better clinical results than others (Gorsuch & Rupp, 1973).

Egan (1948) pointed out that the criteria for speech discrimination test items should include: (1) monosyllabic words; (2) representative occurrance and distribution of fundamental speech sounds in normal speech; (3) consistency in range of difficulty within and between lists; and (4) familiarity to the general populace.

Utilizing three noise conditions, white, department store, and traffic noise, Rossman and Rupp (1975) found the department store noise created more difficult listening than the other two noises.

Studies that have evolved from the early comparative studies have dealt with the effect of discrimination in noise upon children, intensity relationships, types of noise, slope of audiograms, age defects, diseases of the ear, and drug toxicity. It is interesting to note that much research has gone into determining the effect of various conditions on speech intelligibility, but there has been no clear understanding of the scores expected for various populations.

It is very interesting to note that with children, deterioration of scores occurred with increase in the background noise levels (Coleman & Lovrien, 1965).

Larson, Peterson, and Jacquot (1974) also found in comparing children five to six years of age with normal-hearing young adults, the children showed significantly poorer hearing in the presence of noise at S/N ratios of 20, 15, and 10 dB.

Intensity Relationship

When the articulation gain functions were first determined, recordings were used; the different materials indicated that various levels above the threshold provide different scores. After reaching a certain intensity level above threshold, the PB max was reached. Clinicians have long known that a rollover effect appears with an increase in the intensity while determining the discrimination score. In studying Meniere's disease, Clemis and Carver (1967) determined that a 32–40 dB SL be used for all (DS) testing. Jerger and Jerger (1971; 1975) have tried to relate the rollover effect in differentiating the loci of disorders of higher order on the auditory nerve or cortex. They found that no reliable results could be obtained.

Slope of Audiogram

Since an audiogram is plotted for each clinic patient or each person being tested for a hearing problem, it would only seem logical that the audiogram should be suggestive of a possible related discrimination score. Hutton et al. (1961) studied age and four audiometric shapes of mild sensorineural hearing loss cases. The groups were divided into nonpresbycusic, ages 20–59, and presbycusic, ages 60 and above. The shapes were flat, gradually falling, sharply falling, and abrupt types. The results of these comparisons on multiple-choice intelligibility tests were that the presbycusic had poorer discrimination than the nonpresbycusic group. The best discrimination scores for the younger age group were in the gradually falling curve, and the poorest in the sharply falling curve. For the older group, highest scores were shown in the abrupt-type curve and the lowest in the sharply falling category.

The critical nature of pure-tone thresholds is often more dramatically shown in the noise-induced high frequency hearing loss cases relative to discrimination. We have seen graphically the sensation levels and frequency characteristics of speech sounds and therefore can realize how important each frequency is to discrimination ability (Fletcher, 1953). The other contours and slopes received in pure-tone audiometry have provided quite unusual results, not only in discrimination scores but also in the types of problems clinically found in the unusual auditory disorder.

Noise Types

The noises used in speech audiometry have been somewhat limited until recent years because of an inability to produce variations of the band of frequencies necessary to elicit a given result. Since we find much in the literture about masking and the more efficient types of noise available, other noises have been used to determine their effect on intelligibility (Sanders, 1971).

The original use of complex noise showed an inability to properly mask signals. For a long period of time, white noise became the more useful tool in auditory testing. Since this development we now see the use of cafeteria noise, narrow band noise, pink noise, speech noise, competing messages, and general conversation.

Speech, being a very complex stimuli, has no difficulty being heard by the subject when certain noise is present. It has been found by Sanders that speech noise, a narrow band of frequencies closely approximating the speech spectrum, interferes most with communication. Gjaevenes and Sohöel (1967), using "pink" noise in contrast to white noise, found "pink" to be a preferable masker of speech. As the author suggests, white noise is equal power per cycle bandwidth, and "pink" noise is equal power per octave.

DISCRIMINATION SCORES AND CLINICAL RESULTS

The early results in the clinical determination of hearing loss utilized the speech discrimination materials primarily to show an effect on communication as related to audiometric results. The development of the tests and the mode of presentation did not allow for much consideration of the specific results in categorizing clinical problems. In the preparation of materials, it was detected early that the test had to be sufficiently difficult to provide a means for critically identifying specific disorders.

The use of speech intelligibility has been the cornerstone or an alerting signal that some specific problem exists that requires the administration of additional tests, a more careful observation of the patient, the planning of a very comprehensive rehabilitation program, or all of these.

Much research has been done on various disorders and the results of the patients' responses to speech materials has been reported. It is noteworthy that many people who have similar pure tone audiometric contours have greatly different results in discrimination of speech.

The ideal speech discrimination test for clinical purposes would be one that is sensitive to any deviation from normal speech discrimination ability. Lovrinic et al. (1968) surprisingly suggested that the tests commonly used differ in the ways in which they measure this ability. Using five of the more widely used tests, it appeared that the Harvard PB-50 and the Simultaneous Voice Test were the more sensitive of the tests. The Voice Test appears to have a wider range than the PB-50, possibly showing a finer differentiation between abilities.

The Semidiagnostic Test and the Rhyme Test offer some information useful in aural rehabilitation that is not easily obtainable in the other three measures. Because some of the tests require a written response, a problem may arise for certain subjects. The use of disc recordings creates a time problem for writing. The use of verbal presentations also pointed up a possible problem, since scores differed by as much as 10 percent. In all cases, verbal-response scores were higher, suggestive of a built-in error.

In addition to these problems, the use of the carrier phrase is also believed to be a factor in discrimination testing. Kreul et al. (1969) found there is a difference in the carrier phrase used.

Since we note that there are many factors that can affect the intelligibility scores, including the protocols that are used in its determination, it is gratifying to know that the science of hearing has been able to identify the different types of disorders and the approximate discrimination scores expected.

The normal-hearing individual, utilizing the standard methods of material presentation, would expect to have scores in the range of 92–100 percent. Likewise, conductive hearing loss patients would also perform well on the tests.

With sensorineural hearing loss subjects, we begin to find large variations in the results that may be found in the testing routine. Specific disorders, the age of the patient when the problem began, the cause of the handicap, and the listening ability of the subject, all make for many problems in determining the subject's ability to understand. The range of discrimination scores for sensorineural hearing losses ranges from 30–80 percent. This group would include the end organ peripheral disorders caused by disease, heredity conditions, drug toxicity, noise-induced hearing losses, and other related disabling disorders. The presbycusic patient can be included in this group along with the group characterized by phonemic regression.

The central disorders often give rather bizarre discrimination scores, ranging from 0–100 percent. More specifically, we see poor scores in the ear contralateral to the disorder even though other audiometric scores indicate good hearing.

Another technique in diagnostic tests utilizing speech discrimination tests is by bone conduction. Halbrock (1962) used this technique in determining cochlear reserve. Miller (1964) found by bone conduction that nonorganic problems could be identified. Iwankirvicz (1966) pointed out the importance of bone-conducted discrimination results in finding lesions of the ear, particularly in operative cases.

Stockdell (1974) pointed out the different standard procedures in the use of bone conduction in speech discrimination. Tato and Nifaro (1949) and Robinson and Kasden (1970) found 80 percent scores as a consideration in surgical cases. The use of this method allows the diagnostician additional armament in clinical determination.

All of the research that has attempted to define speech discrimination has not satisfied the clinician, researchers, or educators as critical enough to answer the many questions raised. The main criticism of psychoacoustic measurements is that unless they are presented with competing signals, they are insensitive to quantitative and overall qualitative differences in speech transmission systems.

Chial and Hayes (1974) have suggested, like many others, that monosyllabic word tests used in measurement are "inefficient, arbitrary, insensitive, inconclusive, unreliable, and restrictive." Although Chial and Hayes have strongly suggested some of the problems inherent to psychoacoustic measurements with monosyllable word lists, the literature indicates that the majority of persons who attempt to evaluate the adequacy of listener understanding rely upon these lists. Despite this criticism, the use of phonetically balanced word lists continues to be popular clinically. I think that the challenge that researchers make against established methods of this kind of testing creates a healthy situation that can enable the discovery of a more suitable and definative test for use in these evaluative procedures.

The reader is referred to the appendix of this chapter for a brief review of representative word lists of the more widely used discrimination testing materials. For extensive speech intelligibility word lists the reader is referred to H. Davis and S. R. Silverman (1977) and K. W. Berger (1977).

REFERENCES

Berger, K. W. *Speech audiometry materials*. Kent, Ohio: Herald Publishing House, 1977.

Brandy, W. T. Reliability of voice tests of speech discriminations. *Journal of Speech and Hearing Research,* 1966, *9*, 461–465.

Campbell, R. A. Discrimination test word difficulty. *Journal of Speech and Hearing Disorders*, 1965, *8*, 13–22.

Campbell, R. A. An index of pseudo-discrimination loss. *Journal of Speech and Hearing Research, 1965, 8*, 77–84.

Campbell, R. A. Speech Discrimination Testing Material. Paper presented ASHA Convention, 1973.

Carhart, R. Problems in the measurement of speech discrimination. *Archives of Otolaryngology,* 1965, *82*, 253–260

Carhart, R. Monaural and binaural discrimination against competing sentences. *International Audiology*, 1965, *4*, 5–10.

Carhart, R. Principles of Competing Message Speech Audiometry. 2nd Danavox Symposium.

Chial, M, & Hayes, C. S. A Hearing and Evaluation Method. *Journal of Speech and Hearing Disorders,* 1974, *89,* 270–277.

Clemis, J. D., & Carver, W. F. Discrimination scores for speech in Meniere's disease. *Archives of Otolaryngology*, 1967, *86*, 614–618.

Cohen, M., & Schliefer, A. Factors in reliability of discrimination with hearing aid users. *Journal of Auditory Research*. 1969, *9*, 332–335

Coleman, R. O., & Lovrien, R. P. Speech sound discrimination in noise by children. Abstract *ASHA* October, *1965, 7,* 423.

Cooper, J., & Cutts, B. Speech discrimination in noise. *Journal of Speech and Hearing Research*, 1971, *14*, 332–337.

Creston, J. E., M. Gillespie, & C. Krohn. Speech audiometry: taped vs. live voice. *Archives of Otolaryngology*, 1966, *83*, 14–17.

Davis, H., & Silverman, S. R. (Eds.). *Hearing and deafness*. New York: Holt, Rinehart, and Winston, 1977.

Dennison, Laura B., & Kelly, Ben R., High frequency consonant word discrimination lists in hearing aid evaluation. *Journal of the American Auditory Society*, 1978, *4*, 91–97.

Deutsch, Lawrence J., & Kruger, B. The systematic selection of 25 monosyllables which predict the CID W-22 speech discrimination score. *Journal of Auditory Research*, 1971, *11*, 3.

Egan, J. P. Articulation testing methods. *Laryngoscope*, 1948, *58*, 955–991.

Eldert, E., & Davis, H. The articulation function of patients with conductive deafness. *Laryngoscope*, 1951, *61*, 891–909.

Elpern, B. S. Differences in difficulty among CID W-22 autditory tests. *Laryngoscope*, 1960, *70*, 1560–1565.

Elpern, Barry S. Differences in difficulty among CID W-22 auditory tests. ASHA Convention, 1960.

Elpern, B. S. The relative stability of half-list and full-list discrimination tests. *Laryngoscope*, 1961, *71*, 30–36.

Engelberg, M. Test-retest variability in speech discrimination testing. *Laryngoscope*, 1968, *78*, 1582–1589.

Epstein, A., Giolas, T. G., & Owens, E. Familiarity and intelligibility of monosyllabic word lists. *Journal of Speech and Hearing Research*, 1968, *11*, 435–438.

Epstein, A. et al. Familiarity and intelligibility of monosyllabic word lists. *Journal of Speech and Hearing Research*, 1968, *11*, 435–438.

Fairbanks, G. Test of phonemic differentiation: The Rhyme Test. *Journal of the Acoustical Society of America*, 1958, *30*, 596–600.

Feldman, H. A history of audiology. *Translations Beltone Institute Hearing Research*, 1970, 22, 1–111.

Fletcher, H. and Steinberg, J. C. Articulation testing methods. *Bell System Technical Journal*, 1929, *8*, 807–809.

Fletcher, H. *Speech and hearing in communication*. Princeton: D. Van Nostrand Company, Inc., 1953, p. 57.

Fulton, R. T. Task adaptation and word familiarity of W-22 discrimination lists with retarded children. *Journal of Auditory Research*, 1967, *4*, 353–358.

Giolas, T. G., & Duffy, J. R. Equivalency of CID and revised CID sentence lists. *Journal of Speech and Hearing Research*, 1973, *16*, 549–555.

Gjaenenes, K. & Sohöel, T. Masking of speech by "white" and "pink" wide-band noise. *Journal of Auditory Research*, 1967, *7*, 31–34.

Glaser, R. G., Jr. Hearing aid evaluations using spectral density classified word lists. Ph.D. dissertation, Kent State University, 1974.

Gorsuch, P., & Rupp, R. A comparison of the CID W-22 Lists and the Walter Reed Lists for speech discrimination efficiency in noise for normal-hearing subjects. *Journal of Michigan Speech and Hearing Association,* 1973, *9,* 125–130.

Grubb, P. A phonemic analysis of half-list speech discrimination tests. *Journal of Speech and Hearing Research*, 1963, *6*, 271–275.

Grubb, P. Some considerations in the use of half-list speech discrimination tests. *Journal of Speech and Hearing Research, 1963, 6*, 294–297.

Hahlbrock, K. H., Bone conduction speech audiometry. *International Audiology*, 1962, *1*, 186–188.

Heilman, K., Hammer, L., & Wilder, B. An audiometric defect in temporal lobe dysfunction. *Neurology*, 1973, *23*, 384–386.

Hirsh, I. J., Davis, H., Silverman, S. R., Reynolds, E. G., et al. Development of materials for speech audiometry. *Journal of Speech and Hearing Disorders*, 1952, *17*, 321–337.

House, A. S., Williams, C. E., Hecker, M. H. L., & Kryter, K. D. Articulation-testing methods: Consonantal differentiation with a closed-response set. *Journal of the Acoustical Society of America, 1965, 37*, 158–166.

Hughson, W., & Thompson, E. Correlation of hearing acuity for speech with discrete frequency audiograms. *Archives of Otolaryngology*, 1942, *36*, 526–540.

Huntington, D. A., & Ross, M. The reliability and equivalency of the CID W-22 auditory tests. USAF School of Aerospace Medicine, Report 61–110, February, 1962.

Hutton, Charles. Effects of age and audiometric shape on speech intelligibility. *ASHA*, 1961, *3,* 335.

Iwankirvicz, S. Bone articulation curves. *Voix,* 1966, *10,* 1–4, 26–28.

Jerger, J., & Jerger, S. Diagnostic significance of PB word functions. *Archives of Otolaryngology*, 1971, *93*, 573–580.

Jerger, S., & Jerger, J., Extra-and intra-axial brain stem auditory disorders. *Audiology*, 1975, *14*, 93–17.

Katinsky, S., Lovrinic, J., & Bucheit, W. Cochlear findings in VIII nerve tumors. *Audiology*. 1972, *11*, 212–217.

Keith, R., & Talis, H. The use of speech in noise in diagnostic audiometry. *Journal of Auditory Research,* 1970, *10,* 201–204.

Kruel, J. E., Bell, D. W., and Nixon, J. C. Factors affecting speech discrimination test difficulty. *Journal of Speech and Hearing Research*, 1969, *12*, 281–287.

Larsen, G. W., Peterson, P. B., & Jacquot, W. S. Use of Northwestern University Auditory Test no. 6 for speech discrimination testing with children. *Journal of Auditory Research,* 1974, *14,* 287–292.

LeHiste, I., & Peterson, G. E. Linguistic considerations in the study of speech intelligibility. *Journal of the Acoustical Society of America*, 1959, *31*, 280–286.

LeZak, R. Determination of an intensity level to obtain PB Max. *Laryngoscope*, 1963, *73*, 267–274.

Lovrinic, J. H., Burgi, E. J. & Curry, E. T. A comparative evaluation of five speech discrimination measures. *Journal of Speech and Hearing Research*, 1968, *11*, 372–381.

Lynn, G. Paired PB-50 Discrimination Test: A preliminary report. *Journal of Auditory Research,* 1962, 2, 34–37.

Miller, A. L. The use of masked bone-conducted speech as an aid in the detection of feigned unilateral hearing losses. *Journal of Speech and Hearing Disorders*, 1964, *29*, 333–335.

McClellan, M. E. Aided speech discrimination in noise with vented and unvented earmolds. *Journal of Auditory Research,* 1967, *7,* 93–99.

Morales-Garcia, C., & Poole, J. Masked speech audiometry in central deafness. *Acta Otolaryngology*, 1972, *74*, 307–316.

Nielson, T. E., Hearing Aid Characteristics and Fitting Techniques for Improving Speech Intelligibility in Noise. *Oticon Library*, October 8, 1976.

Olsen, W., Noffsinger, D., & Kurdziel, S. Speech discrimination in quiet and white noise by patients with peripheral and central lesions. *Acta Otolaryngology*, 1975, *80*, 375–382.

Owens, E. Intelligibility of words varying in familiarity. *Journal of Speech and Hearing Research*, 1961, *4*, 113–129.

Resnick, D., Reliability of the twenty-five word phonetically balanced lists. *Journal of Auditory Research*, 1962, 2 5–12.

Robinson, M. & Kasden, S. Bone conduction: Speech audiometry. *Annals of Otology, Rhinology and Laryngology*, 1970, 79, 818.

Rose, D. E., Schreurs, K. K., Keating, L. W., & Miller, K. E. A 10-word speech-discrimination screening test. Paper presented at ASHA Convention, 1974.

Rossman, Reva, & Rupp, R. Speech discrimination in environmental noise for normal-hearing subjects. *Journal of Michigan Speech and Hearing Association,* 1975, *11,* 83–89.

Rupp, R., Phillips, D., Briggs, P., Roseman, R., Goldsmith, M., et al. Speech discrimination norms for CID W-22 word lists in different noise environments. *Journal of Michigan Speech and Hearing Association, 1977, 13*, 59–67.

Schultz, M. C. Suggested improvements in speech discrimination testing. *Journal of Auditory Research*, 1964, 4, 1–14.

Stockdell, K. G. Speech by bone conduction in diagnostic audiometry. *Audecibel*, Summer 1974, 100–110.

Tato, J. M. & Alfaro, A. Speech audiometry—discrimination by bone conduction. *Actas of International Congress of ORL*, 1949, 78–82.

Tillman, T. W., Carhart, R., & Wilver, L. A test for speech discrimination composed of CNC monosyllabic words (NU Auditory Test no. 6). USAF School of Aerospace medicine, June, 1966, Report 55–66.

Tobias, J. V. On phonemic analysis of speech discrimination tests. *Journal of Speech and Hearing Research*, 1964, 7, 98–100.

West, R. *The testing of hearing aids*. Madison: College Typing Co., 1939.

Willeford, J., & Billger, J. Auditory perception in children with learning disabilities. In Katz, J. (Ed.), *Handbook of clinical audiology* (2nd ed.). Baltimore: The Williams & Wilkins Co., 1978.

Young, I., and Harbert, F. Noise effects on speech discrimination score. *Journal of Auditory Research*, 1970, *10*, 127–131.

Appendix: Representative Phonetically Balanced Word Lists

PAL PB-50 Words (Egan, 1948) List 7	CID W-22 Words (Hirsh et al., 1952) List 2A	NU Auditory Test No. 6 (Tillman et al., 1966) List 1
gasp	yore (your)	bean*
woo	bin (been)	boat
though	way (weigh)	burn
act	chest	chalk
dwarf	then	choice
scout	ease	death*
sledge	smart	dime*
sniff	gave	door
fling	pew	fall*
cook	ice	fat*
dope	odd	gap
gun	knee	goose
jug	move	hash*
mud	now	home
plod	jaw	hurl*
fake	one (won)	jail
phase	hit	jar
rash	send	keen
rich	else	king
but	tare (tear)	kite*
pounch	does	knock
whiff	too (two, to)	laud
pig	cap	limb
roar	with	lot
sag	air (heir)	love*
by	and	met

(Continued on next page)

Representative Phonetically Balanced Word Lists (Continued)

PAL PB-50 Words (Egan, 1948) List 7	CID W-22 Words (Hirsh et al., 1952) List 2A	NU Auditory Test No. 6 (Tillman et al., 1966) List 1
am	young	mode*
nine	cars	moon
wire	tree	nag*
aim	dumb	page
shaft	that	pool
south	die (dye)	puff*
woe	show	rag*
chop	hurt	raid*
knit	own	raise*
raid	key	reach*
sin	oak	sell*
cut	new (knew)	shout*
him	live (as verb)	size*
dose	off	sub
quiz	ill	sure
siege	rooms	take
coast	ham	third
grade	star	tip*
fort	eat	tough*
comes	thin	vine*
off	flat	week*
pent	well	which
range	by (bye)	whip
mote	ail (ale)	yes*

*From PB-50 list.

This appendix was adapted from: Egan, J. P. Articulation testing methods. *Laryngoscope,* 1948, *58,* 955–991; Hirsh, I. J., Davis, H., Silverman, S. R., et al. Development of materials for speech audiometry. *Journal of Speech and Hearing Disorders,* 1952, *17,* 321–337; and Tillman, T. W., Carhart, R., & Wilver, L. A test for speech discrimination composed of CNC monosyllabic words (NU Auditory Test no. 6). USAF School of Aerospace Medicine, June, 1966, Report 55–66.

Dean C. Garstecki, Ph. D.

6
Alternative Approaches To Measuring Speech Discrimination Efficiency

It is a formidable task to address the use of alternate tests of speech discrimination ability. A myriad of tests is commercially available for use by audiologists, speech-language pathologists, learning disabilities specialists, reading diagnosticians, and other such professionals. The examiner must be prepared to weigh the merits and shortcomings of a host of standardized and experimental materials, remembering that these tests have been designed for a variety of purposes. The initial step is to select a test or formulate a battery of tests which will best serve to meet predetermined needs.

To lend some organization to this selection process, this chapter will attempt to integrate information gleaned from the routine application of speech discrimination tests with what is generally understood about the speech discrimination process in everyday communication to demonstrate how the void in information might be filled by data from alternate speech discrimination tests. A plan is presented for developing a speech discrimination profile for diagnostic and rehabilitative purposes. As an aid to the completion of such a profile, selected speech discrimination tests are discussed. From this overview, implications for further research in the refinement of existing materials and the development of additional materials can be drawn. Throughout the chapter, the term *discrimination* is used to refer to a receiver's ability to recognize or identify meaningful speech signals, regardless of the conditions in which they are presented.

MAJOR USES OF SPEECH DISCRIMINATION TESTS

Over the past five decades, speech discrimination tests have been used to study the fidelity of communication and amplification systems, integrity of the hearing mechanism, and the need for rehabilitation of the hearing-impaired person. Test materials were first developed for use in analyzing telephone communication systems (Fletcher & Steinberg, 1929). World War II provided further impetus for the development of speech discrimination materials for evaluating communication systems. At about this same time, a set of monosyllabic word lists (PB-50s) developed at the Harvard Psychoacoustic Laboratories was made commercially available for clinical use (Egan, 1948). These early materials gained widespread use and scrutiny. Several investigators (Hirsh et al., 1952) noted ways in which these word lists could be improved. New word lists were generated and redesigned (Silverman & Hirsh, 1955), reevaluated (Lehiste & Peterson, 1959), and further refined (Peterson & Lehiste, 1962; Tillman et al., 1963). With each modification an attempt was made to improve test procedures and/or material. This steady pattern of redesign has continued to the present time, accounting for the proliferation of material.

In clinical practice, monosyllabic word lists have been used to measure speech discrimination ability. At best, results from these tests, when considered without corroborative data, can only be suggestive of the type of aural pathology. For example, in a population demonstrating conductive hearing loss, monosyllabic word discrimination ability will probably not be poorer than 90 percent at a 25 dB or greater sensation level (Alpiner, 1978). When lower scores are obtained, it may suggest the presence of a mixed, sensorineural, or other type of hearing impairment. Retrocochlear involvement is suspected when speech discrimination ability is poorer than 50 percent. However, cochlear involvement may also manifest itself in poor speech discrimination ability (Olsen, Noffsinger, & Kurdziel, 1975). Thus, monosyllabic speech discrimination tests generally have been found to have limited clinical utility.

When determining the benefit to be derived from the use of a hearing aid, an unaided monosyllabic word test score of 70 percent or higher suggests that the hearing aid candidate can expect to benefit from the use of an amplification system, especially in quiet listening conditions (Hodgson & Skinner, 1977). For those people demonstrating less than 70 percent unaided ability, speech discrimination using a hearing aid will vary according to degree of discrimination difficulty, listening conditions, and ability to benefit from speechreading cues. Speech discrimination tests, in general, provide little definitive data as to the benefit that might be derived from hearing aid use under everyday listening conditions; however, comparison of unaided and aided speech discrimination scores may provide an estimate of the relative value of an aid for a hearing-impaired person.

Auditory and auditory-visual speech discrimination test data may be used to determine the need for aural rehabilitation. Oyer and Frankmann (1975) suggest that speech discrimination test results help determine the need for auditory training by identifying the types of sound confusions perceived by the hearing-impaired person. Errors in speech perception can be analyzed for similarity in acoustic properties with target phonemes or words. In addition, one can predict if acoustic confusions could be resolved through training in the recognition of visible speech movements or speechreading. In all, a description of speech discrimination errors is beneficial for the development of a precise auditory or auditory-visual training program.

Speech discrimination tests have been used for these purposes for many years. Test materials have gradually been modified, but for the most part, the most popular test materials continue to be monosyllabic word lists (Martin & Pennington, 1971). These materials are administered whether the examiner's primary interest is in assessing a hearing-impaired person's ability to differentiate among acoustically similar speech units or to process everyday conversation. To understand what types of test materials yield information that is of prescriptive value to the examiner and practical value to the hearing-impaired person, factors which influence everyday speech discrimination should be reviewed.

FACTORS THAT INFLUENCE EVERYDAY SPEECH DISCRIMINATION

Interpersonal oral communication is a complex process in which a message is transmitted from sender to receiver through some channel or medium. The sending–receiving process may occur almost simultaneously. While the sender is transmitting a message, the receiver may be responding with facial expression, body movement, and verbal comment. The receiver also may be sorting background cues integrating relevant information into perception of the message. At minimum, three factors seem to influence everyday speech sound discrimination ability. These include: (a) auditory system sensory capability, (b) sensory input mode, and (c) message redundancy.

Sensory Capability

The physical ability to receive, encode, store, retrieve, and relate previous listening experiences with new experiences with rapidity and accuracy is what is meant by the term sensory capability. The peripheral auditory mechanism and central auditory nervous system work in series to process incoming speech. The complexity of the task is demonstrated by the fact that the receiver must sort differences in speech articulation, dialect, speaking rate, vocal intensity, and other related factors and then decide which of the known phonemes, words, or sentences are most like the perceived stimulus. In part, ability to make these judgments may be dependent upon one's experiential background and understanding of linguistic rules and constructs. Thus, sensory capability is not a structure-specific function, but the integration of auditory system and linguistic processes. As such, this ability would be expected to change with age, developing in the young child's early years and deteriorating in the geriatric adult's later years. It is susceptible to delay in growth, damage, or destruction by a variety of internal and/or external factors. Hearing impairment has a differential effect on this process depending on the age at onset, degree, type, and duration of hearing loss.

Since it is not the purpose of this chapter to consider the cause and effect of various conditions that may affect sensory capability, consideration will be given to dealing with the manifestation of any auditory system dysfunction that might have an influence on speech discrimination ability. To obtain this information, any reliable, standardized speech discrimination measure might be administered. These tests results serve to establish baseline function through a controlled and repeatable task. It is a necessary first step in studying overall speech discrimination ability. An estimate of sensory capability should include measurement of speech discrimination ability under natural (unaided or aided), controlled conditions, e.g., presenting recordings of NU no.6 word lists at 50 dB HL in quiet sound-field and subsequently with a competing message (multi-speaker babble) at 0 dB SN level.

Sensory Input Mode

Speech may be discriminated using several input modes (auditory, visual, tactile) alone or in combination. Since most hearing-impaired persons have functional residual hearing either without or with a hearing aid, their most natural sensory input modes are the auditory and visual channels. Tactile speech communication systems are being applied to a broader segment of the hearing-impaired population (Scott, 1979), but presently they are most often used by those unable to benefit from conventional amplification systems. Speechreading in the visual-only condition is measured for purposes of designing an aural rehabilitation program; however, the relationship between these speechreading test scores and success in everyday communication is generally unknown (Alpiner, 1978). In addition, there are few, if any, communication situations in which only visual speech information is presented.

Auditory-only listening situations are common in everyday communication. Telephone communication is one example of an everyday experience in which only auditory information is transmitted. On occasion, the fidelity and transmission characteristics of the telephone system may inhibit optimal speech signal discrimination. The same may be said of radio signals, public address systems, and citizen's band radio and walkie-talkie communication systems. Besides the limitation of the speech transmission system, the listening environment may further inhibit message perception. Bergman (1964) indicated that one cannot expect a normal result from adding an imperfect instrument to an already defective ear. That is, problems in everyday speech discrimination may be compounded for the hearing-impaired person when wearing a hearing aid, especially under noisy listening conditions. Since these are normally encountered occurrences, it is important to evaluate the hearing-impaired person's ability to discriminate speech in the auditory-only condition. In addition, it is important to estimate the influence of the acoustic properties of the speech transmission system and listening environment on speech signal perception and discrimination. How intelligible can you expect a spoken message to be when it is transmitted over a public address system in a crowded bus terminal? At best, this experience is confusing and frustrating for many hearing-impaired persons.

Auditory-visual speech communication is a comparatively easier task for the hearing-impaired person, who benefits from being able to supplement weak or distorted auditory speech information with visual speech cues. O'Neill (1954) found that as noise increases, the visual modality plays a greater role in speech discrimination. The same might be said in regard to the effect of hearing loss. As the loss increases, speechreading cues will supplement auditory speech discrimination. Estimates of auditory-visual speech discrimination may provide a better indication of the hearing-impaired person's ability to process everyday conversation (Binnie, 1973) than auditory-only tests.

Message Redundancy

LINGUISTIC CONTENT

Natural redundancy of the English language contributes to its overall intelligibility. Two people speaking about a topic that is familiar to each have a relatively easy speech discrimination task. If the amount of message redundancy is reduced, however, the receiver may ultimately be required to understand a spoken message on the basis of recall of previous listening experiences and according to expectations stemming from knowledge of English language constructs. In this sense, everyday speech discrimination may require varying levels of ability depending upon the amount of message material available to process. Understanding of a conversation, lecture, or story presented with related situational cues requires the ability to synthesize all message information and discriminate speech presented in a highly redundant context. A more difficult speech discrimination task might include discrimination of monosyllabic words presented without the sequence of information afforded by context or situational cues. This is representative of a task in which there is low redundancy of information requiring greater analytic skill.

An example of a redundancy continuum is presented in Fig. 6-1. Each decrease in the amount of message content requires an increased ability to discriminate speech on the basis of its acoustic properties alone.

Requires Increasing Skill in Analysis of Speech Information ↓

1. Conversation, lecture, or story presented on a familiar topic in a relevant environment (high redundancy)
2. Conversation, lecture, or story presented on a familiar topic without environmental clues
3. Unrelated sentences
4. Phrases and polysyllabic words
5. Monosyllabic words (low redundancy)

↑ Requires Increasing Skill in Synthesis of Speech Information

Fig. 6-1. Message redundancy continuum ranging from a level of high redundancy requiring greater skill in synthesis of speech information to a level of low redundancy requiring a greater skill in analysis of speech information.

AUDIBILITY

In order for speech to be auditorily discriminated, it must first be auditorily perceived. The level of speech audibility depends upon one or more interacting variables including the physical status of the hearing mechanism. As mentioned earlier, and in other chapters of this text, hearing impairment may have an almost predictable effect of speech discrimination. A second variable, in many instances, is the hearing-impaired person's ability to benefit from use of an amplification system. Successful hearing aid use often results in improved speech discrimination ability. Besides hearing aid use, the acoustic environment, especially reverberation time, has a significant influence on speech intelligibility; however, this influence is minimized by modern hearing aids (Ross & Giolas, 1978). A fourth major variable is competing noise. Background noise is present in most everyday listening situations. Variation in noise level and type will have differing influence on speech discrimination. Noise types have been categorized by Graupe, Causey, and Soffa (1977) as:

1. Short duration noise—door slamming, bell ringing, dog barking, etc.
2. Quasi-stationary noise—fans, surf, speech babble, etc.
3. Nonstationary (speechlike) noise—single speaker, reverberation.

Garstecki and Mulac (1974) found that when a competing message is meaningful speech, discrimination of monosyllables and of colloquial and synthetic sentences varied in normal-hearing young adults and elderly adults with mild-to-moderate sensorineural hearing loss.

In sum, message redundancy is influenced by audibility of the speech signal. Audibility is determined by a variety of factors, which may alone or in combination influence speech discrimination.

VISIBILITY

Several investigators have studied the differences between auditory and auditory-visual discrimination of common words. The results of these studies demonstrate that when subjects look and listen, their word recognition scores are generally better than when they listen alone or look alone (Sanders, 1968; Ross et al., 1972). Erber (1971) reported that hearing-impaired children require a quieter environment than normal-hearing children to achieve maximum auditory-visual identification of words. Since everyday conversation affords opportunity for combined auditory-visual speech discrimination, and not all hearing-impaired people derive the same degree of benefit from this additional information, it would seem that some measure of combined auditory-visual speech discrimination would serve a practical purpose in rehabilitating the hearing-impaired person.

SITUATIONAL CUES

Speechreading studies that have incorporated the use of situational cues (Jeffers & Barley, 1971) demonstrate that it is difficult to know what is being measured and its prescriptive value. One general assumption is that situational cues that are related to a message will increase message redundancy. This alone may be reason to consider the influence of situational cues on everyday speech discrimination. Situational cues appear to provide a referent which may be less ambiguous and less fleeting than a speech signal. They may also be distracting, ignored, or misinterpreted by some hearing-impaired persons (Garstecki, 1979). Auditory situational cues may not be perceived by hearing-impaired adults, especially under noise conditions (Wales, Garstecki, & Privratsky, 1977), and thus may not add to message redundancy. These findings suggest that it may be beneficial to evaluate the hearing-impaired person's ability to use situational cues as an adjunct to everyday speech discrimination.

The amount of linguistic information, audibility, and combined audibility-visibility of a message and the availability of related situational cues all appear to have an influence on everyday speech discrimination. To determine which variables may be of importance to any particular person, a complete understanding of the difficult speech discrimination situation is necessary. Several approaches may be used to elicit this information.

EVALUATION OF SPEECH DISCRIMINATION SITUATIONS

In order to understand the impact that speech discrimination difficulty may have on an individual's everyday communication, it is important to know the conditions under which the difficulty occurs. This information can be obtained from the hearing-impaired person's self-report, case history, or hearing handicap survey. The hearing-impaired person and/or some significant other person, perhaps a parent in the case of a child, should be questioned in regard to problems with speaker, message, communication channel, and receiver variables that may negatively influence message perception. It is also beneficial to know the amount and type of message information that is available to the receiver in typically encountered difficult listening situations. One should be able to use this account of the problem to determine how hearing-impaired individuals might compensate for their loss through the use of visible speech cues, environmental cues, understanding the sequence of action, and other message information.

Most hearing clinic case history and/or interview sessions include consideration of the hearing-impaired person's chief complaint and reason for seeking professional assistance. Relatively little emphasis, however, is directed toward eliciting an accurate and comprehensive description of the ability to communicate in a variety of listening conditions. Hearing handicap survey forms can be used as a means of eliciting this information in detail. A variety of questionnaires have been developed for this purpose. Such instruments can be used to provide a systematic procedure for identifying communication problems associated with hearing loss.

Although these surveys were intended for use in evaluating a person's overall hearing handicap, answers to selected questions can provide insight into the types of speech discrimination problems that are experienced (see Table 6-1). Of the surveys currently available, one of the most comprehensive instruments is the Hearing Performance Inventory

Table 6-1
Selected Questions From a Sampling of Hearing Handicap Survey Forms

Hearing Handicap Survey	Selected Examples of Statements Relating to Speech Discrimination
Scale for Self-Assessment of Hearing (High, Fairbanks, & Glorig, 1964	1. If you are six to twelve feet away from a television set, do you understand most of what is said? 11. When you talk to a bus driver, waiter, ticket salesman, etc., can you understand all right?
Hearing Measurement Scale (Noble & Atherley, 1970)	2. Do you ever have difficulty hearing in the conversation when you're with one other person outside? 5. Do you ever have difficulty hearing conversation at work?
Social Hearing Handicap Index (Ewertsen & Nielsen, 1973)	2. Do you have problems in understanding when members of the family are gathered together? 21. Do you often misunderstand other people's conversation?
Profile Questionnaire for Rating Communicative Performance in a School Environment (Sanders, 1975)	4.a. When I speak to the class as a whole, Mary is able to understand with: (little to great difficulty) b. This happens: (seldom to very often) 6.a. In playground or gymnasium games or activities, she is able to follow verbal directions with: (little to great difficulty) b. This happens: (seldom to very often)
Hearing Performance Inventory (Giolas et al., 1978)	17. You are watching a drama or movie on television. Can you understand what is being said when the speaker's voice is loud enough for you and there *is* music in the background? 21. Can you understand what a man is saying on the telephone when his voice is loud enough?

(Giolas et al., 1978). This 158-item form surveys a wide variety of speaker characteristics and communication situations. Its major drawback is that it requires approximately one hour to administer. Although further revision is planned, it is ready for clinical use, especially for the purposes being addressed in this chapter.

Speech Communication Profile

Having reviewed factors that influence speech discrimination and the variety of discrimination tasks presented in everyday communication, it is not difficult to see the need for a variety of speech discrimination tests. To provide some structure to the collection of information pertaining to speech communication ability, a Speech Communication Profile was developed (see Fig. 6-2). This profile has been used primarily in work with hard-of-hearing adults, although with some modification, it could be used with children. It is essentially a record of the communication problem and audiologic test results. It provides a profile of speech discrimination test information that is useful in determining the need for additional evaluation as well as for establishing a hierarchy of goals and activities for an aural rehabilitation program. Sections 1.0 and 2.0 are used to record audiologic test results and hearing handicap survey (or case history) information, which is necessary to determine the specific nature of the problem and frequency of occurrence. Under Section 1.0, the hearing loss description may be obtained from recent otologic or audiologic reports or through actual audiologic assessment. The description of the hearing handicap is obtained through the patient's self-report. Speech audiometry results (Section 2.0) reflect performance using a standardized test administered to the patient under his most natural listening mode (aided or unaided). Section 3.0 is included to alert the examiner to the need for considering the ability to compensate for an auditory deficit through the use of vision. Together, these three sections yield information pertaining to the patient's sensory capability. Section 4.0 is used for rating the influence of communication channel fidelity on speech discrimination. Section 5.0 provides an account of the influence of message redundancy on understanding speech. The influence of linguistic content can be determined by comparing scores across stimulus conditions from low-content monosyllabic word discrimination to high-content running discourse on a familiar topic. Comparing the differences in scores obtained under quiet versus noise conditions, the effect of noise or speech audibility on message perception can be determined. Performance differences under auditory conditions alone and in combination with visual cues can be observed. Finally, differences in speech discrimination in the presence or absence of situational cues, as well as the level of ability with auditory, visual, and nonverbal cues can be noted. The Speech Communication Profile can be used to portray specific problem areas that might be incorporated in a rehabilitation program. By presenting performance scores across all conditions, it provides the rehabilitative audiologist with information to develop a starting point for improving speech discrimination and overall oral communicative ability.

Name ____________________ Age ________ Date __________

1.0 Introductory Remarks

1.1 Description of hearing loss:

1.2 Description of hearing handicap:

2.0 Speech Audiometry

2.1. Test Equipment and Conditions

2.1.1. Audiometer:

2.1.2. Test Stimulus:

2.1.3. Stimulus presentation: ______ Tape ______ MLV

2.1.4. Primary signal: ______ Rt. Spkr. ______ Left Spkr. ______ R & L Spkrs.

2.1.5. Competing message: ______ Multi-speaker babble ______ Other ______ (specify)

2.1.6. P/CM: ______ O db HL ______ Other—specify ______

2.1.7. Primary signal presentation level: ______ 50 dB HL ______ Other—specify ______

2.1.8. Listening condition: ______ Sound Field ______ Other—specify ______

2.1.9. Listening mode: ______ Unaided ______ Aided

2.1.9.1. Aid make:

2.1.9.2. Aid model/style:

2.1.9.3. Receiver type:

2.1.9.4. Settings:

2.1.9.5. Battery:

2.1.9.6. Earmold:

2.1.9.7. Aided Ear: ______ Right ______ Left ______ Both

2.2. Test Findings

2.2.1. SAT: A = ______

2.2.2. SRT: A = ______

2.2.3. Discrim.—Q: A = ______ A/V = ______

2.2.4. Discrim.—N: A = ______ A/V = ______

3.0 Vision

3.1 Binocular visual acuity: ______ (Snellen chart)

3.2 Description of vision problem:

4.0 Sensory Input Channel Efficiency Rating

4.1. Auditory Channel			(Intelligibility Rating)			
	low				high	
4.1.1. Telephone conversation	1	2	3	4	5	NA
4.1.2. CB Radio conversation	1	2	3	4	5	NA
4.1.3. Walkie-Talkie/Intercom	1	2	3	4	5	NA
4.1.4. Public address system	1	2	3	4	5	NA
4.1.5. Radio broadcast	1	2	3	4	5	NA
4.1.6. Other ______	1	2	3	4	5	—
4.2. Auditory-Visual Channel			(Intelligibility Rating)			
	low				high	
4.2.1. One-to-one conversation	1	2	3	4	5	NA
4.2.2. Group conversation	1	2	3	4	5	NA
4.2.3. Lecture/Oral presentation	1	2	3	4	5	NA
4.2.4. Movie	1	2	3	4	5	NA
4.2.5. Theater	1	2	3	4	5	NA
4.2.6. Television program	1	2	3	4	5	NA
4.2.7. Other ______	1	2	3	4	5	—

Fig. 6-2. Speech Communication Profile. (Continued on next page)

5.0 Auditory Message Perception

5.1. Descriptional of problem:

5.2. Evaluation procedure (including description of test stimuli, competing message type, P/CM level, situation cues, etc.):

5.3. Estimated level of message perception

5.3.1.	Running Discourse—Familiar Topic																
5.3.2.	Running Discourse—Unfamiliar Topic																
5.3.3.	Unrelated sentences																
5.3.4.	Monosyllabic words																

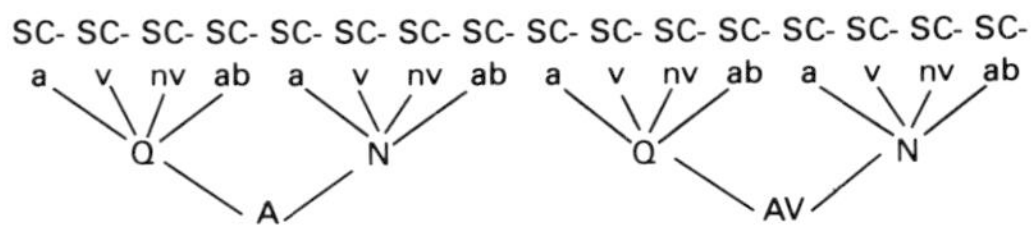

KEY: A = Auditory Channel; A/V = Auditory-Visual Channels; Q = Quiet Condition; N = Noise Condition; SC = Situational Clues (a = auditory; v = visual/picture; nv = non-verbal ab = absent)

Fig. 6-2. (Continued).

ALTERNATE TESTS OF SPEECH DISCRIMINATION

Standardized test materials are not available for measuring speech discrimination under each condition listed in Section 5.0 of the Speech Communication Profile. However, the Profile provides a means of organizing the speed discrimination information that might be obtained. When standardized tests are not available, a general estimate of speech discrimination ability might be made by the administration of a modified standardized test or by experimental test materials. Whenever a nonstandardized test is used, the results must be interpreted with caution. These results may, however, be useful in reaching a qualitative estimate of speech understanding in everyday life (Carhart, 1965).

In selecting an appropriate set of materials, Morgan (1978) and others have stated that tests must be thought of as the standard recording of items, not as the written list of test stimuli. Unless recorded material is used, discrimination scores will be influenced by speaker differences that occur in monitored live-voice presentation. A second concern is the purpose for which a particular set of materials is to be used. Use of speech material standardized only for use with normal-hearing subjects may be appropriate for purposes of diagnostic evaluation. In rehabilitation, it may be of greater interest to note the circumstances under which discrimination ability changes. Quite different material could be chosen in view of the question being asked. Morgan's third concern is that many commonly used test materials have not been standardized under conditions of speech competition. The effects of such competition are not well known; therefore, the primary signal presentation level and the speech-to-competing noise (S/CN) ratio must be documented. A final concern is in regard to what represents a meaningful difference between scores on a given set of materials. In using a single set of materials, the critical measure is test-retest reliability. When several test forms are used, a measure of the difference between forms must be taken into account before a difference in test scores can be attributed to a difference in discrimination ability.

Test results may be dependent upon the type of material used and the presentation level (Egan, 1948). An accurate assessment of phoneme discrimination can be obtained by using nonsense syllables. Monosyllabic words provide phonetic as well as semantic information resulting in larger differences in the relative difficulty of discriminating words. In comparison with nonsense syllables, monosyllabic words are generally easier to discriminate. The relative ease in discrimination of different types of materials will increase as the amount of linguistic information is increased and extralinguistic cues are added. Thus, polysyllabic words can be discriminated on the basis of temporal as well as phonemic and semantic cues. Sentence discrimination is facilitated by the presence of phonemic, semantic, syntactic, and temporal cues (Garstecki & Mulac, 1974). Auditory discrimination of each of these types of materials will be enhanced through combined auditory-visual perception and further increased through the use of situational cues. Although an increase in the amount of linguistic and situational cue information increases redundancy of information, it also increases the likelihood that other aspects of message perception are being measured in the speech discrimination task. However, there are circumstances in audiologic evaluation and aural rehabilitation in which all of this information is useful.

Test Materials

What materials might be used as alternate tests of speech discrimination? As mentioned earlier, the most popular speech discrimination tests are those comprised of monosyllabic word lists. These materials can be used to determine the phonetic confusions experienced by hearing-impaired persons. Unfortunately, test scores are usually reporterd in a "percent correct" form rather than as a description of the phonetic errors. The latter method increases the prescriptive value of the test results.

Monosyllabic word lists are presented under one of two response formats, open- or closed-set. Open-set tests include the Harvard PB–50 lists (Egan, 1948), CID W–22 word lists (Hirsh et al., 1952) and NU Auditory Test no. 6 lists (Tillman & Carhart, 1966). The Harvard PB-50 lists were designed to be "phonetically balanced" in that the phonetic composition of the words in each test list was intended to be representative of the types of sounds found in a sample of 100,000 words in newsprint. The lists fell short of this goal. The CID W-22 word lists were more rigidly balanced using a different set of criteria; Dewey's (1923) newsprint count and frequently occurring speech sounds in New York telephone conversations (French, Carter, & Koenig, 1930).

Lehiste and Peterson (1959) considered the influence of coarticulation factors on speech production in words in designing word lists in which each initial and final consonant and each medial vowel appeared with the same frequency. They later revised their lists to include only those words having a high frequency of occurrence (Peterson & Lehiste, 1962). Tillman and Carhart (1966) revised Lehiste and Peterson's lists to increase the phonemic balance resulting in the development of the NU Auditory Test no. 6. However, studies comparing differenties in performance for each of the tests have demonstrated that different results are obtained when different test materials are administered to the same subjects (Olsen & Matkin, 1979). In sum, open-set discrimination tests may serve as a useful predictor of a person's ability to perceive the acoustic properties of speech signals.

Closed-set materials may be used for essentially the same purpose; however, in the administration of these materials, the respondent is not required to recall previously learned vocabulary in arriving at his response. Word familiarity effects are minimized. Closed-set monosyllabic word discrimination tests also have their place in the audiologist's test battery. Bode and Oyer (1970) comment that although most everyday listening situations require closed-set monitoring skills, many words in connected speech, such as proper nouns, unfamiliar vocabulary, and technical language are not bound by contextual influences. Therefore, both open- and closed-set materials may yield clinically useful information.

Closed-set materials were first developed by Haagen (1945), who observed that subjects often made the same or similar errors on monosyllabic word discrimination tests. Haagen developed a response set in which error responses were used as foils. Haagen found that even though responses to a multiple-item test were not always identical to the responses provided when the same stimulus was presented in an open-set format, scores for the two methods correlated highly with one another. Black and Haagen (1963) further developed these materials by adding items to the original list.

Fairbanks (1958) developed a multiple-choice test in which sets of rhyming monosyllables were presented. Only the initial consonants differed in a set of rhyming words. Because this test was somewhat limited in scope, House (1963) modified Fairbanks's original test to include discrimination of final consonants in monosyllabic words. The revised test was called the Modified Rhyme Test. These word lists are neither phonetically or phonemically balanced, but they have reasonable phonemic similarity. The lists comprising this test have been demonstrated to be statistically equivalent to one another with negligible practice effects when used with a normal-hearing population (House, 1965).

Nixon (1973) investigated the response foils of the Modified Rhyme Test. Young normal-hearing listeners were presented stimulus items in the form of a free response task. In comparing their responses with the foil words, it was found that in many instances, only one or two of the six available response words were possible alternatives to the words heard by the listeners.

Hutton, Curry, and Armstrong (1959) developed the Semi-Diagnostic Test to assess a person's candidacy for aural rehabilitation and to measure progress through the rehabilitation program. Although the test has not been evaluated extensively, it offers a closed-set response format for monosyllable discrimination of pairs. The listener's task is to identify two correct monosyllables from a choice of four words which differ only in vowels or consonants. Besides providing an estimate of auditory discrimination, the test is designed to assess visual and combined auditory-visual discrimination ability. Responses can be scored in a percent correct form and/or they can be analyzed for phonetic confusions.

Clarke (1965) developed the Phonetically Balanced Rhyme Test, which consisted of three individual tests of phoneme identification in pre-, inter-, and post-vocalic positions. However, the clinical applicability of this test has not been established.

Schultz and Shubert (1969) used CID W-22 words in a Multiple Choice Discrimination Test (MCDT). They believed that by using highly familiar words the probability of less familiar words being considered as a possible response was reduced. They felt that if their five response choices included less familiar words, then less frequently used words would have a greater probability of being considered. Nixon (1973) showed that the foil words were frequently not among the responses provided by the hearing-impaired population. Therefore, the analysis of the phonetic composition of mistaken words was not meaningful for identification of phonetic confusions.

Pederson and Studebaker (1972) developed the Oklahoma University Closed-Response Test (OUCRT) to evaluate the ability to discriminate among minimally contrasting initial and final consonants as well as medial vowels. The response alternatives varied only in phoneme place of articulation. Since many hearing-impaired people demonstrate difficulty in auditory discrimination of minially paired words differing only in place of articulation, use of this test with the hearing-impaired yields useful prescriptive information.

The most recently developed closed-set test is the California Consonant Test (Owens & Schubert, 1977). The test is composed of 100 items, 36 initial and 64 final consonant words, with three foils for each. This test has been found to be sensitive to the phonetic confusions demonstrated by subjects with high-frequency sensorineural hearing loss (Owens & Schubert, 1977; Schwartz & Surr, 1979). The information provided by this test should enable the audiologist to determine an appropriate remediation approach for subjects who demonstrate phonetic confusions.

Competing Message Tests

Tests presented against a competing message background are regarded as having greater resolving power than those presented in quiet conditions. In addition, they appear to have greater face validity in that they are more representative of conditions experienced in everyday difficult listening situations. At the present time, white noise is a widely used competing noise in the clinical assessment of speech discrimination ability. White noise is characterized by a wide-frequency band of equally distributed sound energy. However, masking noise typically encountered in everyday listening is generally noncontinuous and dynamic. White noise does not appear to be truly representative of the type of competing message that hearing-impaired people must overcome in everyday communication. A competing speech signal may prove to be a more effective masker than white noise when one is concerned with simulating the speech discrimination difficulty that a hearing-impaired person is likely to encounter.

Olsen and Tillman (1968) found that speech discrimination in normal hearing and sensorineurally hearing-impaired subjects deteriorated by 25 percent when a competing speech signal was presented at a +6 dB speech-to-competing-signal ratio as compared to performance under quiet test conditions. Rupp and Phillips (1969) used speech noise and white noise in testing the discrimination abilities of normal hearing subjects. Results indicated that the speech spectrum noise was markedly more interferring than the white noise at the same intensity levels.

Dirks and Bower (1969) found that whether or not competing speech was as intelligible as meaningful speech was of no consequence. Subjects performed similarly under each condition. Trammell and Speaks (1970) found that a competing speech message was less interferring when it was unintelligible or played in a backward mode. Garstecki and Mulac (1974) found that when the competing speech background was presented in a forward mode, it had a greater masking effect than when it was presented in a less intelligible backward mode. Chermak and Zielonko (1977) suggested that children and adults may be differentially influenced by the intelligibility of the competing message. They found that in children, it did not appear to matter whether or not the competing message was meaningful or nonmeaningful. They felt that the child's ability to discriminate speech in a speech-noise background was related to the level of maturation of the child's selective listening strategy and skill development. Certainly, there is a need for additional research on the influence of a competing message in speech discrimination as it relates to everyday communication. At this time, it is reasonable to conclude that it is important to obtain some estimate of a hearing-impaired person's ability to understand speech presented in a speech-noise background.

SPEECH DISCRIMINATION TESTS FOR CHILDREN

Tests for Children

Speech discrimination tests for children are used for differential diagnosis of aural pathology and hearing aid evaluation as well as to study the possible relationship between disorders of speech, articulation, language, reading, and speech discrimination ability. Tests are constructed to contain material within a child's developing language levels and with the need for maintaining the child's motivation and attention during administration. The most popular test materials are open-set monosyllabic word lists and closed-set word-picture pairs.

The Travis-Rasmus Speech Sound Discrimination Test (Travis & Rasmus, 1931) was one of the first discrimination tests developed for use with children. This test incorporated use of paired nonsense syllables for same-different judgment. A similar technique was used by Templin (1943) in the Short Test of Sound Discrimination. Nonsense syllables were used as test stimuli in order to evaluate a child's ability to analyze the distinctive differences in acoustic properties of speech signals without interference of semantic interpretation. Meaningful test words introduce a semantic variable to the speech discrimination task, which the above investigators preferred to avoid.

Haskins (1949) developed one of the first lists of monosyllabic words for children. Words were selected from the International Kindergarten Union vocabulary lists. They were within the vocabulary of young children and were designated the PBK lists. These three lists of 50 words each can be administered in much the same way as other open-set monosyllabic word test materials previously described. One limitation may be that a child's receptive vocabulary level may negatively influence the test results if it is below that of a normal-hearing kindergartener (Olsen & Matkin, 1978).

Wepman (1958) developed a paired-word discrimination test that contains words that may well be above the comprehension level of the five-to-eight year age of the standardization population. The test requires an ability to comprehend the concept of same-different, and the scoring criterion allows only one point to distinguish differences in discrimination age levels (Wiig & Semel, 1976).

One of the first picture discrimination tests was developed by Robbins and Robbins (1948). This test was designed to assess vowel, nasal, fricative, and sibilant consonant discrimination through a picture-pointing task. The Boston University Speech Sound Discrimination Picture Test (Pronovost & Dumbleton, 1953) was similarly designed to evaluate vowel, semivowel, plosive, and fricative discrimination through a selection of pictured word pairings. These authors recommended use of an audio recording of the test stimuli to improve the consistency of test results. Pronovost (1974) recently revised the test to improve pictorial choices.

Myatt and Landes (1963) developed a test as a compromise between those that require large numbers of pictures and those that only require a choice between two pictures per item. Eighty pictures representing monosyllabic words were divided in 20 groups of four words each, some consisting of phonetically dissimilar words, others with marked phonetic similarity, and a third type containing a mix of each of the above types. Using this organization format, the test provides information about the types of discrimination errors as well as the number of errors that are present. By looking at the types of materials that create the greatest discrimination problem, a starting point and progression of training to improve speech discrimination ability can be determined.

The Discrimination by Pictures Test (Siegenthaler & Haspiel, 1966) consists of 48 pairs of monosyllabic words and corresponding pictures which are familiar to preschool-age children. Responses to the test may be analyized for phonetic confusion or for the child's ability to distinguish among acoustically similar word pairs. With only two response choices per item, a high guess factor may increase the probability of a correct response.

Goldman, Fristoe, and Woodcock (1970) developed a test to evaluate monosyllabic word discrimination using a picture-pointing response format and audiotaped presentation of test items in quiet and with a competing school cafeteria noise. The test is designed for use with a population ranging in age from four years to over 70 years. The stimulus items are minimally paired, allowing for a distinctive feature analysis of test results. The noise subtest results provide a measure of auditory figure-ground discrimination, which may be helpful in predicting ability to communicate in noisy conditions.

The Word Intelligibility by Picture Identification Test (Lerman, Ross

& McLauchlin, 1965; Ross & Lerman, 1970) also allows for a a distinctive feature analysis of speech discrimination in a picture-pointing task. This test is useful for evaluation of children with receptive vocabulary ages of four years and older. In clinical use, however, test scores may exceed those obtained using an open-set response format by as much as 20 percent. The test materials also allow for evaluation and comparision of auditory, visual, and combined auditory-visual speech discrimination.

Prather et al. (1971) developed the Washington Speech Sound Discrimination Test for use with a preschool population. The test was designed primarily to assess the relationship between speech discrimination and articulation. It contains subtests that allow for a distinctive feature analysis of results including differentiation between commonly substituted or error phonemes. It also requires less than 15 minutes administration time.

Katz and Elliott (1978) designed an audiotape recorded speech discrimination test containing items within the vocabularies of three-year old inner-city children. The Northwestern University–Children's Perception of Speech (NU–CHIPS) test consists of 50 monosyllabic words, which are easily pictured and presented in a closed-set, picture-pointing task. It has been demonstrated to be easy to administer and highly reliable.

Sentence Tests

Relatively few speech discrimination tests have been developed using sentence materials. For clinical purposes, the CID Everyday Speech Sentences developed by Grant Fairbanks and a Working Group of the Armed Forces–National Research Council Committee on Hearing and Bio-Acoustics (Davis & Silverman, 1970) have been used for informal evaluation purposes. Although these sentences have high face validity, no standardized test has been developed using this material. Sentences are grouped in sets of ten. Responses are scored on the basis of the listener's ability to recognize 50 key words incorporated within the sentences. This set of sentences was orginally developed for purposes of validating existing discrimination test materials.

Berger (1969) embedded phonetically similar key words within sentences in the Kent State University Speech Discrimination Test. Any one of five key words in each sentence can be used meaningfully and correctly in the sentence. Subjects are instructed to identify the correct key word presented in a sentence context. The test material is presented using audiotape or monitored live voice. Scoring is based on a percent correct basis.

To control for word familiarity, word and sentence length, and syntactical structure in sentence discrimination, Jerger, Speaks, and Trammell (1968) developed synthetic sentence materials. Although they are not meaningful sentences, the word sequence within a sentence follows normal rules of English syntax. Sentences are presented in a closed-set response format usually with a competing message of continuous discourse at 0 dB signal-to-noise ratio.

Kalikow et al. (1977) developed the Speech Perception in Noise (SPIN) test materials to measure sentence discrimination. Sentences were recorded in twelve-speaker background babble with primary and competing messages on separate channels to permit variation in P/CN ratio. Half of the 500 sentences (50 per form) were constructed to end in monosyllabic nouns of high predictability and the remaining half ending with nouns of low predictability. Scoring was based on the subjects' ability to correctly identify the final word in an open-set response format. Preliminary research findings suggest that the SPIN Test results may provide a more realistic estimate of speech discrimination ability under everyday listening conditions than other more traditionally employed measures (Hutcherson et al., 1979).

Auditory-Visual Speech Discrimination

A number of clinical studies have demonstrated that combined auditory-visual speech perception is superior to either auditory or visual speech perception alone. O'Neill (1954), Sumby and Pollack (1954), Erber (1969), Ewertsen and Nielsen (1971), and others have found that auditory-visual word recognition in noise is improved over auditory-alone recognition. Studies by Sanders (1968), Ross et al. (1972), and others have examined auditory-visual word recognition ability in hearing-impaired children, finding better ability than under either mode alone. Binnie (1973) indicated that the sensation level at which the best auditory-visual speech perception is achieved may serve as the starting level for an auditory training program.

Few investigators have used sentence materials as stimuli in assessment of auditory-visual speech discrimination because they are so difficult to score reliably. Some use is being made of speechreading sentence material as an estimate of auditory-visual speech discrimination. Dodds and Harford (1968) and Ewertsen, Nielsen and Nielsen (1970) have used lipreading tests in an auditory-visual presentation mode to estimate the level of everyday communication ability.

Thorton and Erber (1978) used sentence materials to measure the ability of moderate to severely hearing-impaired children to perceive speech under a combined sensory input mode. Their results suggest that sentences could be used in grouping hearing-impaired children for instructional purposes according to general level of speech perception ability. This information could also be used as a predictor of success in a mainstreamed educational environment.

Byman (1974) suggests that because speech perception involves the simultaneous processing of auditory, visual, and situational cues in relation to linguistic constraints, these processes must be evaluated using material that measures the utilization of all of this information. Garstecki (1979) discusses procedures used to evaluate auditory-visual sentence perception in the presence of auditory and visual situational cues. Overall findings suggest that the hearing-impaired person, the elderly adult in particular, may benefit from training in the use of situational cues to complement auditory-visual speech information. He also recommends that sentence materials be evaluated for key word visibility and topic familiarity before being used for assessment or remediation purposes.

SUMMARY

The purpose of this chapter was to provide an overview of alternate ways to measure speech discrimination ability. The need for alternate tests is evidenced by the wide variety of speech discrimination tasks encountered in everyday communication. Some tasks require the ability to perceive auditory information alone, while others require the integration of auditory and visual information. Some messages are more intelligible than others because of their inherent acoustic power, visually contrastive speech movements, or linguistic and extralinguistic redundancy. To better understand the hearing-impaired person's speech discrimination ability on all levels, a battery of appropriate tests must be applied. It behooves the examiner to select test materials that are appropriate for the population under study. Every effort should be made to use standardized test materials to provide a reliable and valid estimate of a person's discrimination ability. Nonstandardized test results or test results obtained from a population different from the standardizing population must be cautiously interpreted and only regarded as an estimate of ability. Ideally, test results should provide a maximum amount of prescriptive information to the examiner and practical information to the hearing-impaired person.

REFERENCES

Alpiner, J. G. *Handbook of adult rehabilitative audiology.* Baltimore: The Williams and Wilkins Company, 1978.

Berger, K. Speech discrimination task using multiple choice key words in sentences. *Journal of Auditory Research,* 1969, *9,* 247–262.

Bergman, M. The present status of auditory training and speech conservation. In *Auditory rehabilitation in adults,* 1964 pp. 85–95. Proceedings of a seminar held in Cleveland, Ohio.

Binnie, C. A. Bi-sensory articulation functions for normal hearing and sensorineural hearing loss patients. *Journal of the Academy of Rehabilitative Audiology,* 1973, *6,* 43–53.

Black, J. W., & Haagen, C. M. Multiple-choice intelligibility tests, Forms A and B. *Journal of Speech and Hearing Disorders,* 1963, *28,* 77–86.

Bode, D. L., & Oyer, H. J. Auditory training and speech discrimination. *Journal of Speech and Hearing Research,* 1970, *13,* 839–855.

Byman, J. Testing of auditory and audio-visual speech perception related to everyday communication. *Scandanavian Audiology* (Suppl. 4), 1974, pp. 58–66.

Carhart, R. Problems in the measurement of speech discrimination. *Archives of Otolaryngology,* 1965, *82,* 253–260.

Chermak, G. D., & Zielonko, B. Word discrimination in the presence of competing speech with children. *Journal of the American Audiology Society,* 1977, *2,* 188–192.

Clarke, F. R. Technique for evaluation of speech systems. Final report from Stanford Research Institute on Contract DA 28-043 AMC-00227 (E), 1965. Prepared for U.S. Army Electronics Laboratories, Ft. Monmouth, New Jersey.

Davis, H., & Silverman, S. R. *Hearing and deafness.* New York: Holt, Rinehart and Winston, 1970.

Dewey, G. *Relative frequency of English speech sounds.* Cambridge: Harvard University Press, 1923.

Dirks, D. D., & Bower, D. R. Masking effects of speech competing messages. *Journal of Speech and Hearing Research,* 1969, *12,* 229–245.

Dodds, E., & Harford, E. Application of a lipreading test in a hearing aid evaluation. *Journal of Speech and Hearing Disorders,* 1968, *33,* 167–173.

Egan, J. P. Articulation testing methods. *Laryngoscope,* 1948, *58,* 955–991.

Erber, N. P. Interaction of audition and vision in the recognition of oral speech stimuli. *Journal of Speech and Hearing Research,* 1969, *12,* 423–425.

Erber, N. P. Auditory and audiovisual reception of words in low-frequency noise by children with normal hearing and by children with impaired hearing. *Journal of Speech and Hearing Research,* 1971, *14,* 496–512.

Ewertsen, H. W., & Nielsen, H. A comparative analysis of the audiovisual auditive and visual perception of speech. *Acta Otolaryngologica,* 1971, *72,* 201–205.

Ewertsen, H. W., & Nielsen, H. Social hearing handicap index. *Audiology,* 1973, *12,* 180–187.

Ewertsen, H. W., Nielsen, H., & Nielsen, S. Audio-visual speech perception. *Acta Otolaryngologica, Supplement 263 (Stockholm),* 1970, pp. 229–230.

Fairbanks, G. Test of phonemic discrimination: The rhyme test. *Journal of the Acoustical Society of America,* 1958, *30,* 596–600.

Fletcher, H., & Steinberg, J. C. Articulation testing methods. *Bell System Technical Journal,* 1929, *8,* 807–809.

French, N. R., Carter, C. W., & Koenig, W. The words and sounds of telephone conversations. *Bell System Technical Journal,* 1930, *9,* 290–324.

Garstecki, D. C. The use of situational cues in visual communication. In M. A. Henoch (Ed.), *Aural rehabilitation for the elderly.* New York: Grune & Stratton, Inc., 1979.

Garstecki, D. C., & Mulac, A. Effects of test material and competing message on speech discrimination. *Journal of Auditory Research,* 1974, *3,* 171–178.

Giolas, T. G., Owens, E., Lamb, S. H., & Schubert, E. D. Hearing Performance Inventory. *Journal of Speech and Hearing Disorders, 1979, 44,* 169–195.

Goldman, R., Fristoe, M., & Woodcock, R. W. *Goldman-Fristoe-Woodcock test of auditory discrimination.* Circle Pines, Minn.: American Guidance Service, 1970.

Graupe, D., Causey, G. D., & Soffa, M. Applications of times series identification and filtering theory to hearing aids. *Hearing Aid Journal,* 1977, *11,* 22–24.

Haagen, C. H. *Intellgibility measurement: Twenty-four word multiple-choice tests.* New York: Psychological Corporation, 1945.

Haskins, J. A phonetically balanced test of speech discrimination for children. Unpublished Master's thesis, Northwestern University, Evanston, Illinois, 1949.

High, W. S., Fairbanks, G., & Glorig, A. Scale of self-assessment of hearing handicap. *Journal of Speech and Hearing Disorders,* 1964, *29,* 215–230.

Hirsh, I. J., Davis, H., Silverman, S. R., Reynolds, E. G., et al. Development of materials for speech audiometry. *Journal of Speech and Hearing Disorders,* 1952, *17,* 321–337.

Hodgson, W. R., Skinner, P. H. *Hearing aid assessment and use in audiologic habilitation.* Baltimore: The Williams and Wilkins Company, 1977.

House, A. S., Williams, C. E., Hecker, M. H., Kryter, K. D. Psychoacoustic speech tests: A modified rhyme test. Technical Documentary Report ESD–TDR–63–403, U.S. Air Force System Command, Hanscon Field, 1963.

House, A. S., Williams, C. E., Hecker, M. H., & Kryter, K. D. Articulation testing methods: Consonantal differentiation with a closed response set. *Journal of the Acoustical Society of America,* 1965, *37,* 158–166.

Hutcherson, R. W., Dirks, D. D., & Morgan, D. E. Evaluation of the speech perception in noise (SPIN) test. *Otolaryngol. Head, Neck Surg.,* 1979, *87,* 239–245.

Hutton, C., Curry, E. T., & Armstrong, M. B. Semi-diagnostic test materials for aural rehabilitation. *Journal of Speech & Hearing Disorders,* 1959, *24,* 319–329.

Jeffers, J., & Barley, M. *Speechreading (lipreading).* Springfield, Illinois: Charles C. Thomas Publishers, 1971.

Jerger, J., Speaks, C., Trammell, J. A new approach to speech audiometry. *Journal of Speech and Hearing Disorders,* 1968, *33,* 318–328.

Kalikow, D. N., Stevens, K. N., & Elliott, L. L. Development of a test of speech intelligibility in noise using sentence materials with controlled word predictability. *Journal of the Acoustical Society of America,* 1977, *61,* 1337–1351.

Katz, D., & Elliott, L. L. Development of a new children's speech discrimination test. Paper presented at the Annual Convention of the American Speech and Hearing Association, San Francisco, California, 1978.

Lehiste, I., & Peterson, G. E. Linguistic considerations in the study of speech intelligibility. *Journal of the Acoustical Society of America,* 1959, *31,* 280–286.

Lerman, J. W., Ross, M., & McLauchlin, R. M. A picture-identification test for hearing-impaired children. *Journal of Auditory Research,* 1965, *5,* 273–278.

Martin, F. N., & Pennington, C. D. Current trends in audiometric practices. *ASHA, 1971, 13,* 671–677.

Morgan, D. E. Speech discrimination materials. Paper presented at the Annual Convention of the American Speech and Hearing Association, San Francisco, California, 1978.

Myatt, B. D., & Landes, B. A. Assessing discrimination loss in children. *Archives of Otolaryngology,* 1963, *77,* 359–362.

Nixon, J. C. Investigation of the response foils of the modified rhyme hearing test. *Journal of Speech and Hearing Research,* 1973, *16,* 658–666.

Noble, W. G., & Atherley, G. R. C. The hearing measurement scale. *Journal of Auditory Research,* 1970, *10,* 229–250.

Olsen, W. O., & Matkin, N. D. Speech audiometry. In D. Rose (Ed.), *Audiological assessment.* Englewood Cliffs, New Jersey: Prentice-Hall, Inc., 1978.

Olsen, W. O., & Tillman, T. W. Hearing aids and sensorineural hearing loss. *Annals of Otology, Rhinology and Laryngology,* 1968, *77,* 717–726.

Olsen, W. O., Noffsinger, D., & Kurdziel, S. Speech discrimination in quiet and in white noise by patients with peripheral and central lesions. *Acta Otolaryngologica,* 1975, *80:* 375–382.

O'Neill, J. J. Contributions of the visual components of oral symbols to speech comprehension. *Journal of Speech and Hearing Disorders,* 1954, *19,* 429–439.

Owens, E. & Schubert, E. D. Development of the California Consonant Test. *Journal of Speech and Hearing Research,* 1977, *20,* 463–474.

Oyer, H. J., & Frankmann, J. P. *The aural rehabilitation process—a conceptual framework analysis.* New York: Holt, Rinehart and Winston, 1975.

Pederson, O. T., & Studebaker, G. A. A new minimal contrasts closed-response-set speech test. *Journal of Auditory Research,* 1972, *12,* 187–195.

Peterson, G. E., & Lehiste, I. Revised CNC lists for auditory tests. *Journal of Speech and Hearing Disorders,* 1962, *27,* 62–70.

Prather, E., Addicott, M. A., Miner, A., & Sunderland, L. *Washington speech sound discrimination test.* Danville, Illinois: The Interstate Printers and Publishers, Inc., 1971.

Pronovost, W. *The Boston University speech sound discrimination picture test.* Cedar Falls, Iowa: Go-Mo-Products, 1974.

Provonost, W., & Dumbleton, C. A. A picture-type speech sound discrimination test. *Journal of Speech and Hearing Disorders,* 1953, *18,* 258–266.

Robbins, S. D., & Robbins, R. S. *Speech sound discrimination tests.* Boston: Expression Co., 1948.

Ross, M., & Giolas, T. G. Auditory management of hearing-impaired children. Baltimore: University Park Press, 1978.

Ross, M., & Lerman, J. Picture identification test for hearing impaired children. *Journal of Speech and Hearing Research,* 1970, *5,* 47–72.

Ross, M., Kessler, M. E., Phillips, M. E., & Lerman, J. W. Visual, auditory and combined mode presentations of the WIPI test to hearing impaired children. *Volta Review,* 1972, *74,* 90–96.

Rupp, R., & Phillips, D. The effect of noise background on speech discrimination function in normal-hearing individuals. *Journal of Auditory Research,* 1969, *9,* 60–63.

Sanders, D. A. Auditory training within a communication framework. In *Proceedings of the 43rd Meeting of the Convention of American Instructors of the Deaf.* Washington, D.C.: U.S. Government Printing Office, pp. 254–258.

Sanders, D. A. Hearing aid orientation and counseling. In M. C. Pollack (Ed.), *Amplification for the hearing-impaired.* New York: Grune & Stratton, Inc., 1975, pp. 370–372.

Schultz, M. C., & Schubert, E. D. A multiple choice discrimination test (MCDT). *Laryngoscope,* 1969, *79,* 382–399.

Schwartz, D. M., & Surr, R. K. Three experiments on the California Consonant Test. *Journal of Speech and Hearing Disorders,* 1979, *44,* 61–72.

Scott, B. Development of a tactile aid for the profoundly hearing impaired: Implications for use with the elderly. In M. A. Henoch (Ed.), *Aural rehabilitation for the elderly.* New York: Grune & Stratton, Inc., 1979, pp. 83–107.

Siegenthaler, B. & Haspiel, G. Development of two standardized measures of hearing for speech by children. U. S. Department of Health, Education and Welfare, Project No. 2372, Contract No. OE–5–10–003, 1966.

Silverman, S. R., & Hirsch, I. J. Problems related to the use of speech in clinical audiometry. *Annals of Otology, Rhinology, and Laryngology,* 1955, *64,* 1234–1244.

Sumby, W. H., & Pollack, I. Visual contributions to speech intelligibility in noise. *Journal of the Acoustical Society of America,* 1954, *26,* 212–215.

Templin, M. A study of sound discrimination ability of elementary school pupils. *Journal of Speech and Hearing Disorders,* 1943, *8,* 127–132.

Thornton, N. E., & Erber, N. P. Auditory-visual speech perception by hearing-impaired children. Paper presented at the Annual Convention of the American Speech and Hearing Association, San Francisco, California, 1978.

Tillman, T. W., & Carhart, R. *An Expanded Test for Speech Discrimination Utilizing CNC Monosyllabic Words, Northwestern University Auditory Test No. 6.* USAF School of Aerospace Medicine, SAM–TR–66–65, 1966.

Trammell, J. L., & Speaks, C. On the distracting properties of competing speech. *Journal of Speech and Hearing Research,* 1970, *13,* 442–444.

Travis, L. E., & Rasmus, B. The speech sound discrimination abilities of cases with functional disorders of articulation. *Quarterly Journal of Speech,* 1931, *17,* 217–226.

Wales, J., Garstecki, D., & Priviatsky, K. Assessment of the aged adult's ability to use everyday communication cues. Paper presented at the Annual Convention of the American Speech and Hearing Association, Chicago, Illinois, 1977.

Wepman, J. *Auditory discrimination test.* Chicago: University of Chicago Press, 1958.

Wiig, E. H., & Semel, E. M. *Language disabilities in children and adolescents.* Columbus, Ohio: Charles E. Merrill Publishing Company, 1976.

Steven C. White, Ph.D.

7

Speech Protocols in the Assessment of Sensory and/or Peripheral-Neural Lesion Sites

A major responsibility of the audiologist is to provide and interpret data that identifies the site of lesion in the aberrant auditory system. Differentiating cochlear from retrocochlear pathology is a significant portion of this obligation, due to the importance of appropriate medical and aural rehabilitative procedures associated with disorders of the sensorineural pathways. It has been long reported that speech intelligibility testing, particularly speech discrimination testing, is useful in differentiaing sensorineural sites of lesion. For example, Shambaugh (1967, p. 697) included speech discrimination testing as one of the most useful early diagnostic tests for tumors within the internal auditory meatus, and Carhart (1965, p. 258) reported that a moderate reduction in discrimination is a frequent symptom in Meniere's disease.

The assessment of the sensorineural mechanism may be complex and consist of routine pure-tone audiometry, speech audiometry, and immittance measurements (Jerger, 1975; Feldman & Wilbur, 1976) in conjunction with any of a number of the following tonal tests: tone decay (Carhart, 1957; Olsen & Noffsinger, 1974), short increment sensitivity index (SISI) (Jerger, Shedd, & Harford, 1959), alternate binaural loudness balance (ABLB) (Jerger & Harford, 1960; Hood, 1969), Bekesy audiometry (Jerger, 1960), and brief tone audiometry (Wright, 1968; Sanders et al., 1971). It is when the findings of a battery of such tests are collated and analyzed that speech discrimination and immittance measurements may also be considered special tests.

It is the purpose of this chapter to review relevant literature that refers to speech audiometry in the evaluation of sensory and/or neural lesion sites. Specifically, the effect of intensity on speech discrimination performance, phonetically balanced maximum (PB max) speech discrimination scores in the auditory test battery, PB max in noise, and presbycusis will be examined.

THE EFFECT OF INTENSITY ON SPEECH DISCRIMINATION

Speech Discrimination and Recruitment

Following Fowler's (1936) report of a procedure for determining the presence of recruitment, Dix, Hallpike, and Hood (1948) unequivocally demonstrated the relationship of recruitment to end-organ pathology. Because of Dix, Hallpike, and Hood's indisputable findings, a test of recruitment became, in essence, a test for cochlear dysfunction. Unfortunately, the relationship of recruitment to speech discrimination was not clear at that time of the study and, therefore, it was the subject of a number of investigations. Davis's (1948) articulation score and articulation function concepts were often used to describe speech discrimination ability.

As early as 1942, Huizing maintained that recruitment, referred to at that time as regression, effected speech intelligibility. Subsequently, he stated in 1948 that recruitment limited the intensity range of speech, since the thresholds for hearing shifts in perceptive deafness while the upper limit of speech intelligibility remains about the same as that for normal-hearing people.

In 1949, Dix, Hallpike, and Hood reported that speech intelligibility of single words and of sentences reached a maximum and then declined as intensity increased in the soundfield in two patients with Meniere's disease, but improved with intensity in two patients with neurofibroma of the eighth nerve. They then stated that

> *. . . it can thus be said of Meniere's disease that while recruitment of loudness is the rule, recruitment of intelligibility, which might be expected, may be conspicuously absent. In fact, the opposite would appear to occur, namely, that as loudness increases intelligibility falls off*". (p. 534, italics from original)

Dix, Hallpike, and Hood felt that the speech discrimination curves offered differentiating features of end-organ lesions from nerve-fiber lesions. Interestingly, only three years earlier Walsh and Silverman (1946) reported that if a patient's articulation score increases proportionately with intensity, i.e., as with the normal ear, the patient had normal cochlear function.

Eby and Williams (1951) described the results for 32 patients with

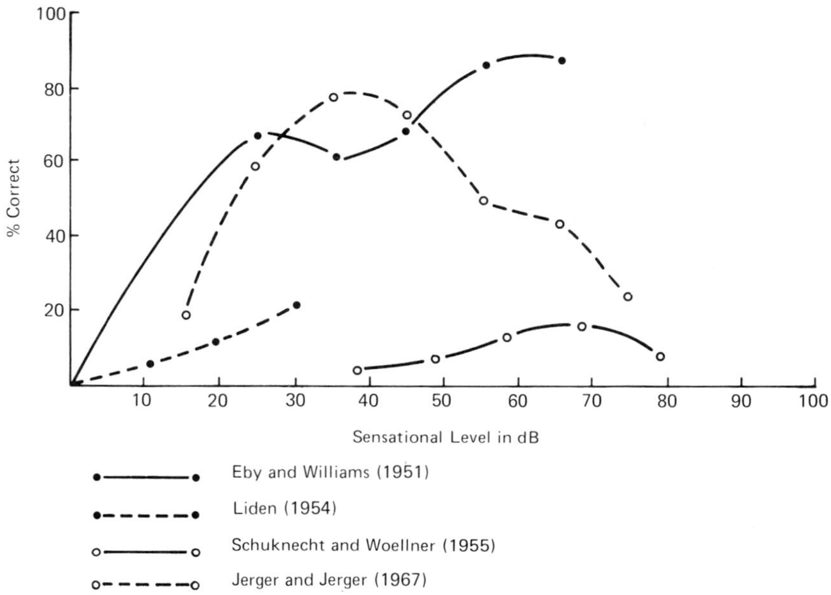

Fig. 7-1. Articulation curves for patients with eighth nerve pathology.

Meniere's disease and 16 patients with a variety of eighth nerve pathology. They found that in five of the six cases of nerve fiber pathology, speech discrimination improved with intensity using live-voice Harvard PB-50 word lists. An example of an articulation function from their report is given in Fig. 7-1, where a score of 90 percent correct was obtained at a 65 dB sensation level (SL). Conversely, in 15 of the 17 cases of cochlear pathology, they found that maximum speech discrimination was achieved at a low sensation level and that the score declined with increases in intensity. Figure 7-2 contains an adaptation of their illustration of a patient with Meniere's disease. The PB max for this subject was only 52 percent at 10 dB SL and 34 percent at 30 dB SL.

Eby and Williams (1951) also evaluated the dynamic range of speech reception threshold to most comfortable loudness (SRT and MCL) for speech and found that the average was 18.42 dB in the cases with Meniere's disease and 28.57 dB in the cases of nerve fiber damage. They concluded that ". . . discrimination deafness is an expression of the same fundamental disorder which is responsible for recruitment" because of the ten decibel difference. (p. 412)

An R-type (recruitment) articulation curve (Fig. 7-3) was postulated in 1952 by Huizing and Reyntjes as separate from either the C-type (conductive) or P-type (perceptive) first described by Davis (1948) and Silverman (1950). Huizing and Reyntjes reported that the recruiting ear exhibits

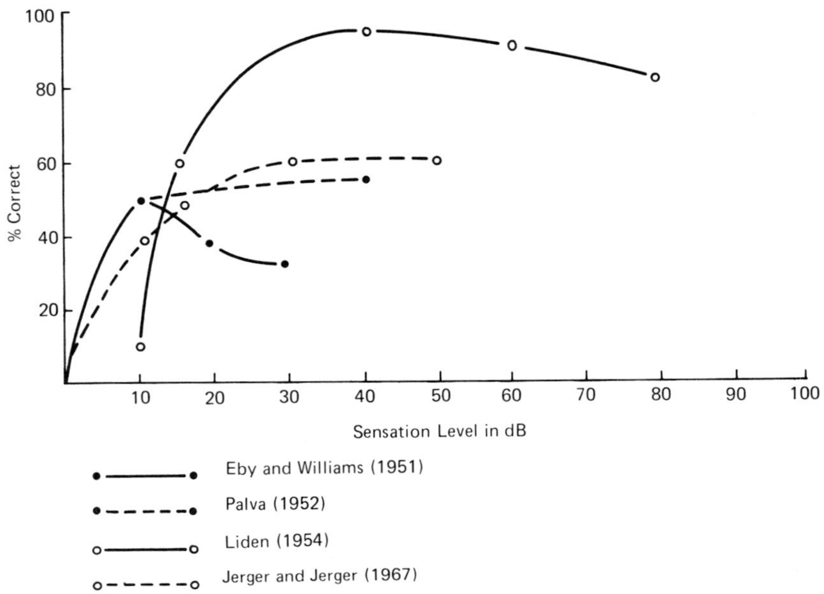

Fig. 7-2. Articulation curves for patients with cochlear pathology.

a rapid fall in articulation score once the optimum listening level is passed. They reported that it was the recruitment phenomenon that caused the steep rise in loudness perception but that the articulation score did not continue to improve since there is a "resonance-hump" as seen in the R-type curve.

In their classic study of the relationship of difference limen and loudness recruitment, Hirsch, Palva, and Goodman (1954) included a section concerned with speech discrimination and recruitment. Using lists consisting of 50 difficult words, scores were obtained either at a 40 dB SL, at a comfortable level if that was greater than 120 dB SPL, or at a level of 10 or 20 dB SL. They interpreted their findings in patients with Meniere's disease as being consistent with Huizing and Reyntjes's concept that a low discrimination score at a high intensity is a fairly reliable indication of recruitment, especially when the hearing loss for speech is more than 20 dB Hearing Level (HL).

Hedgecock (1955) reviewed the earlier work of Hubermann, who in 1890 had observed abrupt onset of loudness for speech in boilermakers; Gradeningo, who proposed an index vocalis for speech discrimination at relative distances in 1912; and Pohlman and Vermillion, who in 1933 had found that certain hearing losses yield rapid increases in loudness for speech that did not result in the expected increases in intelligibility. Hedgecock, as did Eby and Williams (1951), corresponded the relation-

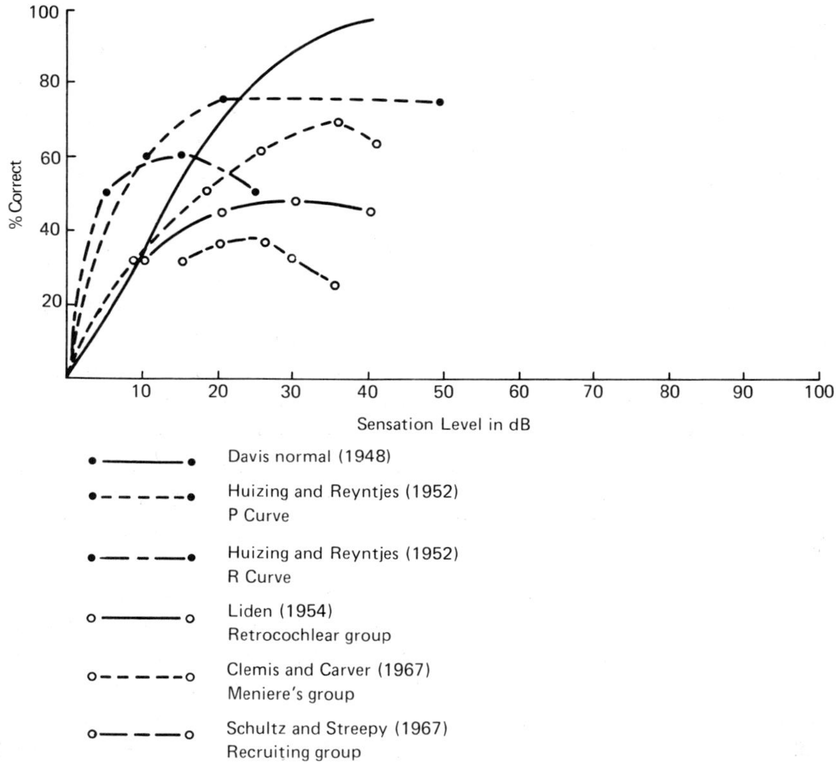

Fig. 7-3. Mean articulation curves for group data. Curves from Davis (1948) and Huizing and Reyntjes (1952) presented for comparison.

ship to the then current practice of relating the intensity span from speech threshold to the MCL. He stated that the range for normal ears was 50 dB while it was as little as 10–15 dB in ears with marked recruitment. The pure tone correlate of this procedure (Hood & Poole, 1965) was found to be successful and further research on the relationship of MCL to sensorineural pathology continues in currrent literature (Kamm et al., 1978).

Palva (1952), in an *Acta Octalaryngologica* supplement (101), reviewed a great number of cases with a variety of pathologies and reported the effect of loudness recruitment on discrimination using Finnish speech stimuli. For example, his case no. 78 (Fig. 7-2) had shown recruitment by ABLB in the right ear and no improvement in speech discrimination with an increase in intensity as well. Similar to Hirsh et al. (1954), he found that in cases where the hearing loss was severe, the speech intelligibility was poor at high intensities. Conversely, when the hearing loss was mild, he found no reduction in speech discrimination.

In 1954, Liden introduced his monograph concerned with Swedish speech audiometry. Chapter 8 of his study begins with a paradoxical statement, at least from today's terminological standpoint: "Walsh and Silvermen demonstrated that a high articulation score points to a good cochlear function, and as a result the discrimination loss has become a symptom of differential diagnostic interest. The greater the discrimination loss, the poorer the nerve function" (Liden, 1954, p. 88). The quote appears contradictory, but in fact, Liden's findings were clear. Liden reminded the reader that it must be remembered that a cochlear loss could be considered a nerve-type (p. 102). In the experimental section of the clinical evaluation of the speech discrimination test, he reported results of tests on 26 ears with either Meniere's disease or endolymphatic hydrops. The cases all had recruitment, but most formed a plateau at maximum for speech discrimination with only two of the cases showing Huizing and Reyntjes R-type (see Fig. 7-2). A speech audiogram from a Meniere's case used to illustrate his findings is found in Fig. 7-1. Note the plateau beginning at a 20 dB SL and that the maximum percent correct score did not improve better than 60 percent. The average discrimination score for the endolymphatic group was 62 percent.

Liden (1954) also reviewed seven cases with surgically confirmed tumors and eight with other pathologies such as tuberculous meningitus. The two groups differed dramatically in terms of the articulation curves. All seven tumor cases demonstrated poor speech discrimination, especially relative to the pure-tone findings, with the average PB max score being 20 percent. Liden presented a group of curves that summarized all the groups investigated and the average articulation curves for each relative to threshold. The curve for the retrocochlear group is presented here (Fig. 7-3) to highlight the graded differences among the normal from the cochlear (recruitment and Meniere's) from the retrocochlear group. With Liden's Swedish speech materials, findings were the first reported relating severely reduced speech discrimination scores to retrocochlear pathology.

Palva, in 1957, reviewed a number of then contemporary tests suggested for the presence of recruitment. He stated that, in his experience, poor speech intelligibility was in good agreement with loudness balance measures of recruitment in cases with moderate or severe losses. He recommended the use of speech audiometry and fixed frequency Bekesy audiometry as the two closely associated with detecting the presence of recruitment.

Schultz and Streepy (1967) reported 20 articulation gain functions for subjects with recruitment as identified by ABLB results. They used half W-22 lists at 5 dB random steps from 15–30 dB SL. Their findings revealed: (1) 13 of the subjects obtained maximum discrimination scores of less than 50 percent; and (2) the average curve showed no plateau, regressing immediately from its peak. Figure 7-3 illustrates the average maximum score at 25 dB SL as well as the decrease in percent correct with the increase in intensity. They argued that the presence of recruitment indicated the need for a complete articulation function since a standard sensation level could not be found for PB max.

The same year, Clemis and Carver (1967) reported that a reliable estimate of PB max could be determined if both a 32 and 40 dB SL were used. They tested ten patients with unilateral Meniere's using the NU Auditory Test no. 6 (Tillman & Carhart, 1965) and found a mean articulation function (Fig. 7-3) that was slowly rising and had the maximum score at 32 dB SL. They felt that the curve ". . . clearly demonstrates that persons afflicted with Meniere's disease find discriminating speech very difficult" (p. 616). They distinguished two trends for articulation functions within their groups: one where the scores improved to 40 dB SL, and another that "curled over" at 40 dB SL or less.

The appearance of reduced speech discrimination scores (i.e., speech discrimination loss) appeared to be consistent with recruitment and, therefore, cochlear pathology. Except for those provided by Liden (1954), the data from the preceding clinical and research seemed clear, but three papers published in the mid-fifties, including Liden's, suggested that retrocochlear pathology could also cause poor speech discrimination scores.

Liden (1954), in his treatise on Swedish speech audiometry, was probably the first to report that normal discrimination was not found in patients with acoustic tumors, although he did feel that speech could be used as a stimulus to identify recruitment. In an experiment evaluating the variations of symptoms in 14 patients with Meniere's disease and seven with endolymphatic hydrops, he found that the discrimination test provided guidance in the evaluation of cochlear function, since variation in scores, especially when assessing the articulation function, could be related to the presence or absence of recruitment. Conversely, the results for seven cases with acoustic tumors all indicated poor discrimination with an average PB max score of 20 percent (see Fig. 7-1), although tolerance was somewhat better than the group with Meniere's disease. When the groups were compared at a common threshold, the retrocochlear group (acoustic tumors and neuritis) showed poorer discrimination and function with intensity increases than did the Meniere's group.

Schuknecht and Woellner (1955) described two cases with pathological diagnoses of acoustic neuronoma. The first patient had a PB max score of 16 percent, using the Harvard PB-50s. The articulation function (Fig. 7-1) illustrated reduced score with increasing intensity. The second patient had a PB max score of 0 percent.

The antithesis of a positive relationship of poor speech discrimination and its relationship to recruitment was made by Walsh and Goodman

(1955). They found, as had Liden (1954) and Schuknecht and Woellner (1955), remarkably poor discrimination in relation to pure-tone thresholds for subjects with retrocochlear pathology. They reported a speech discrimination range of 0 percent to 58 percent for the recorded Harvard PB-50 lists at 40 dB or more SL for four patients of eighth nerve pathology (two with tumor). Both cases with eighth nerve tumor had scores of 0 percent. They did not find the presence of recruitment in these cases as tested by the ABLB. Walsh and Goodman concluded that ". . . the relation between threshold loss and discrimination for speech does not differentiate between auditory lesions of the cochlear and those central to the cochlea." (p. 8)

Speech Discrimination and Site of Lesion

The determination of presence of recruitment is useful in differentiating cochlear from retrocochlear pathology. There is no need, however, to dismiss the clinical utility of speech discrimination in the diagnosis of site of lesion because it does not necessarily relate to recruitment. Five reports have been published that have established a more sophisticated analysis of the speech articulation function.

Jerger and Jerger (1967) reported results of extensive psychoacoustic procedures on three subjects representative of normal hearing, cochlear disorder (Meniere's disease), and eighth nerve disorder (bilateral acoustic neuronoma). Included were experiments conducted concerning speech identification using conventional PB-50 word lists and synthetic sentences (Speaks & Jerger, 1965). The term *performance-intensity* (PI) function was coined and replaced the formerly used term articulation function. Later, Jerger (1970) would introduce the abbreviation PI–PB function to indicate performance-intensity functions for PB words. The PI functions for PB-50 words (Fig. 7-1) showed a nearly normal PB max and mild deterioration in scores at higher intensity levels for the cochlear subject, but an abrupt drop in scores for the eighth nerve subject (Fig. 7-2) after an 80 percent maximum as stimulus intensity increased. Jerger later referred to this abrupt drop as "rollover" (p. 683). The synthetic sentences were found to be a relatively easy task as to the two subjects representing pathology achieved 100 percent correct scores, and no rollover was observed. Jerger and Jerger summarized by describing the PI function for PB words as yielding a slightly reduced maximum and a slight rollover for a cochlear response pattern, and a moderately reduced maximum and a pronounced rollover for an eighth nerve pattern.

In a study to further explore the diagnostic significance of rollover, results of PI–PB functions obtained from 41 patients with cochlear pathology and 16 patients with retrocochlear pathology were reported by Jerger in 1971. The stimulus lists used were the Harvard PB-50 materials recorded for the study and were presented as half-lists in 10–20 dB steps until a shape of the function was clear. Group data results were consistent with Jerger and Jerger's earlier study (1967). All patients with eighth nerve disorders, regardless of degree of hearing loss, demonstrated pronounced rollover. On the other hand, the cochlear impaired subjects showed little or no rollover even when viewed in terms of degree of slope of hearing loss.

In relating the pure-tone average (PTA) to the PB max, Jerger and Jerger (1971) found the results fairly similar for both cochlear and neural groups and felt that the PB max was, therefore, of limited diagnostic value. However, on the basis of results from the brain stem patients, it was felt that a PB max below 70 percent is remarkable diagnostically if the PTA is less than 20 dB. In a further manipulation of the data, Jerger and Jerger developed three scores: (1) the PB min or the lowest PB score above PB max; (2) the rollover score, which was PB max-PB min; and (3) the rollover index calculated by PB max-PB min/PB max. The overlapping of scores, which was the major objection to the use of PB max, diminished by using the PB min since the rollover was more dramatic for the eighth nerve group. Jerger and Jerger then noted the lack of dependence on the PB max score for the eighth nerve group, whereas the cochlear group was dependent upon a high PB max score. The rollover index took this feature into account and there was no overlapping of scores, with the highest cochlear index being 0.40 and the lowest eighth nerve index being 0.45. Jerger and Jerger were also able to demonstrate that the rollover indices are an excellent tool, with the use of synthetic sentence identification in the presence of an ipsilateral competing message (Jerger et al., 1968).

In 1977, Jerger and Hayes made the use of the rollover concept less dependent upon the audiometric configuration by comparing the PI–PB function to a performance of intensity function for synthetic sentence identification or PI–SSI. Again, the PB-50 words were used as well as the SSI at a 0 dB message-to-competition ratio (Jerger et al., 1968). The PI functions for both lists were found to be in good agreement with flat audiometric patterns, PB functions were poorer than SSI when there was a downward slope toward the high frequencies, and the SSI function fell below the PB function when the contour rose upward from the low to high frequencies. It was explained that the function for the PB words was more dependent upon the high-frequency hearing, while the converse was true for the SSI. These trends were observed less with the eighth nerve-disordered patients, but the distinguishing feature again was the rollover phenomenon for this group.

Also in 1977, Dirks et al., were able to confirm the findings of Jerger and his colleagues. Using another set of PAL PB-50 recordings as stimuli to 89 cochlear impaired ears and eight ears with retrocochlear pathology, the resultant PB max scores showed great overlap. The rollover, however, somewhat differentiated the groups and the rollover index ratio of 0.45 successfully divided the groups. The authors were adament in recommending that individual clinics should establish their own distinguishing rollover ratios for the specific recordings used. They also suggested smaller than 10-dB steps for the PB max search, since the rollover index may be confounded by a score other than an accurate one.

Another interesting publication merits review here. McCandless and Schumacher (1979) reported that facial paralysis patients with absent acoustic reflexes demonstrated PI–PB rollover for CID W-22 words at high-intensity levels. They commented that this phenomenon should be expected to be observed, therefore, in seventh as well as eighth nerve pathologic conditions.

PB Max and the Audiologic Test Battery

The refinement of a test procedure is an important aspect of any science and further improves its value in light of a group of tests which are used as an armamentarium. Speech discrimination, or more specifically PB max, has long been viewed as a basic portion of the test battery. In most instances, however, materials developed in 1948 (Egan) and 1954 (Hirsh, et al.) are still administered only at a specific level (Martin & Forbis, 1978). Due to this approach, the scores for these single level tests have been reported in connection with the audiologic evaluation of patients with either sensory and peripheral neural pathologies. These reports illustrate the need for a complete assessment.

Relative to the test battery approach, Jerger (1960) discussed the response patterns for sites of lesions in the auditory system. He established general principles relating to symtomatology of the lesions: (1) manifestations become more subtle as they progress centrally; and (2) complex auditory stimuli such as speech encounter a "bottleneck" in the eighth nerve and lower brain stem. He presented representative cases, including labyrinthine hydrops and acoustic neuronoma. Hearing loss, mildly abnormal adaptation on Bekesy audiometry (Type II), positive SISI scores, recruitment, and reduced speech discrimination scores were described as characteristic of diseases affecting the cochlea. He pointed out that it was the pathologic state of the sensory mechanism in labyrinthine hydrops that was the cause for the poor speech discrimination, and also offered that discrimination ability was rather high (50 percent) considering that state. He also presented findings for a patient with an acoustic neuronoma. This patient had essentially normal hearing sensitivity, severely abnormal adaptation (Bekesy Type III), no recruitment, and very poor speech discrimination (26 percent), especially in light of the pure-tone thresholds. Here at the eighth nerve level, Jerger reiterated the effect of the bottleneck principle; that is, the severe reduction in transmission of speech stimuli while faint pure-tones can still be heard.

In 1962, Jerger recommended a three-test battery approach consisting of SISI, Bekesy audiometry, and ABLB. Relative to a speech protocol, it is worthwile to read Appendix B, for it is there that the reader learns that speech discrimination was an integral part of the assessment and that the scores were determined at both 30 dB and 50 dB above the 1000 Hz threshold. Although results of this procedure are not discussed, it is apparent that it was an essential test.

Problems with results obtained using an auditory evaluation of patients with eighth nerve lesions are extensive. An early report was presented by Brand and Rosenburg (1963). In 22 patients with either surgically confirmed (20 patients) or suspected (two patients) cerebellopontine angle tumors, they found that auditory results were not always consistent with pathology. They were able to divide their patients into four groups. The first group had total hearing loss, consequently prohibiting auditory assessment. The second group of patients evidenced the expected findings, e.g., 42 dB SRT and 0 percent PB max. On the other hand, the third group of four patients gave misleading findings, such as 90 percent speech discrimination score and positive SISI. Other PB max scores ranged from 64–86 percent in the third group. The last group had positive auditory signs and negative calories, x-rays, and tomography. Because of the wide range of findings, Brand and Rosenberg stressed the need for diagnostic studies in audiology, otology, radiology, and neurology.

Johnson presented a series of reports in 1965, 1968, 1969, and 1973 concerned with considerable auditory data collected from patients with acoustic neuronomas. In his latest report, he included information obtained from Meniere's patients and found that there was overlap in speech discrimination scores for 92 patients with Meniere's disease and for 321 patients with acoustic tumors (See Table 7-1). Fifty-five percent of the tumor patients, however, had scores of 30 percent or below, while less than 7 percent of the Meniere's patients had findings in that range. Johnson interpreted the differences in scores as being clinically significant; however, he concluded that a battery of tests, rather than an individual one, is useful for differential diagnosis.

A report on auditory test findings in patients with acoustic neuronomas was given by Shapiro and Nanuton (1967), which contained the message that results should be treated with extreme caution. Speech discrimination scores of 40 dB SL were reported for the first group, which had total hearing loss prohibiting auditory assessment. The second group of

Table 7-1
Speech Discrimination Scores in Patients with Retrocochlear Pathology

Investigation	# of Patients	Low	Medium	High
Shapiro & Naunton (1967)	9	3 (0–30%)	3 (32–80%)	3 (82–100%)
Tillman (1969)	23	13 (0–26%)		10 (28–100%)
Sanders et al. (1974)	27	35% (0–20%)	40% (22%–80%)	25% (82%–100%)
Johnson (1973)	321	176 (0–30%)	59 (32–60%)	86 (62%–100%)
Liden & Korsan-Bengsten (1973)	DNR	64% of patients	—	25% of patients
Thomsen & Terkeldsen (1975)	24 of 125	10 (0–20%)	10 (20–80%)	3 (80–100%)
Clemis & Mastricola (1976)	121	50% (0–28%)	—	50%(30–100%)

patients evidenced the expected findings, e.g., 42 dB SRT and 0 percent PB max. Nine of the 14 patients were administered hearing tests (Table 7-1). Three patients responded in each of the following percent correct ranges: 0–30 percent, 32–80 percent, and 82–100 percent. They too emphasized the need for a complete battery of audiologic, radiologic, vestibular, and laboratory tests, since multiple auditory tests results failed to reveal a consistent pattern.

Tillman (1969) described audiologic test findings for two groups of 23 patients each. One group represented acoustic tumors and the other, labyrinthine hydrops. He considered five individual tests, including one for speech discrimination. He operationally defined 26 percent correct and below scores as a probable indication of retrocochlear lesion, while scores above 26 percent would suggest a cochlear lesion. On the basis of that criterion, 57 percent of the tumor group would have been appropriately identified but, unfortunately, 17 percent of the hydrops would have been mistakely established (See Table 7-1). The test battery as a whole, Tillman concluded, probably would detect a vast majority of the peripheral retrocochlear lesions, since 78 percent of the patients in his study with tumors had results on two or more tests that suggested retrocochlear disorder, while none had such results in the hydrops group.

One hundred and twenty-seven patients were the subjects for a review of results from eight tests of audiologic evaluation by Sanders, Josey, and Glasscock (1974). Twenty-seven of the subjects had medical evidence of acoustic tumor, and 26 of these had surgical confirmation. The other 100 patients had revealed diagnosis of cochlear pathology. They also found an inverse relationship between the scores for the cochlear and the neural groups (Table 7-1). Thirty-five percent of the neural group had scores in the 0–20 percent range, while only 6 percent of the cochlear group did. On the other hand, 59 percent of the cochlear group had scores between 82 and 100 percent, while 25 percent of the neural group had scores in that range. Obviously, there was an overlap of group scores although a tendency for very poor scores was more typical in the neural group. Sanders et al. agreed with previous reports by finding that the prediction of site of lesion was considerably improved by attention to a battery of tests rather than to a single test (Brand & Rosenburg, 1963).

Liden and Korsan-Bengsten (1973) also concluded that a battery approach was superior and that while a low speech discrimination score indicated that a lesion may be retrocochlear, a high score does not exclude it. They reported that 64 percent of their cases had poor discrimination, but that 25 percent had good discrimination (Table 7-1).

A 1975 review of the audiologic findings in 24 of 125 cases of acoustic neuromas revealed a wide range of speech discrimination scores by Thomsen and Terkildesen (Table 7-1). Nevertheless, they stated that the speech test was very valuable, especially with patients who demonstrated moderate hearing losses, since the degree of loss alone did not predict the problem. Therefore, they concluded that a reduction in the number of active nerve fibers was suspected.

In 1976, both Sheehy and Inzer and Clemis and Mastricola reported findings on large samples of patients with eighth nerve tumor. Sheehy and Inzer selected 24 cases where audiologic findings were not accurate in predicting neural pathology. They, like others, found a wide range of scores with 18 of the 24 exhibiting scores of 80 percent or better. They strongly recommended the use of the acoustic reflex test since it was the single most positive procedure. Clemis and Mastricola's findings were similar to previous reports regarding a wide range of speech discrimination scores (Table 7-1). They found half of the patients to have scores less than 30 percent and a third to have results above 70 percent. They recommended that the audiologic battery be considered only as a part of a complete otoneurological evaluation.

It is certain that PB max cannot be determined for a patient whose score is less than 90 percent correct in a routine clinical setting relative to the SRT or PTA. It appears that the best protocol is the PI–PB using Harvard PB-50 materials, and that from this, the PB max and the diagnostic sensitivity of the rollover ratio can be used. There is certainly call for such a procedure in light of reports such as that made by Katinsky et al. (1972), where only two of eight patients with surgically confirmed tumors had PB max scores below 76 percent.

THE EFFECT OF NOISE ON SPEECH DISCRIMINATION

Noise has long been known to effect performance in speech discrimination. The differentiation of various sites of lesion by ipsilateral noise during speech audiometry might appear useful, however, this has not yet been documented.

On the bases of his investigation of speech discrimination with a signal-to-noise (S/N) ratio of +10 dB, Palva (1955) reported that there was no relationship between speech scores and recruitment. He even advised against further study of the use of ipsilateral noise as a tool for differentiating sensorineural groups.

Apparently, the configuration of a sensorineural hearing loss may be the determining factor for reduced performance in noise. Ross et al. (1965) reported that subjects with high-frequency hearing loss demonstrated less relative effect of a 2.5 db SPL S/N ratio upon their W-22 discrimination scores than did those with flatter losses.

Carhart and Tillman (1970), Keith and Talis (1972), and Shapiro et al. (1972) all found that either a competing speech signal or various S/N ratios of continuous or modulated noise produced poorer results in speech discrimination for subjects with sensorineural pathology than for normal-hearing subjects.

Katinsky et al. (1972) pointed out severely reduced scores for patients with eighth nerve tumores when the S/N ratio approached 0 dB. Olsen et al. (1975) subsequently urged considerable caution interpreting the observations of Katinsky et al. since Olsen et al. found that other auditory involvements can produce poor speech discrimination ability in white noise. They also stated that a difference score of more than 40 percent obtained by subtracting a noise score from a quiet score might separate sensorineural pathology from normals.

SPEECH DISCRIMINATION AND PRESBYCUSIS

It is now well known that aging may alter the auditory system in numerous ways. Schuknecht (1974) described four major types of presbycusis: sensory, neural, cochlear conductive, and metabolic, all of which may manifest themselves differently during audiologic assessment. Because of this, a wide range of opinions were published relative to speech discrimination and aging.

The germinal paper in this area is that by Gaeth (1948). He reported inordinately poor speech discrimination in relation to pure-tone findings for a group of older subjects. He referred to this phenomenon as phonemic regression. It is now thought to be associated with neural presbycusis (Schuknecht, 1974).

Reduced speech discrimination ability with presbycusis has been further documented. Speech discrimination loss was found to be very severe for 185 subjects ranging from age 60 to 90 irrespective of degree of hearing loss, according to Pestolozza and Shore (1955). Goetzinger et al. (1961) reported that discrimination measured either by the Harvard PB-50 or CID W-22 lists became significantly poorer with age. In 1969, it was revealed by Punch and McConnell that older people with only a minimal hearing loss have poor speech understanding.

Gang (1976) reported positive rollover ratios for six of 32 older subjects and concluded that rollover is contraindicated as a diagnostic tool since results were not consistent. Later, Jerger and Jerger (1976) and Dirks et al. (1977) correctly argued that rollover for some of the elderly subjects is expected, since they would have eighth nerve pathology such as that in neural presbycusis (Schuknecht, 1974).

SUMMARY

It is apparent that sensory and/or periphreral neural lesion sites may effect speech discrimination ability. Coles (1972) recently stated that speech audiometry was highly reliable as an indicator of neural pathology and that it was a very valuable diagnostic tool. Its sensitivity is considerably increased by the use of the rollover index developed by Jerger and Jerger (1971), but the caution of Dirks et al. (1977) must be reiterated: individual facilities should establish their own distinguishing rollover ratios. This is indeed important since, according to Martin and Pennington (1971) and Martin and Forbis (1978), it appears that over 70 percent of audiologists use the CID W-2 lists (Hirsh et al., 1952) rather than the PAL PB-50 lists (Egan, 1948) used in the development and evaluation of rollover. Martin and Forbis (1978) also suggested that less than 5 percent of audiologists develop PI–PB functions, but 68 percent test at a specific sensation level. This is inconsistent with a complete evaluation of the auditory system.

Audiologists must be made aware of the applicability of the speech discrimination test material used and the dependency of scores on intensity. A PI–PB format should be used in differential diagnosis with the aid of a standard form such as that recommended by the British Society of Audiology (1975). Very poor PB max scores should continue to be thought of as a symptom of neural pathology, while good scores should not preclude further eveluation of eighth nerve function and appearance. Audiologic data can remain only a part of a complete evaluation.

REFERENCES

Brand, S., & Rosenburg, P. E. Problems in auditory evaluation for neurosurgical diagnosis. *Journal of Speech and Hearing Disorders,* 1963, *28,* 355–361.

British Society of Audiology Standard forms for results of audiometry. *British Journal of Audiology,* 1975, *9,* insert between 76 and 77.

Carhart, R. Clinical determination of abnormal adaptation. *Archives of Otolaryngology,* 1957 *65,* 32–33.

Carhart, R. Problems in the measurement of speech discrimination. *Archives of Otolaryngology,* 1965 *82,* 253–260.

Carhart, R., & Tillman, T. W. Interaction of competing speech signals with hearing losses. *Archives of Otolaryngology,* 1970, *91,* 273–279.

Clemis, J. D., & Carver, W. F. Discrimination scores for speech in Meniere's disease. *Archives of Otolaryngology,* 1967, *86,* 614–618.

Clemis, J. D., & Mastricola, P. G. Special audiometric test battery in 121 proved acoustic tumors. *Archives of Otolaryngology,* 1976, *102,* 654–656.

Davis, H. The articulation area and the social adequacy index for hearing. *Laryngoscope,* 1948, *58,* 761–778.

Dirks, D. D., Kamm, C., Bower, D., & Betsworth, A. Use of performance–intensity functions for diagnosis. *Journal of Speech and Hearing Disorders,* 1977, *42,* 408–415.

Dix, M. R., Hallpike, C. S., & Hood, J. D. Observations upon the loudness recruitment phenomenon, with special reference to the differential diagnosis of disorders of the internal ear and VIIIth nerve. *Journal of Laryngology and Otology*, 1948, *62*, 671–686.

Dix, M. R., Hallpike, C. S., & Hood, J. D. "Nerve" deafness: its clinical criteria, old and new. *Proceedings of the Royal Society of Medicine,* 1949, *42,* 527–536.

Eby, L. G., & Williams, H. L. Recruitment of loudness in the differential diagnosis of end-organ and nerve fibre deafness. *Laryngoscope,* 1951, *61,* 400–414.

Feldman, A. S., & Wilbur, L. A. (Eds.). *Acoustic impedance and admittance–the measurement of middle ear function.* Baltimore: Williams & Wilkins, 1976.

Fowler, E. P. A method for the early detection of otosclerosis. *Archives of Otolaryngology,* 1936, *24,* 731–741.

Gaeth, J. H. A study of phonemic regression associated with hearing loss. Unpublished doctoral dissertation, Northwestern University, 1948.

Gang, R. P. The effects of age on the diagnostic utility of the rollover phenomenon. *Journal of Speech and Hearing Disorders,* 1976,

Hedgecock, L. D. The measurement of auditory recruitment. *Archives of Otolaryngology,* 1955, *61,* 515–527.

Hirsh, I. J., Davis, H., Silverman, S. R., Reynolds, E., et al. Development of materials for speech audiometry. *Journal of Speech and Hearing Disorders,* 1952, *17,* 321–337.

Hirsh, I. J., Palva, T., & Goodman, A. Difference limen and recruitment. *Archives of Otolaryngology,* 1954, *60,* 525–540.

Hood, J. D. Basic audiological requirements in neuro-otology. *Journal of Laryngology,* 1969, *83,* 695–711.

Hood, J. D., & Poole, J. P. Tolerable limit of loudness: its clinical and physiological significance. *Journal of the Acoustical Society of America,* 1966, *40,* 47–53.

Huizing, H. C. The symptom of recruitment and speech intelligibility. *ACTA Otolaryngology,* 348, *36,* 346–355.

Huizing, H. C., & Reyntjes, J. A. Recruitment and speech discrimination loss. *Laryngoscope,* 1952, *62,* 521–527.

Jerger, J. Audiological manifestations of lesions in the auditory nervous system. *Laryngoscope,* 1960a, *70,* 417–425.

Jerger, J. Bekesy audiometry in the analysis of auditory disorders. *Journal of Speech and Hearing Research,* 1960b, *3,* 257–287.

Jerger, J. (Ed.). *Handbook of clinical impedance audiometry.* New York: American Electromedics Corp., 1975.

Jerger, J. Hearing tests in otologic diagnosis. *ASHA,* 1962, *4,* 139–145.

Jerger, J. F., & Harford, E. R. The alternate and simultaneous balancing of pure tones. *Journal of Speech and Hearing Research,* 1960, *3,* 15–30.

Jerger, J., Harford, E., Clemis, J., & Alford, B. The acoustic reflex in eighth nerve disorders. *Archives of Otolaryngology,* 1974, *99,* 409–413.

Jerger, J., & Hayes, D. Diagnostic speech audiometry. *Archives of Otolaryngology,* 1977, *103,* 216–222.

Jerger, J., & Jerger, S. Psychoacoustic comparison of cochlear and VIIIth nerve disorders. *Journal of Speech and Hearing Research,* 1967, *10,* 659–688.

Jerger, J., & Jerger, S. Diagnostic significance of PB word functions. *Archives of Otolaryngology,* 1971, *93,* 573–580.

Jerger, J., Shedd, J., & Harford, E. On the detection of extremely small changes in sound intensity. *Archives of Otolaryngology,* 1959, *69,* 200–211.

Jerger, J., Speaks, C., & Trammell, J. A new approach to speech audiometry. *Journal of Speech and Hearing Disorders,* 1968, *33,* 318–328.

Johnson, E. W. Auditory test results in 110 surgically confirmed retrocochlear lesions. *Journal of Speech and Hearing Disorders,* 1965, *30,* 307–317.

Johnson, E. W. Auditory findings in 200 cases of acoustic neuromas. *Archives of Otolaryngology,* 1968, *88,* 598–603.

Johnson, E. W. Audiologic diagnosis of acoustic neuromas. *Archives of Otolaryngology,* 1969, *89,* 280–284.

Johnson, E. W. Clinical application of special hearing tests. *Archives of Otolaryngology,* 1973, *97,* 92–95.

Kamm, C., Dirks, D. O., & Mickey, M. R. Effect of sensorineural hearing loss on loudness discomfort level and most comfortable loudness judgements. *Journal of Speech and Hearing Research,* 1978, *21,* 668–681.

Katinsky, S., Lovinic, J., & Buchheit, W. Cochlear findings in VIIIth nerve tumors. *Audiology,* 1972, *11,* 213–217.

Liden, G. Speech audiometry. *Acta Oto-Laryngologica,* (Suppl. 114), 1954.

Liden, G., & Korsan-Bengtsen, M. Audiometric manifestations of retrocochlear lesions. *Scandinavian Audiology,* 1973, *2,* 29–40.

Martin, F. N., & Forbis, N. K. The present status of audiometric practice: a follow-up study. *ASHA,* 1978, *20,* 531–541.

Martin, F. N., & Pennington, C. D. Current trends in audiometric practices. *ASHA,* 1972, *14,* 671–677.

McCandless, G. A., & Schumacher, M. H. Auditory dysfunction with facial paralysis. *Archives of Otolaryngology,* 1979, *105,* 271–274.

Olsen, W. O., & Noffsinger, D. Comparison of one new and three old tests of auditory adaptation. *Archives of Otolaryngology,* 1974, *99,* 94–99.

Olsen, W. O., Noffsinger, D., & Kurdziel, S. Speech discrimination in quiet and in white noise by patients with peripheral and central lesions. *Acta Otolaryngologica,* 1975, *80,* 375–382.

Palva, T. Finnish speech audiometry. *Acta Otolaryngologica,* (Suppl. 101), 1952.

Palva, T. Studies of hearing for pure tones and speech in noise. *Acta Otolaryngologica,* 1955, *45,* 231–243.

Palva, T. Recruitment testing. *Arch Otolaryngologica,* 1957, *66,* 93–98.

Ross, M., Huntington, D. A., Newby, H. A., & Dixon, R. F. Speech discrimination of hearing impaired individuals in noise. *Journal of Auditory Research,* 1965, *5,* 47–72.

Sanders, J. W., Josey, A. F., & Glasscock, M. E. Audiologic evaluation in cochlear and eighth nerve disorders. *Archives of Otolaryngology,* 1974, *100,* 283–289.

Sanders, J. W., Kemker, F. J., & Josey, A. F. Brief tone audiometry in patients with VIIIth nerve tumor. *Journal of Speech and Hearing Research,* 1971, *14,* 172–178.

Schultz, M. C., & Streepy, C. S. The speech discrimination function in loudness recruiting ears. *Laryngoscope,* 1967, *77,* 2114–2127.

Schuknecht, H. *Pathology of the ear.* Cambridge: Harvard University Press, 1974.

Schuknecht, H. F., & Woellner, R. C. An experimental and clinical study of deafness from lesions of the cochlear nerve. *Journal of Laryngology and Otology,* 1955, *69,* 75–97.

Shambaugh, G. E., Jr. *Surgery of the ear.* Philadelphia, W. B. Saunders Co., 1967.

Shapiro, I., & Naunton, R. F. Audiologic evaluation of acoustic neuromas. *Journal of Speech and Hearing Disorders,* 1967, *32,* 29–35.

Shapiro, M. T., Melnick, W., & Ver Meulen, V. Effects of modulated noise on speech intelligibility of people with sensorineural hearing loss. *Annals of Otology, Rhinology, and Laryngology,* 1972, *81,* 241–248.

Sheehy, J. L., & Inzer, B. E. Acoustic reflex test in neuro-otologic diagnosis. *Archives of Otolaryngology,* 1976, *102,* 647–653.

Silverman, S. R. Use of speech tests for evaluation of clinical procedures. *Archives of Otolaryngology,* 1950, *51,* 786–797.

Speaks, C., & Jerger, J. Method for measurement of speech identification. *Journal of Speech and Hearing Research,* 1965, *8* 185–194.

Thomsen, J., & Terkildsen, K. Audiological findings in 125 cases of acoustic neuromas. *Acta Otolaryngologic,* 1975, *80,* 353–361.

Tillman, T. W. Special hearing tests in otoneurologic diagnosis. *Archives of Otolaryngology,* 1969, *89,* 51—56.

Tillman, T., & Carhart, R. An expanded test for speech discrimination utilizing CNC monosyllabic words. Northwestern University Auditory Test no. 6. Technical Report No. SAM-TR-66-55, USAF School of Aerospace Medicine, Brooks Air Force Base, Texas, 1966.

Walsh, T. E., & Silverman, S. R. Diagnosis and evaluation of fenestration. *Laryngoscope,* 1946, *56,* 536–555.

Wright, H. N. Clinical measurement of temporal auditory summation. *Journal of Speech and Hearing Research,* 1968, *11,* 109–127.

Raymond M. Hurley, Ph.D.

8

Speech Protocols in the Central Auditory Nervous System Evaluation

The pioneering work of Bocca and his associates (1954 and 1955) ushered in a new era in auditory assessment and simultaniously squelched the beliefs that lesions of the temporal lobe did not produce auditory symptoms, and/or auditory tests were insensitive to dysfunction at that level due to the bilateral representation of the ears at each temporal lobe. Bocca's use of distorted speech stimuli with cases of temporal lobe pathology documented for the first time the now expected contralateral ear effect, i.e., lesions of the primary auditory cortex are reflected in the performance of the ear contralateral to the disordered hemisphere. The Bocca publications resulted in a sequence of reports that dealt with central auditory nervous system (CANS) evaluation. Using CID W-22 and Rush Hughes materials, Goldstein, Goodman, and Hall (1956) substantiated the contralateral ear effect with four hemispherectomy patients. Matzker (1959) developed a binaural fusion procedure and provided preliminary data on its effectiveness in identifying lesions of the brainstem. Jerger, in a series of early reports (Jerger, 1960a; Jerger, 1960b; Jerger, 1964) summarized results of a test battery using cases with various CANS pathologies, and Katz (1962) shared preliminary data generated by his dichotic format Staggered Spondaic Word (SSW) test.

Since these initial reports, interest in CANS evaluation has had a slow, but steady, growth. Presently, the interest level is of such magnitude that yet another subspeciality of audiology, "neuroaudiology," has emerged. From the outset, central to the majority of CANS evaluation procedures is the use of speech stimuli. Speech forms have been compressed, expanded, filtered, and interrupted. These stimuli have been presented at varying sensation levels (SL) under monaural, dichotic, and competing message conditions.

The intent of this chapter is to review briefly the topographic CANS anatomy and consider clinically relevant evaluation models. Further, past and present CANS test protocols are reviewed and their ultimate success with clinical cases examined.

CANS ANATOMY

As the basic anatomy and physiology of the CANS was given an in-depth treatment in Chapter 3, these topics will receive but a brief review here in order to orient the reader toward an anatomically based CANS evaluation model. The anatomical boundaries of the CANS would appear to vary somewhat, contingent upon who is doing the defining. For this chapter, the CANS is defined as beginning at the postsynaptic side of the cochlear nucleus (CN) at the level of the medulla and pons through the primary auditory cortex and the intrahemispheric association areas in the cerebrum and the interhemispheric pathways connecting the two hemispheres.

As illustrated in Fig. 8-1, all afferent activity transmitted by the cochlear nerve terminates on the cochlear nucleus (CN) with the predominate projection to the ventral CN. There are no documented afferent projections that bypass the CN and synapse at a higher level. Nuclei of the CN are projected to both ipsilateral and contralateral superior olivary complex (SOC) and to both the ipsilateral lateral lemniscus (LL). The largest projections are contralateral to the SOC and LL by the stria of Monakow, to the LL by the stria of Held, and to the trapezoid body. Thus, the SOC is the first level within the CANS where bilateral interaction may occur. Both ipsilateral and contralateral projections constitute the LL, which in turn form the major fiber projection to the ipsilateral inferior colliculus (IC). There are, however, some fibers that synapse on the dorsal LL and either project ipsilaterally within the LL to the IC or cross the midline within the commissure of Probst and project to the contralateral IC. These latter fibers constitute the second level within the CANS where bilateral interaction may occur. All afferent flow synapses on the IC. The ipsilateral afferent projections from the IC constitute the brachium (Peduncle) of the IC and synapse at the level of the thalamus on the medial geniculate bodies (MGB), while a contralateral neural track, the commissure of the IC, provides projections to the contralateral MGB. Again, this is another level within the CANS where bilateral interaction may occur.

The auditory radiations (ARs) connect the MGB to the primary auditory cortex. Specifically, the ARs project first laterally through the internal capsule and then inferiorly to the transverse gyrus of Heschl on the

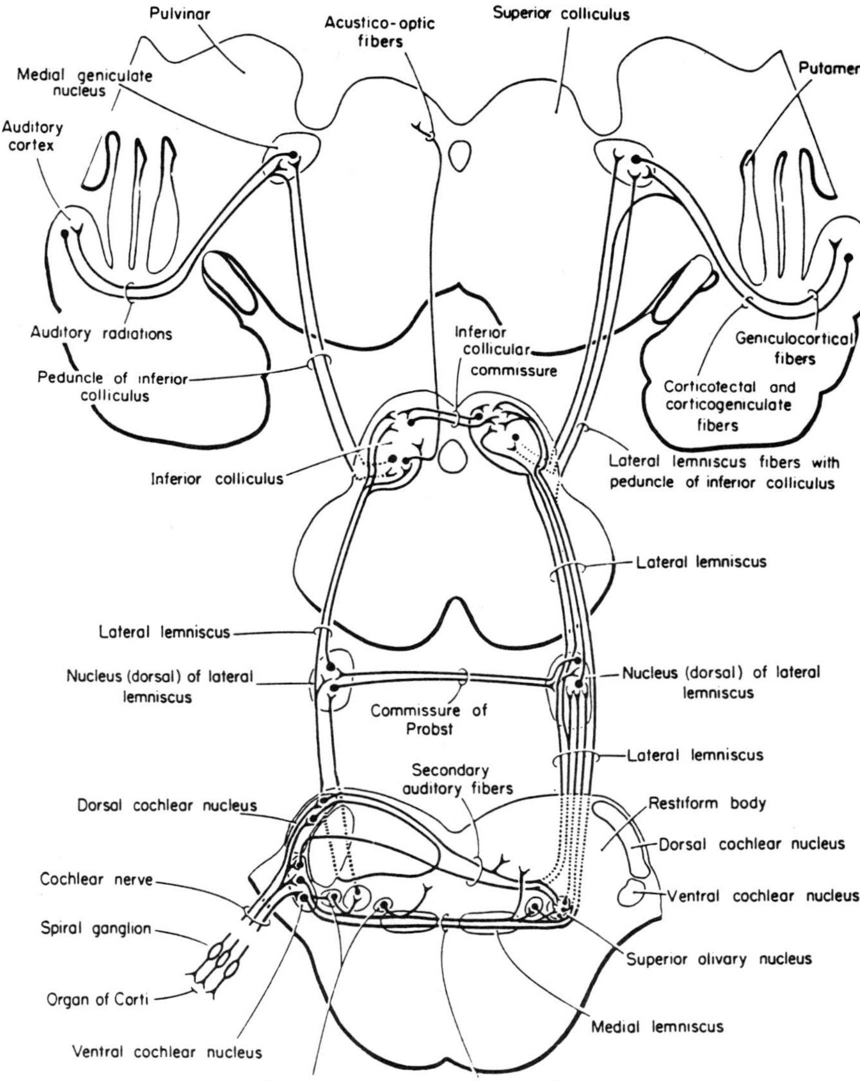

Fig. 8-1. Central auditory nervous system (CANS) from the cochlear nerve to the primary auditory cortex. [From Crosby, E.C., Humphrey, T., & Lauer, W. W. *Correlative anatomy of the nervous system*. New York: Macmillan, 1962. With permission.]

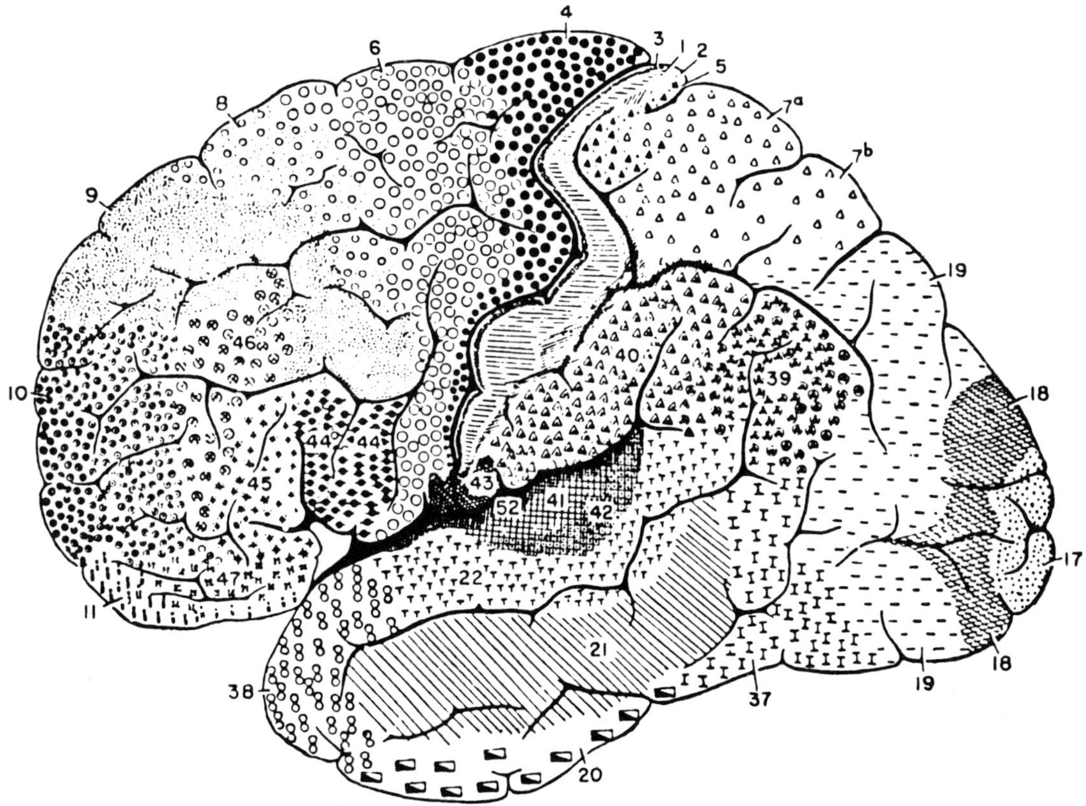

Fig. 8-2. Brodmann's cytoarchitectural fields on the lateral surface of the human cortex. Areas 41 and 42 represent the primary auditory cortex, while areas 22 and 52 represent the auditory association areas. [From Crosby, E. C., Humphrey, T., & Lauer, W. W. *Correlative anatomy of the nervous system*. New York: Macmillan, 1962. With permission.]

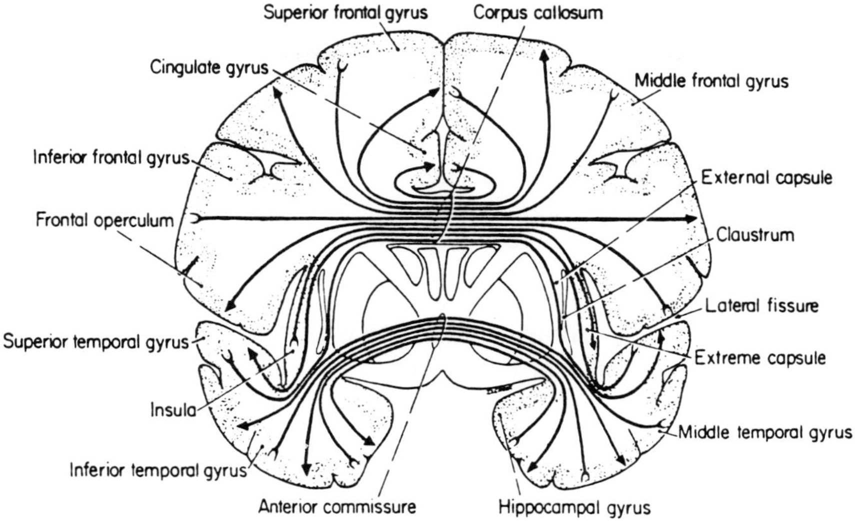

Fig. 8-3. Interhemispheric pathways of the corpus callosum and anterior commissure. [From Crosby, E. C., Humphrey, T., & Lauer, E. W., *Correlative anatomy of the nervous system*. New York: Macmillan, 1962. With permission.]

superior temporal lobe, which lies deep with the lateral fissure (Fissure of Sylvius) and is represented by area 41 on Fig. 8-2. Proximal, but inferior to area 41, is a secondary auditory association area, area 42, which receives a few projections from the MGB. The main auditory association region, area 22, borders the primary auditory cortex and has rich intrahemispheric connections with areas 41 and 42. Area 22, in turn, is connected by association fibers to the frontal lobe, area 44, to the occipitotemporal and to the parieto-angular gyrus, area 39. In brief, Heschl's gyrus has many and varied intrahemispheric association pathway.

Interhemisphere connection, illustrated in Fig. 8-3, is by two sets of commisural fibers. The rostral aspect of the middle and inferior temporal gyri of each hemisphere is linked through the anterior commissure fibers, while the remaining segments of the inferior and middle temporal gyri and the superior temporal gyrus (Heschl's gyrus) are connected through the corpus callosum.

Hemisphere Asymmetry

There is ever increasing anatomical, physiological, and behavioral evidence supporting the concept of functional hemispheric asymmetry for the processing of linguistic and nonlinguistic auditory stimuli. Geschwind and Levistsky (1968), studying 100 adult brains, investigated morphological hemisphere asymmetry in the temporal planun, an area posterior to Heschl's gyrus and extending onto the lateral surface of the temporal lobe. Sixty-five percent of the brains studied had a larger temporal planum in the left hemisphere while 11 percent had a larger temporal planun in the right hemisphere. Subsequently, Wada, Clarke, and Hamm (1975) examined 100 adult and 100 infant brains and found asymmetry in favor of the left hemisphere in 90 percent of the 200 brains studied. Recently, Galaburda, Sanides, and Geschwind (1978) determined through detailed study of four brains that left temporal planun asymmetry is not reflective of a more generalized morphological asymmetry between the hemisphere, but is specific to the planun areas. Collectively, these studies indicate the left temporal planun to be larger than or equal in size to the right temporal planum in 89–90 percent of the brains studied. This percentage is consistent with the estimate that 96 percent of the adult population is left brained for speech and language regardless of handedness.

The morphological asymmetry ties neatly with the evidence of functional asymmetry for various categories of auditory stimuli. Speech stimuli such as consonant-vowels and monosyllables produce a right ear advantage under dichotic presentation. Nonspeech auditory stimuli such as noise, melodies, and tonal pitches have generated a left ear superiority with dichotic presentation. The stimulus-related ear asymmetry results from the CANS being a contralaterally dominant system, as the contralateral projections outnumber the ipsilateral. Further, neuronal conduction time is short through the contralateral CANS network. Thus, the functional ear asymmetry is the product of the contralaterally potent CANS and hemisphere specialization for processing different catagories of auditory signals. In summary, the CANS can be characterized by several general statements: (1) The system is orderly in topographic anatomy with neural units at each level capable of coding and recoding the basic auditory parameters; (2) There are four levels within the system where bilateral interaction can occur; (3) The system is contralaterally dominated; (4) There is binaural representation at each temporal lobe; (5) There appears to be hemisphere specialization for speech and nonspeech auditory stimuli.

EVALUATION MODELS

A logical progression in the study of CANS evaluation includes a transition from anatomical data to clinical test data. An evaluation model that allows clinically determined data to be referred back to a functional or analog CANS model provides this necessary transition. The ideal model is one that has evolved from the stratified anatomy and functional organization of the CANS with the intrinsic capacity to provide direction in localizing CANS dysfunction. Such an idealized model is one which has built-in elasticity to accommodate emerging data on CANS evaluation. Perhaps, the model "best" fitting the above criteria is the one proposed by Carhart (1969), in which he outlines seven points of potential CANS dysfunction:

1. In the cochlear nerves' ipsilateral transmission to the CN
2. In the recoding activity at the CN
3. In the contralateral transmission of ipsilateral flow from the CN the more cephalic CANS areas
4. In the binaural interaction at the level of the SOC
5. In the transmission of the binaural interaction products from the SOC to the MGB and to the auditory radiations
6. In the processing of monaural and/or binaural information at Heschl's gyrus
7. In the intrahemispheric or interhemispheric processing.

A less elaborate model, but none the less rational, is a modified version of Katz's (1978) evaluation model, depicted in Fig. 8-4. As opposed to Carhart's model, the present model places emphasis on localizing the lesion within the stratified levels of the CANS and minimizes the search for pinpoint accuracy in identifying the dysfunction. Specifically, the model divides the CANS into the low brain stem, CN and SOC, the high

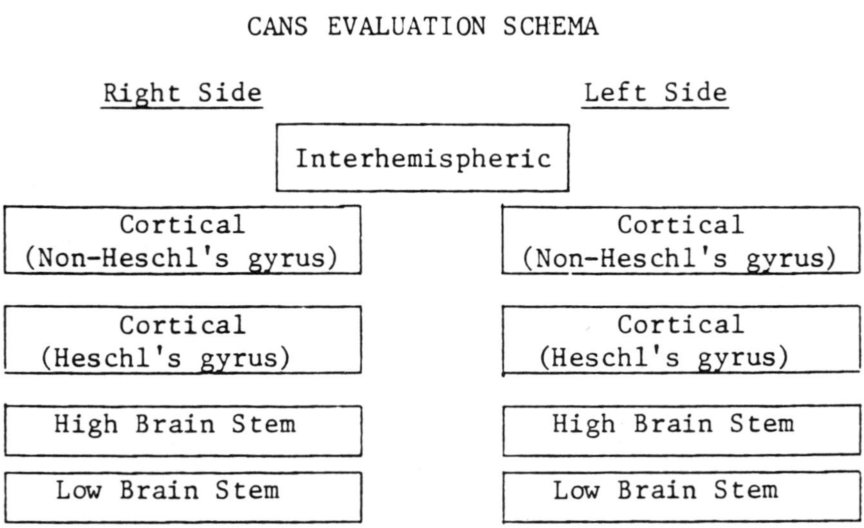

Fig. 8-4. CANS evaluation model patterned after Katz (1978).

brainstem, LL and MGB, and the mid-brain, MGB. The division is based on the premise that lesions of the brainstem, high brainstem and mid-brain should be distinguishable in clinical subjects. Likewise, at the cortical level, lesions of Heschl's gyrus should be differentiated from lesions of auditory association area, which in turn should be differentiated from lesions of the interhemispheric pathways. The Carhart model could be viewed as what the state of the art might become, while the Fig. 8-4 model is potentially the present state of the art.

MONAURAL SPEECH INTELLIGIBILITY PROCEDURES

An integral part of the basic audiometric test battery is an assessment of speech recognition usually measured at a fixed sensation level (SL) with a monosyllabic word test using an open set format. Unfortunately, this basic measure has been ineffective in categorizing various pathologies of the auditory system. In theory, if a purpose of a basic diagnostic evaluation is to determine if additional testing is necessary, then the traditional method of speech recognition assessment with respect to lesions of the CANS has at best produced inconsistent results and, at worst, has been insensitive. The lack of diagnostic potency rests in the very nature of the speech materials and the anatomy and physiology of the CANS. That is, the speech materials have multiple acoustic cues available to the listener for perception in addition to the intrinsic knowledge the listener possesses of the linguistic rules that govern the language. These multiple perceptual factors make speech a redundant signal. The CANS is likewise a redundant system with its ability to provide binaural information at several levels due to the ipsilateral and contralateral projection of each cochlea to each temporal lobe. This neural redundancy within the CANS has been termed internal or intrinsic redundancy, while the speech signal's redundancy is considered to be an external type. The dual redundancy has resulted in the inconsistent sensitivity of undistorted monosyllabic word tests to CANS lesions.

Table 8-1 summarizes speech intelligibility results from several published studies. A review of the table might lead one to conclude that undistorted monosyllabic word tests do produce, on the average, a small but consistent ear effect. On the surface, the trend is in that direction, particularly in the brainstem group, but there is little evidence found in the literature to indicate that these differences are significant. Lynn and Gilroy (1977) subjected their temporal and parietal lobe data to statistical analysis, which showed the differences to be nonsignificant. For their 35 temporal lobe subjects, 80 percent did not demonstrate an ear effect, while 17 percent did show a contralateral ear effect. Of the 28 parietal lobe

Table 8-1
Results of Monosyllabic Ward Tests From Selected Reports of CANS Dysfunction

Study	Ipsi Ear	Contra Ear	N	Etiology/Locale
Brainstem disorders				
Jerger (1960b)	100%	48%	1	Vascular
Jerger (1964)	92%	72%*	7	Vascular
Shaprio (1966)	1st test 56%	60%	1	Pontine glioma
	2nd test 42%	84%		
	3rd test 22%	80%		
Jerger & Jerger (1974)	85.5%*	78%*	16	Interaxial tumors
Katz (1978)	43%*	95%*	7	Unspecified
Cortical disorders				
Jerger (1960a)	92%	88%	1	Glioblastoma
	90%	98%	1	Epilepsy
Jerger (1964)	87%*	64%*	6	Heschl's gyrus
	91%*	82%§	4	Non Heschl's gyrus
Berlin et al. (1965)	90%*	86%*	15	Heschl's gyrus
	90%*	88%*	20	Right temporal lobe
	95%*	94%*	17	Left temporal lobe
Lynn & Gilroy (1977)	98%†	91%†	11	Right temporal lobe
	99%†	89%†	11	Left temporal lobe
	98%†	96%†	14	Right parietal lobe
	96%†	97%†	10	Left parietal lobe
Katz (1978)	90%*	85%*	14	Heschl's gyrus
	97%*	96%*	21	Non Heschl's gyrus

*Mean values
†Approximate mean values

cases, none showed an ear effect. For temporal lobe cases that have involvement of the primary auditory cortex (Heschl's gyrus), Katz (1978) reported a significant difference (0.5 level) between the mean scores for the ipsilateral and contralateral ears, with the contralateral ear being poorer. Katz's (1978) brainstem series also shows a large mean score difference between ears (although no significant information was provided) with the ipsilateral ear producing the poorer performance. In the opposite direction, Jerger and Jerger (1974) show 10 of their 16 intraaxial brainstem lesion series to have bilateral speech recognition scores between 80 and 100 percent while three cases did show a contralateral ear effect and one case an ipsilateral ear effect. No indication is given if any of the ten subjects in the first group had ear difference of ten or more percentage points as an ear difference of this magnitude coupled with normal hearing would warrant further investigation.

In summary, monosyllabic word tests appear to be inconsistent in their ability to reflect CANS dysfunction. At the brainstem level, individual cases have demonstrated symmetrical scores within normal limits, abnormal symmetrical scores, and asymmetrical scores where one ear is normal. In the latter instance, there is considerable disagreement as to which ear will reflect the lesion, the ipsilateral or contralateral ear. At the cortical level, the data appear to be less variable and reflects either normal symmetrical scores or asymmetrical scores, with the ear contralateral to the hemisphere lesion showing the poorer performance.

Potential areas for modification in speech recognition testing include improvement of the sensitivity of the stimuli and/or an alteration of the presentation mode. An example of the former is Campbell's (1965) revision of the CID W-22 materials, which made the lists more homogenous in average difficulty. Margolis and Millin (1971) have further refined the Campbell CID W-22 revision. However, no additional research with these materials has been reported.

The Jergers (1971; 1974; 1975b), in an effort to improve the diagnostic potency of monosyllabic word test(s), have obtained performance-intensity (PI) functions for monosyllabic phonetically balanced (PB) materials with several series of patients with varying types of auditory pathology. In brief, PB half-lists of 25 words are given at several suprathreshold intensity levels until the PI–PB function is well defined. The PI–PB function is examined for the paradoxical rollover phenomenon, i.e., the PI–PB function climbs to a maximum, then decreases substantially at higher intensity levels. The amount of rollover is determined by subtracting the PB minimum from the PB max. PB max is the highest intelligibility score at any intensity level and PB minimum is the lowest intelligibility score achieved at an intensity level above PB max. For brainstem lesions, rollover in excess of 20 percent is considered significant (Jerger & Jerger, 1975b), but it occurs in less than 50 percent of brainstem cases. The Jergers have further refined the PI procedure by using a comparison between the PI–PB function and the PI function for the Synthetic Sentence Identification (SSI) test. This particular facet is discussed later in this chapter.

Rush Hughes–PB Differential

Another avenue used to increase the diagnostic potency of monosyllabic word test is to utilize intrinsically more difficult materials such as the Rush Hughes recordings. In an often cited study, Goetzinger and Rousey (1959) compared CID W-22 and Rush Hughes scores within several age groups demonstrating an approximately 20 per cent difference between the maximum scores on these tests for individuals between 11 and 74 years of age. Above this age limit, the Rush Hughes/W-22 difference increased.

A subsequent report by Goetzinger and Angle (1965) showed that a difference value greater than 30 percent was consistent with a lesion in the contralateral temporal lobe. Consistent with these findings are data provided by Goldstein et al. (1956), who reported a mean difference value of 32 percent for four hemispherectomy patients on the Rush Hughes/CID-W22 comparison. The normative and pathological data for the Rush Hughes/W-22 differential, however, is in need of revalidation as a mismatch existed between the recording groove and the playback stylus in the Goetzinger studies (Stevens, 1978). Specifically, Goetzinger used the "universal microgroove" recording with an oversized 2.5 mil playback stylus. This specific mismatch is known to produce excessive harmonic distortion (Lilly & Franzen, 1968), which raises the possibility that Rush Hughes-W-22 difference values less than 30 percent may be reflective of cortical pathology (Stevens, 1978).

Redundancy Reduction Procedures

The high degree of inconsistency in the effect of CANS lesions on monosyllabic word materials has resulted in attempts to increase the sensitivity of these measures by reducing the inherent redundancy in the materials. The underlying reasoning is that a lesion will decrease the intrinsic neural redundancy, but could still go undetected due to the extrinsic redundancy of monosyllabic word materials. Thus, a further reduction in the available redundancy would improve the sensitivity of the measure to CANS dysfunction. Extrinsic redundancy reduction has been in the form of filtering, interrupting, and time compressing the monosyllabic word materials. While the literature contains citations relevant to the various forms of low-redundancy speech audiometry, the majority of data concern the use of filtered and compressed materials.

FILTERED SPEECH

Bocca, Calearo, and Cassinari (1954) were the first to demonstrate the potency of low-pass filtered speech tests in the identification of CANS lesions. These ingenious investigators used PB disyllabic words that were low-pass filtered below 800 Hz with a right temporal lobe tumor patient. The preliminary results showed a contralateral ear effect. A subsequent series (Bocca et al., 1955) of 18 subjects with temporal lobe dysfunction clearly demonstrated the contralateral ear effect in the majority of the cases studied. The cases for which the low-pass filtered data was equivocal were found at surgery to have tumors that did not involve the primary auditory cortex (Heschl's gyrus).

Jerger (1960; 1964) and others (Berlin et al., 1965; Hodgson, 1967;

Lynn & Gilroy, 1977) have reported on the use of low-pass filtered speech in recognition testing in clinical samples. These data are summarized in Table 8-2.

In these studies, the etiology underlying the CANS dysfunction vary from tumors in the Bocca et al. and Lynn and Gilroy series to localized surgical ablation (Jerger, 1964) to a series of hemispherectomy patients (Berlin et al., 1965; Hodgson, 1967). Although the cut-off frequency varied between 500 and 800 Hz with the rejection rate often unspecified, the data in Table 8-2 reveals a uniformity of results. Specifically, the contralateral ear effect emerges in those patients with involvement of Heschl's gyrus and is absent in patients with lesions distal from Heschl's gyrus. This point is amplified in the data of Jerger, Berlin et al., and Lynn and Gilroy. Of the 34 temporal cases in the Lynn and Gilroy series, 74 percent showed a contralateral ear effect, while 24 percent produced normal symmetrical results. Seventy percent of the parietal lobe groups, however, had normal symmetrical scores with 22 percent demonstrating a left ear effect.

Standardization of low-pass filtered materials has largely been on an individuals–investigator basis. The studies reviewed utilized cut-off fre-

Table 8-2
Results of Low-pass Filtered Tests Obtained From Clinical Cases Reported in the Literature

Study	Ipsi Ear	Contra Ear	N	Etiology/Locale
Bocca et al. (1954)	60%	42%	1	Heschl's gyrus
Bocca et al. (1954)	76%*	54%*	9	Heschl's gyrus
Jerger (1960)	66%*	35%*	2	Heschl's gyrus
Jerger (1964)	48%*	43%*	4	Heschl's gyrus
(Post-OP results)	47%*	30%*	6	Non Heschl's gyrus
Berlin et al. (1965)	57%*	50%*	17	Left temporal lobe
	42%*	46%*	20	Right temporal lobe
	44%*	41%*	15	Heschl's gyrus
Hodgson (1967)	Pre-OP 56%	44%	1	Hemispherectomy
	3 wks. Post-OP 54%	37%		
	3 mos. Post-OP 60%	46%		
Lynn & Gilroy (1977)	52%†	38%†	11	Right temporal lobe
	54%†	44%†	11	Left temporal lobe
	42%	40%†	14	Right parietal lobe
	41%†	51%†	10	Left parietal lobe

*Mean score
†Approximate mean score

quencies from 500–800 Hz with the rejection rate varying from 17dB/octave (Bocca et al., 1954) to 34 dB/octave (Lynn & Gilroy, 1977). Normative values of 70–80 percent (Bocca, 1958) and 47–63 percent (Lynn & Gilroy) have been reported. Individuals considering the construction of low-pass filtered monosyllabic word materials would do well to keep both the cut-off frequency and rejection rate parameters close to those mentioned, and strive to arrive at a cut-off frequency-rejection rate combination that results in mildly to moderately depressed scores with a small variance for normal-hearing subjects.

COMPRESSED SPEECH TESTS

Temporal alteration of speech stimuli as a redundancy reduction measure was originally developed to investigate the normal speech and hearing processes (Fairbanks et al., 1954). Although preliminary work was done with time expansion, time compression and acceleration of speech materials has generated the greatest amount of interest. Calearo and Lazzaroni (1957) were the first to recognize the potential of time acceleration as a technique to reduce the redundancy of speech materials, thereby taxing the processing capacity of the CANS and ultimately resulting in a procedure sensitive to CANS dysfunction. Basically, two techniques have been used to modify the speech materials: time acceleration and time compression. Time acceleration results from increasing the playback speed of the materials; in time compression, the silent intervals within the materials are removed. The former technique causes a frequency shift in the materials while the latter does not. The early European investigators used time acceleration of sentence materials to demonstrate a contralateral ear effect in temporal lobe cases.

The initial research efforts with time-compressed speech (Luterman et al., 1966; Sticht & Gray, 1969) brought equivocal findings. Beasley and his colleagues (Beasley et al., 1972a; Beasley et al., 1972b; Kurdziel et al., 1975; Konkle et al., 1977) have provided the needed normative data. Beasley et al., (1972a) presented Northwestern University Auditory Test no. 6 materials (NU-6) to 96 normal-hearing listeners at SLs between 8 and 32 dB under several time compression rates that ranged from 0–70 percent. These data are depicted in Figure 8-5. Examination of these data shows recognition to increase with higher SLs and decreased time compression. Speech recognition drops precipitously at 70 percent time compression at all SLs. In a following study, Beasley et al.(1972) extended the SL parameter to 40 dB. The mean intelligibility scores obtained at 32 dB and 40 dB SL for the various rates of compression for the two Beasley studies are displayed in Table 8-3. These normative data, however, are not consistent across age. Konkle, Beasley, and Bess (1977) have demonstrated an aging effect with the NU–6 time-compressed materials. A com-

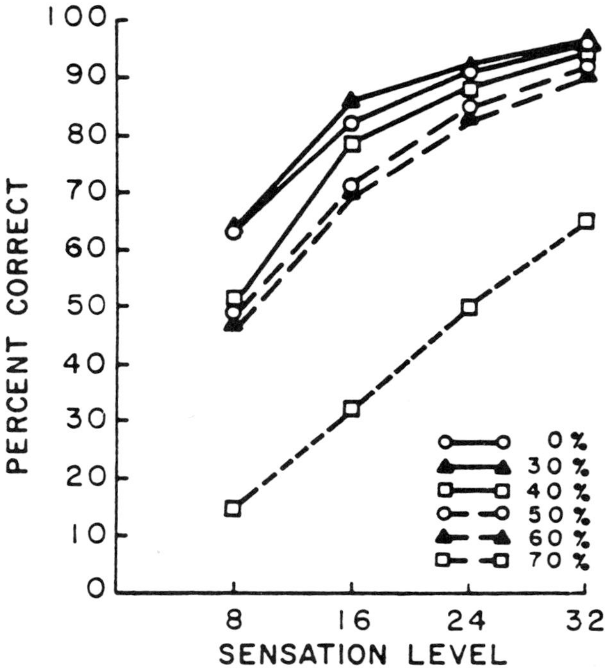

Fig. 8-5. Effects of the percentages of time compression as a function of sensation level. [From Beasley, D. S., Schwimmer, S., & Rintelman, W. F. Intelligibility of time-compressed CNC monosyllables. *Journal of Speech and Hearing Research,* 1972, *15,* 340–350. With permission.]

parison between the Beasley et al.(1972a) and the Konkle et al. (1977) data is found in Figure 8-6. Clearly, when using the time-compressed NU-6 materials, an adjustment for this aging effect must be considered at least for individuals 54 years of age and older. Particularly note the large difference among the age groups at 60 percent time compression.

Presently, time-compressed materials have not been used extensively

Table 8-3
Normal Mean Percent Correct Scores at 32 dB SL and 40 dB for Each Time Compression Condition

SL	Percentage of Time Compression					
	0	30	40	50	60	70%
32 dB	96.4	96.6	94.0	92.3	90.4	65.5
40 dB	98.2	97.4	97.2	95.5	94.2	80.4

Adapted from Beasley et al: Intelligibility of time. Compressed CNC monosyllables. *Journal of Speech and Hearing Research,* 1972a, *15,* 340–350; and Beasley et al: Perception of time-compressed CNC monosyllables by normal listeners. *Journal of Auditory Research,* 1972b, *12,* 71–75.

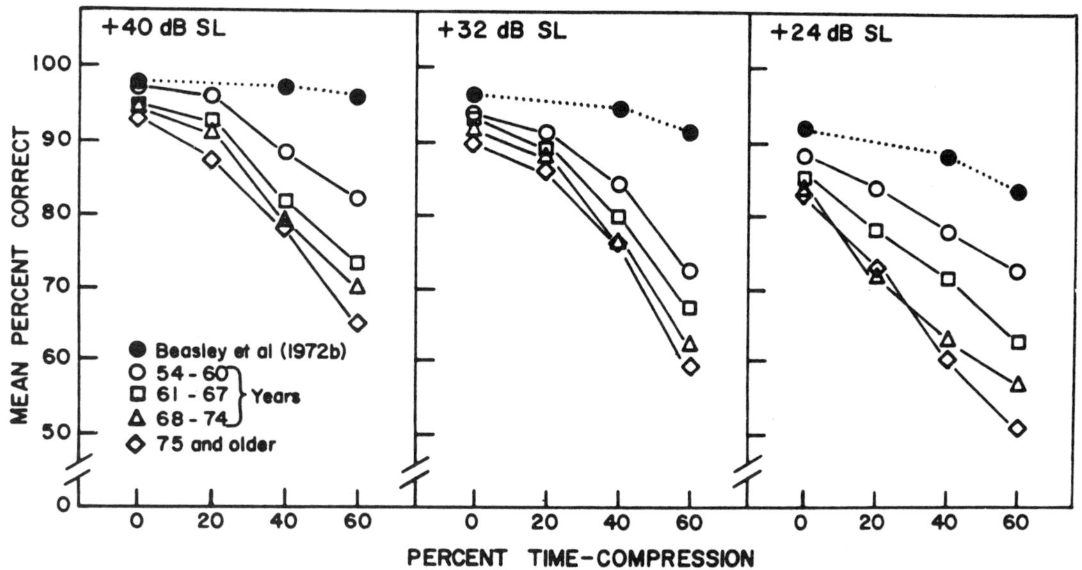

Fig. 8-6. Mean percent correct scores for the four age groups at each time compression and sensation level. [From Konkle, D., Beasley, D., & Bess, F. Intelligibility of time-altered speech in relation to chronological aging. *Journal of Speech and Hearing Research,* 1977, *20,* 108–115. With permission.]

with clinical subjects. Kurdziel, Rintelmann, and Beasley (1975) used the Beasley et al. NU-6 materials to study the effect of sensorineural hearing loss on time-compressed speech recognition functions. The nine subjects with noise-induced sensorineural hearing loss achieved lower recognition scores at each compression rate than normal hearing listeners, but demonstrated essentially the same shape in their performance functions as that derived from normal-hearing listeners; that is, performance decreases with higher compression rates and lower SLs, and increases with lower compression rates and higher SLs. These sensorineural cases in the Kurdziel et al. series show the precipitous decrement in performance at 70 percent time compression noted previously in the Beasley et al. normative series. Within the sensorineural group, individuals varied as to the SLs at which they registered their maximum intelligibility scores. Thus, in cases with cochlear involvement, intelligibility performance for time-compressed materials must be obtained at several SLs.

In a continued effort to provide clinical sample data, Kurdziel and her colleagues (1976) studied 31 cases with known unilateral cortical lesions. A diffuse lesion group was made up of ten cases with cerebrovascular accidents (CVA), one case with a large temporal lobe tumor and four hemispherectomy cases. The discrete lesion series consisted of 15 cases who had undergone resection of the anterior temporal lobe for seizure control and one subject who had a tumor removed from the anterior temporal lobe. Table 8-4, summarizes the performance of these two groups

Table 8-4
Means and Ranges of Intelligibility Scores for the Diffuse Lesion and Discrete Lesion Groups at Each Time Compression Condition

Condition %	N %	Ipsilateral Ear $\overline{X}$ %	Range %	N %	Contralateral Ear $\overline{X}$ %	Range %
Diffuse lesions						
0	15	97.0	84–100	15	94.5	88–100
40	11	94.5	84–100	14	83.2	52–100
60	13	88.7	72–100	15	60.4	30–86
Discrete lesions						
0	16	98.7	96–100	16	98.5	92–100
40	0			0		
60	16	89.6	68–100	16	89.7	64–100

From Kurdziel, S. A., Noffsinger, D., & Olsen, W. Performance by cortical lesion patients on 40 and 60 percent time-compression materials. *Journal of The American Audiological Society,* 1976, *2,* 3–7. Reprinted with permission of The Williams & Wilkins Co., © 1976, Baltimore.

on the Beasley et al. (1972a) materials time compressed to 40 and 60 percent. Clearly, the diffuse lesion group demonstrate a contralateral ear effect at both 40 and 60 percent time compression. At 40 percent time compression, the difference between the ipsilateral and contralateral means is 11.3 percent, while this difference is 28.3 percent for the 60 percent time compression condition. None of the 15 diffuse lesion cases achieved a contralateral ear score of greater than 86 percent at 60 percent time compression. The difference in performance at 0 and 60 percent time compression for the ipsilateral ear was never greater than 16 percent in all but three cases in this group. The contralateral ear difference between 0 and 60 percent time compression for the CVA cases, however, ranged from 22–48 percent, but this difference value for three of the four hemispherectomy cases was approximately 12 percent.

Time-compressed NU-6 materials did not produce an ear effect in the discrete lesion group. In fact, the ipsilateral–contralateral ear difference was never greater than ten percent; paradoxically, five cases registered better contralateral ear scores. A comparison of scores at 0 and 60 percent time compression was eight percent or less in the ipsilateral ear for 15 of the 16 cases and six percent or less within the contralateral ear for 15 of the 16 cases. One case demonstrated a large difference score of 28 percent in both ears.

As with low-pass filtered materials, time-compressed monosyllabic word tests are differentially sensitive to the locale of the lesion within the temporal lobe. The discrete lesion group in the Kurdziel et al. report probably did not have Heschl's gyrus involvement resulting in an intact primary auditory reception center and no contralateral ear effect. The CVA cases in the diffuse group probably had involvement of the Heschl's gyrus area, which results in a contralateral ear effect. The paradoxical finding that three of the four hemispherectomy cases did not produce a marked decrement in their contralateral ear intelligibility scores at 60 percent time compression could be used to argue against the sensitivity of time-compressed monosyllables to lesions involving Heschl's gyrus, since a hemispherectomy by its very nature removes Heschl's gyrus. But, for example, if one or all of those three cases had ipsilateral-contralateral ear difference scores of ten percent at the 60 percent time compression condition, the test would be positive.

Several conclusions may be drawn from the available data on time-compressed monosyllabic word tests: (1) Normal listeners produce normal recognition scores for monosyllables up to and including 60 percent time compression at 32 dB and 40 dB SL; (2) The norms are applicable to the young adult population and may be applicable to those under 54 years of age; (3) Above 54 years of age, an appropriate age adjustment must be made; (4) PI function for time compressed materials should be obtained from an ear suspected of having cochlear involvement; (5) Diagnostic information results from both performance comparisons between and within ears at 0 and 60 percent time compression; and (6) Involvement of Heschl's gyrus will be reflected in a contralateral ear effect at 60 percent time compression.

BINAURAL TEST PROCEDURES

Binaural Fusion Tests

Anatomically, binaural fusion (binaural resynthesis) first occurs in the CANS in the brainstem at the SOC. Matzker (1959) took note of this anatomical arrangement and designed a test based on binaural fusion for the detection of CANS brainstem disorders. The Matzker procedure utilized 41 German bisyllabic PB words, band-passed filtered between 500 and 800 Hz and between 1815 and 2500 Hz, presented at a SL previously determined to produce maximum recognition. Matzker's test protocol called for three presentation conditions: (1) Dichotically with the low-pass filtered band to one ear and the high-pass filtered band to the contralateral ear; (2) Diotically with the low-pass filtered band and high-pass filtered band to each ear; and (3) Same as number one. A normal performance was defined by a low error rate across all three presentations and the presence of a small "learning effect" reflected in recognition score improvement after the initial presentation. An abnormal performance was indicated by a high error rate for the two dichotic conditions, with an improved recognition score for the diotic condition. Matzker believed his test to be sensitive to CANS brainstem pathology, but insensitive to unilateral cortical dysfunction because of binaural representation at each hemisphere. Linden (1964) attempted to replicate Matzker's data using a modified form with the band-pass parameters at 300–600 Hz and 1200–2400 Hz, and altered test and interpretation protocols. Specifically, performance comparisons were among the scores produced by each band presented monaurally and the scores that resulted from the dichotic condition. Linden interpreted his test data to indicate that Matzker's test was not sensitive to CANS dysfunction. But, as Lynn and Gilroy (1972) astutely point out, Linden's conclusion may be unfounded, in that he presented no evidence documenting brainstem pathology in any of his subjects, all of whom may have had only cerebral involvement.

While examination of the Matzker's test continued in Japan (Hayashi et al., 1966; Ohta et al., 1967) Smith and Resnick (1972) were developing a procedure modeled after Matzker's, which they dubbed the Dichotic Binaural Fusion (DBF) test. The DBF test consisted of three Peterson and Lehiste (1962) CNC tests that were band-pass filtered at 360–890 Hz and

Table 8-5
Plus and Minus One Standard Deviation Ranges for 30 Normal-hearing Subjects and 16 Sensorineural Hearing Loss Subjects on the Dichotic Binaural Fusion (DBF) Test

	Diotic	Dichotic # 1	Dichotic # 2
Normals	64.2–78.3%	62.4–78.4%	62.9–75.9%
Sensorineurals	29.0–56.6%	24.9–61.3%	28.2–60.6%

Adapted from Smith, B. B. & Resnick, D. A. An auditory test for asessing brain stem integrity; preliminary report. *Laryngoscope,* 1972, *82,* 414–424.

1750–2220 Hz, presented under three conditions: (1) Dichotically with the low-pass band to the right ear and the high-pass band to the left ear; (2) Diotically to each ear; and (3) Dichotically with the ears being the reverse of number one. Normative values for the DBF test are displayed in Table 8-5 and represent plus and minus one standard deviation of derived means obtained from 30 normal-hearing listeners and 16 listeners with sensorineural hearing. These data indicate that both the normal-hearing and sensorineural-hearing loss groups produce a consistent range of scores difference between highest and lowest, three presentation conditions, although in absolute performance the sensorineural group's scores are poorer by 15 to 35 percent. Smith and Resnick extended their preliminary data to include a clinical sample of three patients with temporal lobe lesions and four patients with brainstem lesions. As the significant measure of the DBF procedure is the comparison between diotic and dichotic conditions, the derived data from these series are presented in this difference form (see Table 8-6). Negative values indicate that the dichotic performance

Table 8-6
Difference Values Obtained by Subtracting the DBF Dichotic Conditions From the Diotic Conditions for Three Temporal Lobe Cases and Four Brainstem Cases

		Diotic–Dichotic #1	Diotic–Dichotic #2
Temporal lobe cases	1	– 6.0%	6.0%
	2	8.0%	4.0%
	3	– 12.0%	– 6.0%
Brainstem case	1	26.0%	28.0%
	2	26.0%	20.0%
	3	18.0%	16.0%
	4	12.0%	34.0%

Adapted from Smith, B. B., & Resnick, D. M. An auditory test for assessing brain stem integrity; preliminary report. *Laryngoscope,* 1972, *82,* 414–424.

was better than the diotic performance. For the temporal subjects, these difference values are either very small or negative, while for the brainstem subjects, these difference values are considerably larger, ranging from 18–34 percent. Smith and Resnick's DBF procedure would appear to easily separate brainstem pathology from cortical pathology. Further, the procedure is straightforward and void of complicated scoring procedures. The DBF, however, still awaits independent validation with cases having discrete lesions of the brainstem and cases having discrete temporal lobe lesions.

Noffsinger et al., (1972) included a binaural fusion procedure as part of an auditory test protocol used in assessing the effects of multiple sclerosis on auditory function. NU-6 materials were band-pass filtered at 250–750 Hz and 1250–1750 Hz. The dichotic-diotic technique of Smith and Resnick was utilized. Noffsinger et al. report a recognition score of 80 percent as the average performance achieved by normal-hearing listeners in either the dichotic or diotic presentation mode. This expected value is close to the normal range reported by Smith and Resnick. The Noffsinger et al. binaural fusion procedure produced four test conditions: (1) Diotic to right ear; (2) Diotic to left ear; (3) Dichotic with the low-pass band to right ear and the high-pass band to left ear; and (4) Dichotic with the low-pass band to left ear and the high-pass band to right ear. Of the 36 multiple sclerosis cases given the procedure, only eight had abnormal performance, and only one of the eight had an abnormal score for the dichotic conditions. For scoring, a dichotic score of 60 percent or less was considered abnormal, as was a difference of ten percent between the ears on any of the four test conditions.

Lynn and Gilroy in their prolific effort to document the effect of CANS lesions on various auditory measures have used two fusion-like procedures in their test battery. The first is Ivey's (1969) modification of the Matzker test, which consists of selected spondaic words band-pass filtered at 500–700 Hz and 1900–2100 Hz. The expected performance range for dichotic presentation is 74–100 percent. With temporal lobe cases (Lynn & Gilroy, 1972; Lynn et al., 1972; Gilroy & Lynn, 1974), the results have been within normal limits. When there has been secondary involvement of the brainstem, however, binaural fusion results have been abnormal.

The second fusion-like technique utilized by Lynn and Gilroy (1977) is their Rapidly Alternating Speech Perception (RASP) test, which involves the oscillation of speech between the ear every 200–300 msec. Normal listeners achieved a RASP recognition score of 90–100 percent as did cases with unilateral cerebral pathology. Six low brainstem cases with pontine lesions and five with intraaxial lesions produced a mean RASP recognition score of 38 percent. Nine cases with upper brain disorders had an average performance of 83 percent, which is very close to the normal range. The RASP procedure would appear to be most sensitive to lesions of the lower brainstem at the level of the pons.

Masking Level Difference

Another binaural phenomenon that has been explored in clinical samples is the masking level difference (MLD). The MLD is a psychoacoustic phenomenon involving a binaural release from masking reflected in a threshold and/or recognition improvement when a phase reversal is imposed on the signal (S) or the masker (N). The magnitude of the MLD is the difference between a homophasic condition and two antiphasic conditions. A homophasic condition is created when there is no interaural phase difference for the signal or the masker; that is, the binaurally presented signal and noise are in phase between themselves at the ears. In MLD nomenclature, this homophasic condition is signified by SoNo with the "o" indicating interaural phase agreement. An antiphasic condition is created when either the signal or the masker undergo a 180° phase change while the unaltered stimulus retains its phase relationship between the ears. For example, a 500 Hz tone is being presented binaurally in phase while a narrow band of noise centered at 500 Hz is simultaneously being presented binaurally resulting a SoNo condition. Next, the 500 Hz tone's binaural phase relationship is altered such that the tone is 180° out of phase between the ear. This condition is designated by SπNo with "π" indicating the phase reversal. The reverse of the above would be the masker being 180° out of phase between the ears and the 500 Hz tone in phase between the ears, producing a SoN condition. MLD values are computed thusly: (1) SoNo – SπNo = MLD value; or (2) SoNo – SoNπ = MLD value. Normal MLD values for spondaic words are approximately 8 dB for the SπNo condition and 7 dB for the SoNπ condition (Carhart et al., 1968; Olsen et al., 1976; Olsen & Noffsinger, 1976). Olsen and his colleagues report that 96 percent of their 62 normal-hearing subjects achieved a MLD of 6 dB or greater at the SπNo condition and 4 dB or greater at the SoNπ condition.

Speech recognition measures have been obtained under MLD conditions. Cullen and Thompson (1974) presented Petersen and Lehiste (1965) CNC materials to 14 normal-hearing listeners under SoNo, SπNo, and SoNπ conditions. The CNC materials were presented at 60dB SPL and the masker at 63dB SPL. On the average, the SoNo condition resulted in a recognition score of 40 percent. The mean MLD for the SπNo condition was 31 percent and 23 percent for the SoNπ condition. The plus or minus one standard deviation range was approximately 16 to 40 percent and approximately 14 to 32 percent for the SπNo and SoNπ conditions, respectively.

Olsen, Noffsinger, and Carhart (1976) presented MLD data obtained from a variety of clinical groups that ranged from conductive loss to cochlear impairment to retrocochlear involvement to cortical lesions. The data was evaluated in terms of the number of subjects in each clinical group that produced a MLD value below that achieved by 95 percent of the normal-hearing group. These data are summarized in Table 8-7. For the SπNo condition, approximately one half of the subjects in the conductive loss, presbycusic, and multiple sclerotic groups had MLDs below the cut-off value; while 75 percent of the eighth nerve tumor group and 85 percent of the Menieres disease group had MLDs below the cut-off limit. The SoNπ condition showed that 30–40 percent of the conductive loss, Meniere's disease, eighth nerve tumor, presbycusic, and multiple sclerotic groups had MLDs below the cut-off value. Note that for both MLD conditions, the cortical lesion group, on the average, produced MLD values within normal limits.

In addition to normal-hearing subjects, Cullen and Thompson (1974) studied speech recognition MLDs in four subjects who had undergone resection of the superior temporal gyrus. MLDs for the SoNπ condition ranged from 20.0–29.8 percent and for the SπNo condition ranged from 21.0–36.4 percent. Obviously, cortical lesions do not affect the MLD mechanism.

The MLD findings in these and other studies (Schoeny & Carhart, 1971; Noffsinger et al., 1972; Olsen & Noffsinger, 1976) have demonstrated that MLD function is disrupted by cochlear and brainstem pathology. The MLD phenomenon results from a phase correlation process within the CANS and is mediated below the thalamic level. Anatomically, the SOC is the leading candidate to be the seat of the MLD mechanism. With respect to the application of MLD testing to CANS evaluation, the

Table 8-7
Number of Subjects With Spondee MLDs Equal To or Below the Cut-off Value for the SπNo and SoNπ Conditions

Groups	N	Number of Subjects Below Cut Off Spondee MLD: SπNo ≤ 5dB	Number of Subjects Below Cut Off Spondee MLD: SoNπ ≤ 3dB
Normal	50	3	3
Conductive loss	10	5	3
Noise trauma	50	16	11
Meniere's disease	20	17	9
Eighth nerve tumor	20	15	9
Presbycusis	20	10	6
Multiple sclerosis	100	58	41
Cortical lesion	20	1	0

Adapted from Olsen, W. O., Noffsinger, D., & Carhart, R. Masking level differences encountered in clinical populations. *Audiology,* 1976, *15,* 287–301.

potency of this procedure lies in its presumed anatomical basis and the differential response of brainstem and cortical lesions to the MLD paradigm. A significantly reduced spondee MLD in the face of normal hearing sensitivity and normal speech recognition scores would be the diagnostic cue to separate brainstem lesion from cortical pathology.

Staggered Spondaic Word Test

While his contemporaries were investigating CANS assessment through redundancy reduction techniques, Katz (1962) chose to utilize a dichotic format in pursuing the development of his Staggered Spondaic Word Test. With the SSW, Katz opted to rely on the presentation technique and not the materials as the sensitizing feature of his test. Spondaic words were chosen as the stimuli because of their high degree of recognition; Katz hoped that the contaminating effects of cochlear involvement could be thereby circumvented. Specific information concerning the early phases of the SSW development can be found in Katz (1962; 1968); and Brunt (1972). Scoring and interpretation guidelines are provided in Katz (1977a) and Brunt (1978).

The present form of the SSW, list EC, consists of four practice items and 40 test items made up of two overlapping spondees per presentation. The presentation paradigm is illustrated in Table 8-8. The SSW test format produces four scoreable items for each presentation: (1) Right noncompeting (R-NC); (2) Right competing (R-C); (3) Left competing (L-C); and (4) Left noncompeting (L-NC). Quantitative information is derived from three scores: a condition score, an ear score, and a total performance score. In order to negate the effect of reduced speech recognition on the SSW interpretation, the amount of error as reflected by a standard monosyllabic word test is subtracted from the raw SSW data, resulting in a corrected SSW (C-SSW) score. Justification for this speech recognition correction, according to Katz, results from the high positive correlation (.86 for 61 subjects), between the total SSW performance and the speech recognition scores of subjects with sensorineural hearing loss (Katz, 1977b). The use of this correction procedure has not, however, been uni-

Table 8-8
SSW Presentation Paradigm

	Noncompeting	Competing	Noncompeting
Right ear	Day (R–NC)	Light (R–C)	
Left ear		Lunch (L–C)	Time (L–NC)

versally accepted (Lynn & Gilroy, 1977). Normative values for the C-SSW are presented in Table 8-9. All the normative values are in percent of error with the negative values (overcorrection category) resulting from speech recognition scores being poorer than the SSW scores. These normative values are valid for individuals between 11 and 60 years of age.

In addition to the quantitative information provided by the direct comparison of each subject's performance to the normative data standards in Table 8-9, supplementary information exists in the SSW raw data in the form of "response bias" that can be utilized to locate intrahemispheric lesions (Katz, 1977). Response bias takes the form of an ear effect, an order effect, and a reversal effect. An ear effect is determined through direct comparison of the error rates for the right ear first (REF) and left ear first (LEF); that is, the number of errors produced when the presentation sequence began in the right ear versus the number of errors produced when the presentation sequence began in the left ear. An order effect refers to an error comparison of the first spondee and the second spondee, regardless of which ear was in the lead or lag position. For the ear and order effects, an error rate difference of five or greater is considered significant (Katz, 1977a). Katz (1977b) indicates that a trend is beginning to emerge, suggesting that subjects with significantly more errors on REF have posterior temporo-parietal involvement, while subjects with fronto-temporal involvement have significantly more errors on LEF. Further, a higher error score on the second spondee, an order effect, is believed to be consistent with posterior temporo-parietal involvement as opposed to a higher error score on the first spondee, which is associated with an anterior temporal lobe involvement (Katz, 1978). According to these response indicators, the profile of an individual with an anterior temporal lobe tumor would be a high error score on LEF and a high error score on the first spondee. Presently, the localization trend developing for ear and order effects lack independent verification.

Reversals are a reordering of the half spondee presentation sequence by the person being tested. For example, if the test presentation was "up-

Table 8-9
Normative C–SSW and A-SSW Values

	Over-corrected	Normal	Mildly Abnormal	Moderately Abnormal	Severely Abnormal
Total score	−5	−4–5	6–15	16–35	36–100
Ear score	−7	−6–10	11–20	21–40	41–100
Condition score	−10	−9–15	16–25	26–45	46–100

From Katz, J. (Ed.) *The SSW test manual.* St. Louis: Auditec of St. Louis, 1977. Reprinted with permission.

stairs, down-town," but the subject responded out of sequence, "down-town, up-stairs," this would constitute a reversal. Reversals may hold potential as another indicator of intrahemisphere localization. Katz and Pack (1974) examined the reversal patterns for 17 subjects with cortical lesions distal to Heschl's gyrus and essentially normal performance on the SSW. Thirteen of these 17 patients had a significant number of reversals and cortical involvement in the pre-and postcentral gyrus areas that border the central fissure (Fissure of Rolando) or in the anterior temporal lobe. Again, reversals appear to be very potent indicators for localizing lesions at the cortical level, but lack independent confirmation at this writing.

Katz (1978) states that the SSW is differentially sensitive to involvement of the various anatomical levels within the CANS. Specifically, Katz outlines distinctly different SSW profiles for low brainstem involvement, high brainstem involvement, and cortical involvement with and without Heschl's gyrus involvement. Katz refers to these latter two as auditory reception (AR) and nonauditory reception (NAR), respectively. Using the C-SSW values and an ipsilateral-contralateral ear comparison, Katz (1978) contrasts the mean performance profile of three low brainstem cases with the mean performance profile of four high brainstem cases. In brief, the profile for the three lower brainstem cases was an overcorrected score for the ear ipsilateral to the involved side and a score within normal limits for the contralateral ear. In contrast, the profile produced by the four high brainstem cases was a severely abnormal score for the ear ipsilateral to the involved side and a score within normal limits for the contralateral ear.

In a series of reports, Katz (Katz & Pack, 1974; Katz, 1977; Katz, 1978) has presented data on the SSW profile differences between AR and NAR cases. A composite of each profile is illustrated in Table 8-8. These data represent the mean and standard deviations for 21 AR cases and 23 NAR cases. Clearly, the AR and NAR provide distinctly different SSW profiles with little or no overlap in the contralateral ear comparisons. Typically, the AR case will produce ipsilateral ear scores in the normal or mild categories, while the contralateral ear scores fall within the moderate to severe categories, particularly in the contralateral competing score. Based on the data in Fig. 8-7, NAR cases will produce, on the average, normal scores except for the contralateral competing condition where the worse performance is only mildly abnormal. Independent support for these AR and NAR profiles comes from the work of Lynn and Gilroy (1972), who presented data on five patients with posterior temporal lobe tumors and five patients with anterior temporal lobe tumors. Presumably, the anterior or inferior temporal lobe tumors spared Heschl's gyrus, while the posterior temporal lobe tumors involve the Heschl's gyrus area. Mean

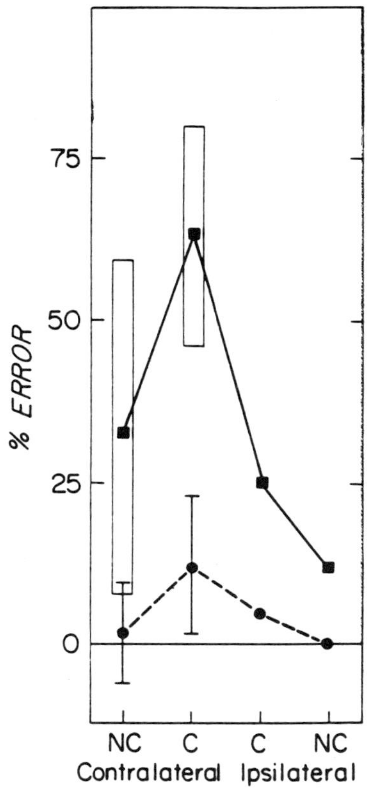

Fig. 8-7. Mean and standard deviation scores in percent of error, for 21 auditory reception (AR) cases and 23 nonauditory reception (NAR) cases. [From Keith, R., (Ed.). *Central auditory dysfunction*. New York: Grune & Stratton, 1977. With permission.]

and standard deviation error values for these ten patients are summarized in Table 8-10. The overall trend reflected in the Lynn and Gilroy data is consistent with the data provided by Katz, although two of the anterior temporal lobe cases produced contralateral competing scores in the moderate and severe categories.

In a later report, Lynn and Gilroy (1977) presented data on 22 cases of surgically verified temporal lobe tumors. The approximate mean error scores for these 22 temporal lobe cases are displayed in Table 8-11. The contralateral ear effect is very dramatic, as these subjects performed consistently poorer for both the competing (C) and noncompeting (NC) conditions in the ear contralateral to the disordered hemisphere. Lynn and Gilroy analyzed their data to determine if significant difference occurred between the ipsilateral and the contralateral ear for the competing and

Table 8-10
Approximate Mean Error Values for the Four SSW Conditions From Five Patients with Posterior Temporal Lobe Tumors and Five Patients with Anterior Temporal Lobe Tumors

		Contra Ear		Ipsi Ear	
		NC	C	C	NC
Posterior temporal lobe tumors	Mean	49.2	86.0	10.8	8.5
	SD	29.9	15.3	30.7	14.4
Anterior temporal lobe tumors	Mean	10.4	28.6	10.8	5.0
	SD	10.6	24.0	9.2	5.4

Adapted from Lynn, G. E., & Gilroy, J. Neuro-audiological abnormalities in patients with temporal lobe tumors. *Journal of the Neurological Sciences,* 1972, *17,* 167–184.

noncompeting conditions. In their temporal lobe series, the ipsilateral and contralateral ears were significantly different for both the competing condition (.01 level) and the noncompeting condition (.05 level for the right temporal lobe group and .01 level for the left temporal lobe group). Though not stated, it appears that these temporal lobe series consisted mainly of cases with posterior involvement, as there were significant ipsilateral–contralateral ear differences, and the illustration case referred to as "typical" of the series was one with a right posterior temporal lobe tumor. With a larger temporal lobe lesion sample of 34, Lynn and Gilroy (1977) reported that 85 percent produce abnormal scores in the contralateral ear on the competing SSW condition, but only 53 percent of the cases had abnormal contralateral ear scores for the noncompeting SSW condition.

In the same publication, Lynn and Gilroy summarized their findings obtained from a series of 24 cases with deep parietal lobe tumors involv-

Table 8-11
Approximate Mean Values, in Percent of Error, for the Four SSW Conditions of 11 Patients With Right Temporal Lobe Tumors and 11 Patients with Left Temporal Lobe Tumors. Significance Indicators Are for ContralateralVersus Ipsilateral Ear Comparisons

	Contra Ear		Ipsi Ear	
	NC	C	C	NC
Right temporal lobe tumors	16*	40†	6	2
Left temporal lobe tumors	22†	54†	12	4

*05 level of significance
†.01 level of significance
Adapted from Lynn, G. E., & Gilroy, J. Evaluation of central auditory dysfunction in patients with neurological disorders. In R. Keith (Ed.) *Central auditory dysfunction.* New York: Grune & Stratton, 1977, pp. 177–218.

ing the corpus callosum. In contrast to the temporal lobe series discussed above, the deep parietal tumor group did not show a contralateral ear effect on the SSW, but for three of the four SSW conditions, a significant (.05–.01 level, depending on condition) left ear effect emerged regardless of the disordered hemisphere. The left ear's performance for this series, particularly the competing condition, was consistently poorer than the performance of the right ear. Table 8-12 summarizes the approximate mean performances for these parietal cases. The left ear effect occurs in the deep parietal group because the tumor interrupts the interhemisphere callosal transmission to the dominant decoding left hemisphere, while suppression of the noncallosal ipsilateral route to the left hemisphere is produced by the more effectively transmitted contralateral signal coming from the right ear. In short, the effect produced by interruption of the interhemisphere callosal pathway is manifested in the ear ipsilateral to the hemisphere dominant for speech and language. Normally, under dichotic presentation the speed of transmission is faster by the contralateral route, and assuming a left hemisphere dominant for speech, the left ear stimulus would cross over via the callosal fibers to the left hemisphere for decoding, while the right ear stimulus is transmitted via the faster contralateral route directly to the left hemisphere. Examining for the frequency of the left ear effect in corpus callosum cases, Lynn and Gilroy (1977) found 78 percent of their 28 cases produced left ear effects on the SSW competing condition, but only 25 percent of these 28 cases produced abnormal left ear performance on the SSW noncompeting condition.

In summary, the available data show the SSW to be sensitive to dysfunction at various levels within the CANS. Unfortunately, not all investigators have utilized the same SSW scoring technique. In particular, the "response bias" aspect of the SSW protocol has not been universally

Table 8-12
Approximate Mean Values, in Percent of Error, for the Four SSW Conditions of 14 Patients With Right Parietal Lobe Tumors and 11 Patients With Left Parietal Lobe Tumors. Significance Indicators are for Right Ear Versus Left Ear Comparisons

	Right Ear		Left Ear	
	NC	C	C	NC
Right parietal lobe tumors	2	5	41*	11*
Left parietal lobe tumors	6	15	42*	12

*.05 level of significance
†.01 level of significance

Adapted from Lynn, G. E., & Gilroy, J. Evaluation of central auditory dysfunction in patients with neurological disorders. In R. Keith (Ed.), *Central auditory dysfunction*. New York: Grune & Stratton, 1977, pp. 177–218.

used, and is in need of further study. Without question, however, the SSW is very sensitive to lesions involving Heschl's gyrus with the ear contralateral to the affected hemisphere showing a significantly higher error rate than the ipsilateral ear. Likewise, the SSW is sensitive to disruption in the interhemisphere pathways. The difficulty, however, arises when the ear showing the abnormal performance is the left ear, as lesions of the right posterior temporal lobe and lesions involving the corpus callosum produce left-ear effects.

SENTENCE TESTS

Synthetic Sentence Identification Test

In 1965, Speaks and Jerger published their initial findings concerning the Synthetic Sentence Identification (SSI) test. The rationale and methodology involved in the SSI development may be found in the original article and subsequent publications (Speaks et al., 1966; Jerger et al., 1968). Briefly, Speaks and Jerger, noting the difficulties in both material and methodology associated with more traditional approaches to speech recognition testing (i.e., monosyllabic word materials, open-set format, and auditory vocal response mode) diverted from these classical protocols to a test composed of third order approximate sentences of uniform length and presented in a closed-set format. The selection of synthetic sentences was partially motivated by the developers' interest in suitable research materials. Synthetic sentence materials and a closed-set format were utilized to circumvent the listeners' reliance on their knowledge of the rules of grammar and syntax to aid in their perception of sentence-length materials. Inherently, synthetic sentences have less redundancy than natural sentences. The SSI test protocol does not require a verbal response from the subject. Therefore, the probability of tester error is considerably reduced. Currently, the SSI score is derived from the presentation of ten synthetic sentences. Various scramblings of these basic ten sentences are used to obtain recognition scores under differing test conditions. Table 8-13 displays the ten basic sentences used in the SSI procedure.

Used as a test for the assessment of CANS dysfunction, the SSI protocol includes the presentation of these materials with ipsilateral and contralateral competing messages. The competing message is connected discourse. Individual performances are assessed by presenting the materials at several message-to-completion ratios (MCRs) under conditions of contralateral competing message (CCM) and ipsilateral competing message (ICM). The SSI materials are presented at 50 dB SPL for both the CCM

Table 8-13
Ten Basic Synthetic Sentences That Make Up the SSI Test

1.	Small boat with a picture has become
2.	Built the government with the force almost
3.	Go change you car color is red
4.	Forward march said the boy had a
5.	March around without a care in your
6.	That neighbor who said business is better
7.	Battle cry and be better than ever
8.	Down by the time is real enough
9.	Agree with him only to find out
10.	Women view men with green paper should

and ICM conditions, while the competing message is varied in intensity per ten sentence set to obtain the various MCRs. The CCM condition specifies MCRs at 0, −20, and −40 dB, i.e., the SSI materials at 50 dB SPL and the competing message at 50, 70, and 90 dB SPL. The ICM condition is assessed at MCRs of +10, 0, −10 and −20 dB, i.e., the SSI materials at 50 dB SPL and the competing message at 40, 50, 60, and 70 dB SPL. Regardless of the MCR, a normal performance on the CCM condition ranges between 90 and 100 percent identification (Jerger, 1973; Keith, 1977). Normative data for the ICM condition are summarized in Table 8-14. Both the approximate means and ranges of the Jerger and the Keith data are in agreement. Historically, the SSI has not been administered to CANS dysfunction cases with peripheral hearing loss due to the possible contaminating effects of cochlear involvement on the performance profile. Keith's (1977) search of the literature indicates there is no information on CANS cases with pure-tone averages greater than 25 dB HL.

Jerger (1973) outlined the expected SSI performance patterns associated with brainstem and with temporal lobe dysfunction. Brainstem disorders are characterized by poor ICM performance in the ear contralateral to the involved side unless the lesion crosses the midline; in that case, the

Table 8-14
Means and Ranges of Performances in the SSI–ICM for Normal-hearing Subjects Reported by Jerger (1973) and Keith (1977)

MCR	Jerger	Keith
+10	100	100
0	93 (84–100)	94.5 (84–100)
−10	80 (71–92)	90.0 (78–100)
−20	55 (45–68)	61.0 (47–75)

ICM would be depressed bilaterally. CCM performance with brainstem lesions is typically normal. Temporal lobe disorders produced reduced, performance on both the ICM and CCM conditions with the poorest performance in the ear contralateral to the disordered hemisphere, or in the case of the ICM condition, both ears may show abnormal scores. In the 1973 report, Jerger provided clinical cases whose SSI profiles were consistent with the above interpretation. Subsequently, Jerger and Jerger (1974) presented data on patients with interaxial brainstem tumors that were either surgically and/or radiographically defined. In all eleven cases, the SSI–ICM performance was abnormal. In fact, the SSI–ICM was the only audiometric measure (pure-tone, Bekesy, acoustic reflex, PB max, and SSI–CCM) that was consistently abnormal. Five of the 11 cases had abnormal SSI–ICM scores in only one ear and the remaining six had abnormal scores in both ears. Each of the 11 cases had an abnormal score on the ear contralateral to the tumor locale. Furthermore, in the six cases with bilaterally abnormal SSI–ICM scores, the contralateral ear was always poorer than the ipsilateral. The SSI–CCM condition, however, was considerably less powerful in identifying the interaxial tumors. Eight of the 11 cases had SSI–CCM scores that ranged from 90 to 100 percent across the MCRs. In the three cases for which the SSI–CCM was abnormal, the abnormal score was recorded by the ear contralateral to the side of the tumor.

In a following publication, Jerger and Jerger (1975a) studied ten cases with interaxial brainstem lesions and ten cases with temporal lobe lesions. Again, the interaxial brainstem cases showed abnormal performance on the SSI–ICM in the ear contralateral to the lesion. For these brainstem cases, the SSI–CCM scores were bilaterally normal. The series of ten temporal lobe lesion cases performed, as a group, in a predictable manner, as these cases showed abnormal SSI–ICM scores bilaterally, while the SSI–CCM scores were abnormal in the ear contralateral to the involved hemisphere.

Based on the above reports, the SSI using the ICM and CCM conditions is capable of identifying lesions of the brainstem and lesions of the temporal lobe. Unfortunately, the procedure does not appear to be in wide use, which results in limited clinical information. If the Jergers' preliminary data are borne out with additional clinical cases, the SSI will be a potent identifier of CANS lesions, particularly those affecting the brainstem.

Competing Sentence Test

Willeford (1968; 1978) has developed sentence materials aimed at CANS assessment at the cortical level. The Competing Sentence Test (CST) utilizes "real sentences" presented in a dichotic mode with an

Table 8-15
Sample CST Natural Sentences

Primary (35 dB SL)	Competing (50 dB SL)
My brother is a tall boy.	Your mother is a good cook.
The roast beef is very good.	Please pass the salt and pepper.
I was late to work today.	This watch keeps good time.

From Willeford, J. A. Competing sentences for diagnostic purposes. Unpublished paper, 1968. With permission.

open-set response format. Natural or real sentences were selected as stimuli by Willeford in hopes that these materials could be used to assess an individual's decoding capacity for spoken language. Each sentence was constructed to minimize the listener's ability to decode the whole sentence based on the correct perception of a single key word. Table 8-15 contains samples of these CST sentences. For clinical usage, these "natural sentences" are presented in a simultaneous mode with the "primary message" presented at 35 dB SL re: pure-tone average to one ear and the "competing message" at 50 dB SL re: pure-tone average to the contralateral ear. Subjects are instructed to ignore the "competing message" but to attune to the "primary message." Normally, the test protocol includes 25 presentations per ear. List equivalency between the "primary sentences" and the "competing message" has been demonstrated (Ivey, 1969). In addition, Ivey showed these sentence materials and test paradigms produce identification scores of 98 percent or greater in normal-hearing adults, Lynn and Gilroy (1977) have confirmed the high identification potential of the CST with 20 normal-hearing subjects, who all scored 100 percent.

Lynn and Gilroy, in a series of publications (Lynn & Gilroy, 1972; Lynn & Gilroy, 1975a; Lynn & Gilroy, 1975b; Lynn & Gilroy, 1977) have shared their experience with the CST materials. They have demonstrated that the CST produce distinctly different results in cases with posterior temporal lobe tumors as opposed to cases with anterior/inferior temporal lobe tumors (Lynn & Gilroy, 1975). Table 8-16 summarizes the Lynn and Gilroy CST data obtained from ten cases with posterior temporal lobe tumors and from six cases of anterior/inferior temporal lobe tumors. Within the posterior temporal lobe group, six cases achieved 100 percent identification scores in the ipsilateral ear while being unable to identify any of the CST sentences in the contralateral ear. Only one case produced normal bilateral scores. Two cases, however, showed the greatest score reduction on the ipsilateral ear, which was the left ear. Both of the above two cases had deep temporal lobe tumors that impinged upon the interhemispheric pathways; recall that these types of lesions had produced "left ear effects" on the SSW test. Again, lesions of the anterior/inferior

Table 8-16
Approximate Means and Ranges of CST Scores for Ten Patients With Posterior Temporal Lobe Tumors and Six Patients With Anterior/Inferior Temporal Lobe Tumors

	Posterior Temporal		Anterior/Inferior Temporal	
	Ipsi Ear	Contra Ear	Ipsi Ear	Contra Ear
Mean	84.0	33.0	100	96.7
Range	0–100	0–100	100	90–100

Adapted from Lynn, G. E., & Gilroy, J. Effects of brain lesions on the perception of monotic and dichotic speech stimuli. In M. Sullivan (Ed.), *Proceedings of a symposium on central auditory processing disorders*. Omaha: University of Nebraska Press, 1975, pp. 47–83.

temporal lobe produce essentially symmetrical scores within normal limits. In a later publication, Lynn and Gilroy (1975) presented additional data on a sample of 22 temporal lobe cases. Each of these 22 cases achieved an ipsilateral ear score of 100 percent and a significantly (.01 level) reduced contralateral ear score. In a larger sample of 35 temporal lobe patients, Lynn and Gilroy (1977) report abnormal CST scores in the contralateral ear of 57 percent of these cases, and in the ipsilateral ear of only six percent of the cases. Thirty-eight percent of the cases had normal contralateral ear scores.

Parietal lobe tumors produced the previously discussed "left ear effect" on the CST. Lynn and Gilroy's series of 24 parietal lobe tumors, 14 right and 10 left hemisphere, had significantly (.05 level) poorer left ear scores, regardless of the involved hemisphere. The mean right ear scores were approximately 90 percent, while the mean left ear score was no better than 60 percent. In the parietal lobe cases studied by Lynn and Gilroy, 48 percent had poorer left ear scores on the CST and only four percent of these cases demonstrating abnormal right ear scores. Forty-eight percent of this parietal lobe tumor sample had bilateral normal scores. Thus, the CST is sensitive to lesions in the posterior temporal lobe, which are represented by the contralateral ear effect. Lesions of the anterior/inferior temporal lobe, however, are not disruptive to the processing of CST materials. Furthermore, deep parietal lobe lesions affect interhemisphere transmission, and the lesions are mirrored in a left ear effect or may produce equivocal findings on the CST.

SUMMARY

Although speech audiometry protocols have played and will continue to play a major role in the assessment of CANS integrity, the procedures are not infallible and vary in their sensitivity to the level of the lesion within the CANS. Traditional monosyllabic word tests lack the inherent composition to independently determine if further testing or a battery of special tests, is necessary for an individual who may have CANS dysfunction at the cortical level. Any given case can present essentially normal hearing for pure-tone and spondaic word stimuli with speech discrimination scores for monosyllable materials of 98 percent and 92 percent. Such an audiometric profile would, on the average, go unnoticed. Katz (1978) has shown that a five percent difference in speech discrimination scores between ears was significant in cases with posterior temporal lobe lesions. The illustration case has a six percent ear difference and intelligibility scores that are within normal limits. Clearly, additional research is needed to improve the sensitivity of this basic audiometric measure. To this end, Jerger and Hays (1977) have recommended that PI–PB and PI–SSI functions be obtained in order to use the PI relationship between the two speech recognition measures as additional diagnostic information. These authors show a case with a temporal lobe tumor in which the easier SSI materials produce a PI function that consistently remains below the PI–PB function. Obviously, time constraints in a clinical setting often preclude the possibility of obtaining complete PI functions for every patient, but the effort to improve the potency of a basic audiometric measure is well placed.

Another area in need of additional research is the effect of cochlear involvement on CANS tests. Katz advocates the subtraction of the amount of monosyllabic word error from the raw SSW score in order to provide some degree of correction for cochlear distortion. Lynn and Gilroy believe that reduced speech intelligibility scores in CANS cases result from multiple factors and not simply from cochlear distortion. Thus, these investigators argue against a correction factor for intelligibility errors. Recently, Miltenberger, Dawson, and Raica (1978) evaluated 70 subjects with varying degrees of sensorineural hearing loss and pure-tone configuration on four CANS procedures: (1) CST; (2) low-pass filtered monosyllables; (3) binaural fusion procedure; and (4) RASP. Fifty-four (77 percent) of the 70 subjects produced abnormal scores on one or more of the four CANS tests, a sobering commentary on the contaminating effects of sensorineural hearing loss on these CANS tests. Unfortunately, the SSW was not administered to these 70 subjects.

The single most consistent finding is the contralateral ear effect in cases with lesions of the posterior temporal lobe. Even this contralateral ear effect, if the ear in question is the left ear, can be equivocal, as both lesions of the right temporal lobe and lesions of the corpus callosum are reflected in the performance of the left ear. In an attempt to settle this quandry, Katz has developed a test based on the premise that nonlinguistic auditory stimuli is decoded in the non-dominant hemisphere for speech

Table 8-17
Test Procedures According to the Level Within the CANS at Which They Are Independent Indicators of Dysfunction

CANS Level	Tests
Low brainstem	1. Binaural Fusion 2. SSI–ICM 3. RASP 4. MLD 5. PB Rollover
High brainstem	1. Binaural Fusion 2. MLD 3. SSI–ICM
Hemisphere	1. SSW 2. CST 3. Low pass monosyllables 4. Compression speech 5. SSI–CCM 6. Rush Hughes–PB Difference 7. Dichotic CVs 8. CES*
Interhemispheric	1. SSW 2. CST 3. CES*

*Katz's Competing Environmental Sound Test

and language. The Competing Environmental Sound (CES) test is presently undergoing further clinical study.

On balance, speech audiometry protocols designed for CANS assessment have demonstrated themselves capable of identifying dysfunction within the CANS. Table 8-17 provides a summary of the CANS protocols reviewed in this chapter. Each test is listed according to the anatomical level within the CANS at which it is diagnostically sensitive when viewed as an independent indicator. Granted, no single test should be used in isolation; however, the potency of any diagnostic test is to some degree related to its ability to independently determine the presence or absence of a disorder. With this criteria as a guide, the CANS test versus anatomical levels pairings were made.

Much of the controversy surrounding the CANS protocols presented in Table 8-17 will surely be resolved in the next decade as the ranks of "neuro-audiologists" grow. Certainly, the significant lack of detailed neurological information that in the past accompanied clinical reports of CANS dysfunction has changed, as this type of vagueness does not suffice in the age of CAT scans, etc. The efforts of the Jergers, Katz, and Lynn and Gilroy exemplify the tone of the future. Brainstem evoked response (BSER) is beginning to show promise as a procedure for identifying lesions of the CANS brainstem complex. However, BSER emergence does not necessarily signal the end of speech protocol development aimed at CANS brainstem lesions. Correlative studies between BSER and CANS tests results can only lead to further refinement of CANS speech protocols. Furthermore, the sheer cost differential between the hardware necessary for auditory electrophysiology and the software of the CANS speech protocol tapes is sufficient motivation for continued research and development of appropriate techniques utilizing speech stimuli.

REFERENCES

Beasley, D. S., Schwimmer, S., & Rintelmann, W. F. Intelligibility of time-compressed CNC monosyllables, *Journal of Speech and Hearing Research,* 1972a, *15,* 340–350.

Beasley, D., Forman, B., & Rintelmann, W. Perception of time-compressed CNC monosyllables by normal listeners. *Journal of Auditory Research, 1972b, 12,* 71–75.

Berlin, C. I., Chase, R. A., Dill, A., & Hagepanos, T. Auditory findings in patients with temporal lobectomies. Paper given before the American Speech and Hearing Association, Chicago, Illinois, 1965.

Bocca, E. Clinical aspects of cortical deafness, *Laryngoscope,* 1958, *68,* 301–309.

Bocca, E., Calearo, C., & Cassinari, V. A new method for testing hearing in temporal lobe tumors. *Acta Otolaryngologica,* 1954, *44,* 219–221.

Bocca, E., Calearo, C., Cassinari, V., & Migliavacca, F. Testing "cortical" hearing in temporal lobe tumors. *Acta Otolaryngologica,* 1955, *45,* 289–304.

Brunt, M. The Staggered Spondaic Word Test. In J. Katz (Ed.), *Handbook of clinical audiology,* Baltimore: Williams & Wilkins, 1972, pp. 334–356.

Brunt, M. The Staggered Spondaic Word Test. In J. Katz (Ed.), *Handbook of clinical audiology* (2nd ed.). Baltimore: Williams & Wilkins, 1978, pp 262–275.

Calearo, C., & Lazzaroni, A. Speech intelligibility in relation to the speed of the message, *Laryngoscope,* 1957, *67,* 410–419.

Campbell, R. Discrimination word difficulty. *Journal of Speech and Hearing Research,* 1965, *8* 13–22.

Carhart, R. Special hearing tests for otoneurologic diagnosis. *Archives of Otolaryngology,* 1969, *89,* 64–67.

Carhart, R., Fillman, T. W., & Dallos, P.J. Unmasking for pure tones and spondees: Interaural phase and time disparities. *Journal of Speech and Hearing Research,* 1968, *11,* 722–734.

Cullen, J. K., & Thompson, C. L. Masking release for speech in subjects with temporal lobe resection. *Archives of Otolaryngology,* 1974, *100,* 113–116.

Fairbanks, G., Everitt, W. L., & Jaeger, R. P. Methods for time or frequency compression–expansion of speech. Transactions of *I.R.E.-P.G.A.* AU-2, 1954: pp. 7–12.

Galaburda, A. M., Sanides, F., & Geschwind, N. Human brain: Cytoarchitectonic left–right asymmetrics in the temporal lobe. *Archives of Neurology,* 1978, *35,* 812–817.

Geschwind, N., & Levitsky, W. Human brain: Left–right asymmetries in temporal speech region. *Science,* 1968, *161,* 186–187.

Gilroy, J., & Lynn, G. E. Reversibility of abnormal auditory findings in cerebral hemisphere lesions. *Journal of the Neurological Sciences,* 1974, *21,* 117–131.

Goetzinger, C. P., & Rousey, C. L. Hearing problems in later life. *Medical Times,* 1959, *87,* 771–780.

Goetzinger, C. P., & Anglell, S. Audiological assessment in acoustic tumors and cortical lesions. *Eye, Ear, Nose and Throat Monthly,* 1965, *44,* 39–49.

Goldstein, R., Goodman, A., & King, R. Hearing and speech in infantile hemiplegia before and after left hemispherectomy. *Neurology,* 1956, *6,* 869–875.

Hayashi, R., Ohta, F., & Morimoto, M.. Binaural fusion test: a diagnostic approach to the central auditory disorders. *International Audiology,* 1966, *5,* 133–135.

Hodgson, W. R. Audiological report of a patient with left hemispherectomy. *Journal of Speech and Hearing Disorders,* 1967, *32,* 39–45.

Ivey, R. G. Tests of CNS auditory function. Unpublished master's thesis, Colorado State University. 1969.

Jerger, J. Observations on auditory behavior in lesions of the central auditory pathways. *Archives of Otolaryngology,* 1960a, 71, 797–806.

Jerger, J. Audiological manifestations of lesions in the auditory nervous system. *Laryngoscope,* 1960b, *70,* 417–425.

Jerger, J. Auditory tests for disorders of the central auditory mechanism. In W. Fields & B. Alford, (Eds.), *Neurological aspects of auditory and vestibular disorders.* Springfield, Illinois: Charles C. Thomas, 1964, pp. 77–93.

Jerger, J. Diagnostic Audiometry. In J. Jerger (Ed.), *Modern developments in audiology.* New York: Academic Press, 1973, pp. 75–115.

Jerger, J., & Jerger, S. Diagnostic significance of PB word functions. *Archives of Otolaryngology,* 1971, *93,* 573–580.

Jerger, J., & Jerger, S. Auditory findings in brain stem disorders. *Archives of Otolarynogology,* 1974, *99,* 342–350.

Jerger, J., & Jerger, S. Clinical validity of central auditory tests. *Scandanavian Audiology,* 1975a, *4,* 147–163.

Jerger, S., & Jerger, J. Extra-and intra-axial brain stem disorders. *Audiology,* 1975b, *14,* 93–117.

Jerger, J., Speaks, C., & Trammel, J. A new approach to speech audiometry. *Journal of Speech and Hearing Disorders,* 1968, *33,* 318–327.

Katz, J. The use of staggered spondaic words for assessing the integrity of the central auditory nervous system. *Journal of Auditory Research,* 1962, *2,* 327–337.

Katz, J. The SSW test—an interim report. *Journal of Speech and Hearing Disorders,* 1968, *33,* 132–146.

Katz, J. *The SSW test manual.* St. Louis: Auditec of St. Louis, 1977.

Katz, J., The staggered spondaic word test. In R. Keith (Ed.), *Central auditory dysfunction.* New York: Grune and Stratton, 1977, pp. 103–121.Katz, J. Clinical use of central auditory tests. In J. Katz (Ed.), *Handbook of clinical audiology* (2nd ed.). Baltimore: Williams & Wilkins, 1978, pp. 233–243.

Katz, J., & Pack, G. New developments in differential diagnosis using the SSW test. In M. Sullivan (Ed.), *Central auditory processing disorders.* Omaha: University of Nebraska Press, 1974, pp. 85–107.

Keith, R., Synthetic sentence identification. In R. Keith (Ed.), *Central auditory dysfunction,* New York: Grune & Stratton, 1977. pp. 73–101.

Konkle, D., Beasley, D., & Bess, F. Intelligibility of time-altered speech in relation to chronological aging. *Journal of Speech and Hearing Research,* 1977, *20,* 108–115.

Kurdziel, S. A., Rintelmann, W. F., & Beasley, D. Performance of noise-induced hearing-impaired listeners on time-compressed CNC monosyllables. *Journal of the American Audiological Society,* 1975, *1,* 54–60.

Kurdziel, S. A., Noffsinger, D., & Olsen, W. Performance by cortical lesion patients on 40 and 60 percent time-compressed materials. *Journal of the American Audiological Society,* 1976, *2,* 3–7.

Linden, A. Distorted speech and binaural speech resynthesis test. *Acta Otolaryngologica,* 1964, *58,* 32–48.

Lilly, D., & Franzen, R. Reproducing styli for speech audiometry. *Journal of Speech and Hearing Research,* 1968, *11,* 817–824.

Luterman, D. M., Welsh, O. L., & Melrose, J. Responses of aged males to time-altered speech stimuli. *Journal of Speech and Hearing Research,* 1966, *9,* 226–230.

Lynn, G. E., & Gilroy, J. Neuro-audiological abnormalities in patients with temporal lobe tumors. *Journal of the Neurological Sciences,* 1972, *17,* 167–184.

Lynn, G. E., & Gilroy, J. Effects of brain lesions on the perception of monotic and dichotic speech stimuli. In M. Sullivan (Ed.), *Proceedings of a symposium on central auditory processing disorders.* Omaha: University of Nebraska Press, 1975, pp. 47–83.

Lynn, G. E., & Gilroy, J. Central aspects of auditions. In J. L. Northern (Ed.), *Hearing disorders.* Boston: Little, Brown & Co., 1976, pp. 102–116.

Lynn, G., & Gilroy, J. Evaluation of central auditory dysfunction in patients with neurological disorders. In R. Keith (Ed.), *Central auditory dysfunction.* New York: Grune & Stratton, 1972a, pp. 177–218.

Lynn, G. E., Benitez, J. T., Eisenbrey, A. B., Gilroy, J., et al. Neuro-audiological correlates in cerebral hemisphere lesions; temporal and parietal lobe tumors. *Audiology,* 1972, *11,* 115–134.

Margolis, R., & Millin, J. P. An item-difficulty based speech discrimination test. *Journal of Speech and Hearing Research,* 1971, *14,* 865–873.

Matzker, J. Two new methods for the assessment of central auditory functions in cases of brain disease. *Annals of Otology, Rhinology, and Laryngology,* 1959, *68,* 1185–1197.

Miltenberger, G. E., Dawson, G. J., & Raica, A. N. Central auditory testing with peripheral hearing loss. *Archives of Otolaryngology,* 1978, *104,* 11–15.

Noffsinger, D., Olsen, W. O., Carhart, R., et al. Auditory and vestibular aberrations in multiple sclerosis. *Acta Otolaryngologica,* 1972, *303,* 1–63.

Ohta, F., Hayashi, R., & Morimoto, M. Differential diagnosis of retrocochlear deafness; binaural fusion test and binaural separation test. *International Audiology,* 1967, *6,* 58–62.

Olsen, W. O., & Noffsinger, D. Masking level differences for cochlear and brain stem lesions. *Annals of Otology, Rhinology, and Laryngology,* 1976, *85,* 820–825.

Olsen, W. O., Noffsinger, D., & Carhart, R. Masking level differences encountered in clinical populations. *Audiology,* 1976, *15,* 287–301.

Peterson, G. E., & Lehiste, I. Revised CNC lists for auditory tests. *Journal of Speech and Hearing Research,* 1962, *27,* 62–70.

Schoeny, Z. G., & Carhart, R. Effects of unilateral Ménière's disease on masking-level differences. Journal of the Acoustical Society of America, 1971, *50,* 1143–1150.

Shapiro, I. Progression of auditory signs in pontine glioma. *Laryngoscope,* 1969, *79,* 201–212.

Smith, B. B. & Resnick, D. M. An auditory test for assessing brain stem integrity; preliminary report. *Laryngoscope,* 1972, *82,* 414–424.

Speaks, C. & Jerger, J. Method for measurement of speech identification. *Journal of Speech and Hearing Research,* 1965, *8,* 185–194.

Speaks, C., Jerger, J., & Jerger, S. Performance-intensity characteristics of synthetic sentences. *Journal of Speech and Hearing Research,* 1966, *9,* 305–312.

Stevens, J. H. Monosyllabic speech tests. In J. Katz (Ed.), *Handbook of clinical audiology* (2nd ed.). Baltimore: Williams & Wilkins, 1978, pp. 244–251.

Sticht, T. G., & Gray, B. B. The intelligibility of time-compressed words as a function of age and hearing loss. *Journal of Speech and Hearing Research,* 1969, *12,* 443–448.
Wada, J., Clarke, R., & Hamm, A. Cerebral hemispheric asymmetry in humans. *Archives of Neurology,* 1975, *32,* 239–246.
Willeford, J. A. Sentence tests of central auditory dysfunction. J. Katz (Ed.), *Handbook of clinical audiology* (2nd ed.) Baltimore: Williams & Wilkins, 1978, pp. 252–261.
Willeford, J. A. Competing sentences for diagnostic purposes. Unpublished paper, 1968.

Thomas F. Hemeyer, Ph. D.

9

Speech Protocols in Determining Dynamic Range

The purpose of this chapter is to discuss dynamic range. Several other measures involved in the determination of dynamic range, or closely related to the concept of dynamic range, will also be discussed. The chapter will be divided into three main sections: (1) identification, definition, and explanation of the concepts to be discussed; (2) discussion of clinical methods used to determine the measures involved; and (3) consideration of the clinical and rehabilitative application of the concepts and measures discussed.

IDENTIFICATION AND EXPLANATION OF RELEVANT CONCEPTS

Dynamic Range

Dynamic range (DR) can be defined as the usable range of hearing with respect to intensity. This concept is usually applied to the understanding of speech, and thus the definition might be stated in a more limited sense as the usable range of hearing with respect to speech. An operational definition of DR would be the intensity range between a person's spondee threshold (ST) and his or her tolerance level (TL) (alternate names for TL will be indicated later).

The DR can be expressed as a decibel (dB) range, as from 50 dB HL (ST) to 100 dB HL (TL). It can also be expressed as a single dB notation that indicates the intensity range involved: TL − ST = DR. In the example cited, this would be 100 dB HL (TL) – 50 dB HL (ST) = 50 dB DR. The latter method of citing a person's DR is probably more common.

The rationale behind DR is not at all profound. It is assumed that a person's ST represents the lowest intensity level at which a person can understand speech. Any speech signal less intense than the ST is considered below that person's usable range of intensity for the understanding of speech. It is also assumed that any speech stimuli presented above a person's TL is so loud that the person will also find it not usable (and probably take whatever steps are necessary to see that it is discontinued). The person's usable range of hearing, or DR, is thus the range from his or her ST to his or her TL.

Norms for the DR of normal hearers will be dependent upon the norms for their STs and TLs. If the customary use of the 0–25 dB HL range as normal hearing is used (a practice the author does not endorse, but will use here), then normal hearers' STs can occur anywhere from 0–25 dB HL. It is assumed that testing will not be done below 0 dB HL.

Norms for speech TLs, which will be discussed more fully under the TL heading, range from about 80–110 dB HL (Davis, 1946; Dudich et al., 1975; Hemeyer & Rupp, 1970: McElhone, 1971; Olson & Hipskind, 1973; Schmitz, 1969; Stephens & Anderson, 1971). A typical TL might be indicated as 100 dB HL.

The typical DR would then be about 100 dB (ST = 0 dB HL; TL = 100 dB HL). The minimum normal DR would be about 55 dB (ST = 25 dB HL, TL = 80 dB HL). The maximum normal DR would be about 110 dB (ST = 0 dB HL; TL = 110 dB HL). It should be noted, however, that the ranges indicated are based on averaged data. Even in a normal population, ranges may exceed those indicated, particularly at the upper limits. TLs in excess of 120 dB HL are cited in the literature (McElhone, 1971), and clinical experience sometimes reveal TLs in excess of 100 dB HL.

It should also be noted that the only reason a DR of 55 dB might be considered normal is because a hearing level of 25 dB HL is usually considered normal. A DR as narrow as 55 dB is really atypically small. In general, it would be helpful to think of a normal DR as about 100 dB; the further one moves from this size DR, the more atypical a person becomes (although the limits of "normal" are wide).

Tolerance Level

Of all audiological measures commonly obtained in clinical practice, perhaps none are subject to greater variation due to clinician differences in definition and testing procedure than TL and the most comfortable loudness level (MCL). In the following discussion of TL, a definition preferred by this author will first be given, then alternate terminology will be discussed.

TL can be defined as the intensity level at which a person first finds a sound (in this case speech) to be intolerably loud. It is the level above which a person cannot stand to listen to a sound. It is not necessarily, nor likely, the same as a person's threshold of pain (or TP, the intensity level at which a person experiences pain); TL would be below TP. TL is also not necessarily, nor likely (in the author's opinion) the same as the level at which a person first feels that a sound is louder than he or she would choose to listen to it over a prolonged period of time. TL would be higher than the point where a sound is first louder than ideal.

Considerable variation exists in the definitions and names applied to the TL concept. Unfortunately, the variations in definitions and names do not usually relate meaningfully to each other. Two audiologists might use the same label, but each may have a quite different definition. On the other hand, two audiologists might use different labels but have quite identical definitions.

Some of the terms used are uncomfortable loudness level (UCL or ULL), loudness discomfort level (LDL), threshold of discomfort (TD), discomfort level (DL), and tolerance level (TL). The first two listed (UCL and LDL) are probably most commonly used.

Definitions of TL (or whatever the term used may be) are also variable, as evidenced by instructions given to patients. They range from an intensity level that is louder than one would choose to listen to for some length of time (Dudich et al., 1975) to an intensity level where any additional increase will be intolerable (Martin, 1975). The variations in definitions are reflected in the range of average TLs obtained as cited under DR.

Actually, as was the case with bone conduction symbols, it is probably as important to establish some uniformity as it is to adopt any "correct" definition or terminology. If either logic or clinician preference strongly favored one term or one definition, the variability would not likely exist. Here, the author can only indicate the nature of the situation and proceed to use the term and definition he prefers. An alternate term and definition will be given reflecting an alternate approach.

This author prefers TL because it seems to have a more concrete definition and its terminology seems to more clearly indicate that the upper limit of usable hearing is what is wanted. Consistency does exist that the DR is the range from a person's ST to some measure of the limit of usable hearing (as TL, UCL, LDL, or TD). If a person's most comfortable loudness level (MCL) is 50 dB HL, then theoretically 55 or 60 dB HL would be above the level he or she would *choose* to listen to for some length of time. Yet it does not appear that a 55 or 60 dB HL response is what the clinician wants or gets when using the "choose to listen to" definition.

TL was defined in the first paragraph of this section of the chapter. An alternate term and definition might be UCL (selected because it is commonly used and parallels MCL): the intensity level at which a person first finds a sound louder that he would care to listen to for some length of time, that is, uncomfortably loud.

Since the various terms used for the upper limit of the DR have not previously been systematically differentiated, the norms that were given for TL (DR section) were given without differentiation with respect to terminology used (TL, UCL, ULL, LDL, TD, DL). Throughout this chapter, the notation TL is used even when summarizing literature where alternate names have been employed. The reader will recall a TL of 100 dB HL was suggested as typical, but a range from 80–110 or 80–110+ dB considered normal.

If the term and definition used for the upper limit of the DR suggested in this chapter were adopted (i.e., TL), the norms for TL would change from *averages* from 80–110 dB HL to *averages* more like 100 dB HL. It is expected that some normal-hearing people would still achieve a TL of 80 dB HL, but that this would now be the lower limit of normal rather than an average for any normal-hearing group.

Most Comfortable Loudness Level, Most Comfortable Loudness Range

An intensity level within the DR that is often obtained and that is helpful to know is the listener's MCL. MCL measures are also subject to lack of standardization. In the case of MCL, however, the terminology and the basic concept and definition have been quite uniform, at least until recently, but variability has arisen in actual testing procedure. Although testing procedures are dealt with in a subsequent section of the chapter, it is necessary to discuss first some aspects of testing procedures in order to adequately cover the concept of MCL.

MCL can be defined as the intensity level at which a person would most like to listen to speech. This definition, at least in terms of the concept expressed, is widely accepted. Variability in MCLs obtained is seen, however, when results from three testing procedures are compared. The methods are ascending method, descending method, and bracketing with forced comparisons.

Variations related to use of an ascending and descending method are best illustrated in a study done by Ventry and Johnson (1978). In this study, an ascending versus a descending approach to MCL determination was compared in 100 subjects with sensorineural hearing losses. In the ascending method, the instructions were: "As soon as the words become loud enough to be most comfortable to listen to, raise your finger . . .." In the descending method, the instructions were: "As soon as the words become soft enough to be most comfortable to listen to, raise your finger . . .." Test–retest data was collected for both methods to check on reliability.

The mean results from the ascending method were 62.8 dB HL (retest, 60.4 dB HL). The mean results from the descending method were 83.0 dB HL (retest, 83.4 dB HL). While both methods produced consistent results, the results produced by each method were markedly different.

A third approach in determining MCLs is a bracketing approach where the patient is given two intensity levels to compare (such as 40 dB and 50 dB) and asked which he or she prefers. Based on the patient's response (assuming 50 dB is preferred to 40 dB), additional pairs are presented (as 50 dB and 60 dB) until an MCL is determined (Hemeyer & Rupp, 1970). In this procedure, 5 dB steps (or even less) might be used instead of 10 dB steps. While this method has not been carefully compared to the ascending and descending method discussed above, it appears that it would yield results somewhere between the ascending and descending approach. (Results from Smith & Rupp, 1973, and McCarthy, 1977, seem to support this conclusion.)

Citing marked fluctuations in MCL results even prior to the Ventry and Johnson study, Berger (1971), Berger and Lowry (1971), and Smith and Rupp (1973) suggested that MCL might more realistically be considered in terms of a most comfortable loudness range rather than an MCL. Smith and Rupp's rationale was stated as follows:

> Considering MCL variability and the possibility that by requiring the patient to make a subjective determination of one MCL, we may be disregarding the complex flexibility of the hearing mechanism and psychological set of the patient in an attempt to report a single clinical measure. It would seem more realistic if this variability was initially recognized as a range (i.e., MCL-Range) so that we could examine a possible range of intensity spread rather than only generalize it as a single intensity value.

The concept of MCR appears to have merit and appears to be gaining in popularity. It appears to offer excellent potential for site of lesion differentiation (to be discussed later). MCR can be defined as an intensity range within which a person is able to listen comfortably to speech. The lower limit (less intense limit) of the MCR might be given the acronym LLMCR and defined as the lowest intensity at which a person is comfortable listening to speech. The upper limit (more intense limit) of the MCR might be given the acronym ULMCR, and defined as the highest intensity level at which a person is comfortable listening to speech.

It should be noted that terminology viewing the MCL as a range occurred prior to the Berger (1971), Berger and Lowry (1971), and Smith and Rupp (1973) references cited previously. The concept referred to was different, however. Watson (1944), for example, who is often credited as the first person to identify and discuss the MCL concept, used the term "range of comfortable loudness" (RCL). He defined RCL as we currently define DR; that is, the range between the "level at which conversational voice can be repeated and the point at which it becomes disagreeably loud and painful." Bangs and Mullins (1953) use the terminology RCL to mean the range from a person's MCL to his or her TL. McCarthy (1977) uses the term comfortable loudness range (CLR) to mean the area from the minimum comfortable intensity to the TL.

Even when Berger (1971) and Berger and Lowry (1971) suggest the term MCR, they do not specify it quite as rigidly as it has been defined here, although the concept appears similar. They really indicate the measure we call MCL should be labelled MCR because of its variability. The concept of MCR as defined in this chapter is most like that used by Smith and Rupp (1973) and by Jerger and Jerger (1974). The latter investigators used only pure tones.

Again, it is not clear what terminology is most logical or "correct." The terms employed in this chapter allow reference to any of the ranges indicated above. Watson's RCL equals the current DR. Bangs and Mullins's RCL equals the range from the current MCL to the TL. McCarthy's CLR equals the range from LLMCR to TL.

The norms for the speech MCL of normal hearers range from about 30 dB HL (Ventry et al., 1971) to 55 dB HL (Dudich et al., 1975). These norms represent averages and individual normal-hearing subjects might well obtain higher or lower MCLs. It appears that 40–50 dB HL is probably a good average to associate with MCL of speech for normal hearers.

The amount of work done with MCR with normal-hearing subjects is quite limited and norms can be tentative at best. Based on data from Smith and Rupp (1973), the range of an average MCR is from approximately 30 dB HL (LLMCR) to about 55 dB HL (ULMCR). This range is precisely that indicated as the range of MCLs from various other studies. Smith and Rupp (1973) found their subjects' MCLs to be closer to their ULMCRs than to their LLMCRs.

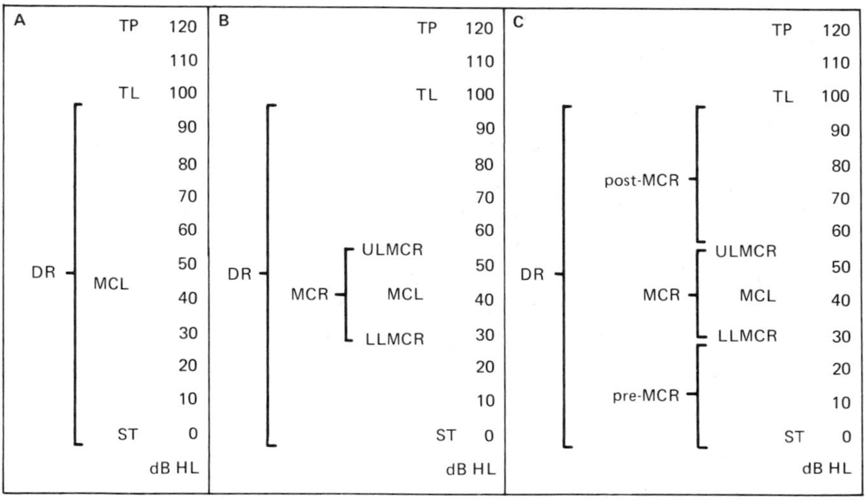

Fig. 9-1. An illustration of DR and related concepts. (A) Traditional DR concepts (DR, SRT, MCL); (B) Traditional DR concepts with MCR added; (C) Same as 1B with pre-MCR and post-MCR added.

Synthesis

Figure 9-1 summarizes DR and related concepts and is broken down into three parts: A, B, and C. The A section summarizes traditional DR terminology. In section B, the concept of MCR is added. In section C, two additional notations are added: pre-MCR and post-MCR.

These final two terms allow identification of each section of the DR. Their definition is quite clear. The pre-MCR is the range between a person's ST and his or her LLMCR. The post-MCR is the range between a person's ULMCR and his or her TL.

The concepts that most directly comprise DR have now been considered. Two additional areas that closely relate to DR will also be discussed before clinical procedures are covered. The two additional areas are recruitment and acoustic reflex. It should also be noted that while the current chapter is concerned with speech, the same terminology, principles, and discussion apply to pure tones as well.

Recruitment

Recruitment is a concept closely associated with DR. Recruitment can be defined as an abnormally small DR. Recruitment can also be defined as an abnormal increase in loudness as a function of suprathreshold increases in intensity. That is, recruitment means loudness grows abnormally fast as the dB level of a sound is increased.

To illustrate recruitment, an example is helpful. Assume a normal-hearing 20-year-old man has an ST of 5 dB HL and a TL for speech of 85 dB HL in both ears. His DR for speech is 85 − 5 = 80. Assume we see this person 20 years later and that he now has 65 dB HL thresholds and ST in the right ear (RE). His left ear (LE) still has a 5 dB ST. His LE DR is still 80 dB. His RE DR is 85 − 65 = 20 dB.

In his healthy LE, this person goes the psychological loudness span from speech just barely intelligible to speech intolerably loud in 80 dB. In his RE he goes the same psychological span in only 20 dB. What takes 80 dB in his LE is compressed to a range of 20 dB in his RE (a marked difference). This means that on the average, each 1 dB increase in intensity in his RE causes the same loudness as each 4 dB increase in intensity in his LE. We can therefore say that loudness in his pathological ear is growing abnormally fast as a function of suprathreshold increases in intensity. This person has recruitment.

In the example just cited, the exclusive cause of recruitment was an elevated threshold level. The DR was reduced from 80 dB in the healthy ear to 20 dB in the pathological ear by a 60 dB drop in threshold. It is important that this fact be noted. It illustrates that even severe recruitment can occur even when no change in TL takes place. Some people have a tendency to assume that recruitment automatically implies a lowered (less intense) TL as compared to normal. While it may in some cases be partially related to a lowered TL, this is definitely not a requisite for recruitment. People can have severe recruitment with normal and even elevated TLs.

Whether or not recruitment in cochlear losses is usually or often accompanied by (i.e., partialy caused by) lowered TLs is an area of dispute. Recruitment can definitely exist with normal TLs. It is disputed whether or not this is the typical case in recruitment or whether TLs are often lowered in addition to the elevation in STs.

While several studies can be cited which relate to the above controversy, two studies will be used to illustrate the problem. Hood and Poole (1966) presented an extensive and frequently cited study on TLs. They used tones rather than speech as stimuli, but the data apply to the principle under discussion. The average TL (LDL) of 100 normal hearing subjects was about 98 dB HL. The average TL of 100 subjects with Meniere's disease (all of whom had recruitment via the ABLB test) was 100 dB HL. Meniere's disease is a cochlear loss where some people feel the TL is particularly affected. Similar results with fewer subjects are available, however, from other studies where sensorineural losses were not confined to Meniere's. It can be seen that based on Hood and Poole's results, TLs seem not to be changed by cochlear losses.

In marked contrast to the Hood and Poole study is a study by Schmitz (1969). Schmitz determined TLs (LDL, the same terminology used by Hood & Poole) for 20 normal and 20 sensorineural (cochlear) loss subjects. While mean TLs were not reported because so many of the normal-hearers' TLs exceeded equipment output limitations, the data are clear: "Seventy percent of the normal subjects had an LDL at or above 120 dB SPL, whereas 90 percent of the pathological subjects had LDL's below 108 dB." Schmitz used speech stimuli, but the radical difference between the Hood and Poole and the Schmitz findings cannot seemingly be accounted for on that basis. Similar discrepancies exist in the literature with similar stimuli.

It is also interesting to note that Hood and Poole used subjects with unilateral Meniere's disease, whereas Schmitz used subjects with bilateral cochlear losses. Again, however, a review of other studies suggest this is not a crucial difference regarding the contradictory results obtained.

The above illustrates, in dramatic fashion, why it is not clear what happens to TLs in people with cochlear losses. The Hood and Poole data are impressive in view of the large number of subjects they used. Also in support of the Hood and Poole conclusion, and the contention that TLs are not usually significantly reduced in cochlear losses, is the observation that hyper-recruitment is often not even included as a typical ABLB outcome (as in Carver, 1978). Hyper-recruitment should occur in unilateral cochlear cases where TLs are significantly lowered. The seeming lack of a need for a hyper-recruitment category seems to suggest it does not frequently occur to a significant extent.

With respect to TLs in people with cochlear losses, the author is inclined to agree with McCandless (1976): "In most subjects, especially those with cochlear pathology, the upper usable tolerance limits (functional tolerance thresholds) are about the same as in the normal ear." It is also interesting to note in this statement that where McCandless seeks terminology to reflect the upper limit of the DR, he relies on "tolerance"-related terminology.

In the section on DR, normal DRs were indicated as being anywhere from 55–110 dB or 55–110+ dB. Since recruitment shows up as a reduced DR, any DR less than 55 dB is evidence of recruitment. The narrower the DR, the greater the recruitment. It should be recalled, however, that an average normal DR of 100 dB was indicated, particularly when the term

TL was used for the determination of the upper end of the DR. A patient having a DR of 60 dB, while falling within normal DR limits, is at a disadvantage as compared to someone having a wider DR.

Acoustic Reflex, Acoustic Reflex Threshold

Several studies have been done comparing the acoustic reflex threshold (ART) to TLs or MCLs. While pure tones or noise have usually been the stimuli used, since the ART as compared to TLs has received so much attention, this area of investigation will be summarized here. While it is beyond the scope of this chapter to thoroughly discuss the acoustic reflex (AR), it will be defined and its relationship to TLs and MCLs considered.

The AR, used synonomously with stapedial reflex, is a bilateral contraction of the stapedius muscles in response to moderately intense and intense auditory stimuli. The lowest intensity which initiates an AR in normal-hearing subjects is usually somewhere between 70 and 100 dB HL (median = 82.2 dB HL) (Northern, 1975). The purpose of the AR is not clear; several theories have been proposed. The more popular and traditional theories indicate the AR serves some type of protective function.

The relationship between the ARTs and TLs for both tones and speech varies, depending upon the study one examines. Some representative results from various studies will be cited to illustrate the variation. Berger et al. (1979), Niemeyer (1971), and Olson and Hipskind (1973) all found ARTs to occur, on the average, below TLs (by about 13, 10–20, and 4–8 dB, respectively). Dudich et al. (1975) and Kallstrom and Carstensen (1978) found TLs to occur, on the average, below ARTs (by about 8 and 5 dB, respectively). McCandless (1976) and McCandless and Miller (1972) conclude that ARTs and TLs are in very good agreement with each other. Beedle and Harford (1973) and Berger et al. (1979) conclude that ARTs and TLs are not in very good agreement, and that trying to predict TLs from ARTs, or vice versa, is extremely hazardous. Berger et al. (1979) did bring out a point worth menioning: average ARTs and TLs may be similar, but this does not mean they correlate. Indications of correlations in ART versus TL studies are not common.

With respect to the relationship between ARTs and MCLs, the situation is less confusing (because fewer studies have been done), but not much more enlightening. While MCLs consistently occur below ARTs (Dudich et al., 1975; Preves & Orton, 1978), correlation coefficients are not indicated to demonstrate to what extent these measures vary in a correlated manner.

Perhaps if the conflicting results cited above demonstrate anything, they demonstrate the need for more uniform definitions and testing procedures in the area of TLs. The results suggest TLs and ARTs occur in the same general intensity range, but the extent to which they correlate is not clear.

CLINICAL METHODS

Dynamic Range

Since DR was defined as a person's TL minus the ST, clinical methods for obtaining the DR are those involved in the methods used to obtain STs and TLs. Procedures for determining STs were covered in chapter 4 and will not be reviewed here. It will suffice to say here that the first step in obtaining the DR for speech is to obtain a valid ST. The procedure for determining TL will be covered below. Once the TL has been determined, DR = TL − ST.

TL And MCL—MCR: General Considerations

Since some of the clinical procedural considerations in obtaining TL are common to MCL and MCR, some of the information at the beginning of this section will apply to both TL and MCL–MCR. Then more specific methods will be indicated for TL and MCL–MCR separately.

It has previously been indicated that standardized procedures have not been established for TL or MCL–MCR testing. Variation that exists might be divided under three headings: Instructions, stimuli, and testing procedures. Each will be considered.

INSTRUCTIONS

The problems with instruction variation are most pronounced with TL determination and relate back to its varying definitions. Unfortunately, little research has been done investigating the effects of test instructions based on alternate definitions. Testing procedures suggested in this chapter will be based on the definitions previously given.

Hochberg (1975) did investigate the effects of instructing subjects to listen for "comfortable speech loudness versus comfortable speech intelligibility" on MCL results. Hochberg found that when instructed to listen for comfortable speech intelligibility subjects chose, on the average, a 4.96 dB higher intensity level than when instructed to listen for comfortable speech loudness.

STIMULI

Even when the focus of attention for TL and MCL–MCR determination is limited to speech, variation exists with respect to speech stimuli used. Connected discourse (cold running speech), questions, PB words, spondee words, and digits have all been used. Both recorded and live-voice stimuli are used. In a clinical setting, the majority (70–73 percent) of audiologists use cold running speech for both MCL and TL determination. The next most frequent stimuli are spondee words (Martin & Pennington, 1971). A recorded version of the John Fulton Lewis, Jr., radio broadcast "Top of the News" is a frequently used cold running speech stimulus.

Little, if any, investigation has taken place to determine if variations in speech stimuli result in different TL or MCL–MCR result. One would expect that variation of this type might not have appreciable effects, although the intensity variations in connected discourse might pose a problem if not controlled.

Schmitz (1969) controlled for intensity variation by using a recorded passage that had no more than ± 2 dB intensity variation on a VU meter and which had all major pauses edited out. This, however, creates a secondary problem in rendering the speech not natural and probably more difficult to understand.

TESTING PROCEDURES

Various psychophysical methods have been used to determine TLs and MCLs: method of limits, method of constant stimuli, method of adjustment, and a Bekesy tracking method. In the method of limits, the examiner adjusts the stimulus based on feedback he receives from the patient. In the method of constant stimuli, the patient must respond (as yes or no) to every stimulus presented; a predetermined number and type of stimuli are usually presented in random order. In the method of adjustment, the patient adjusts the stimulus himself to meet some criteria he has been given. In the Bekesy tracking method, the patient presses the Bekesy control button in keeping with the instructions. The various methods may overlap but they are listed separately because each has been used, labelled as such, in TL or MCL–MCR determination.

Studies investigating procedural effects have not been numerous but some have been done. Morgan et al. (1974) compared three psychophysical methods with respect to TL determination: a programmed method of constant stimuli, a method of adjustment, and a tracking method. They found the method of constant stimuli and the tracking method produced higher (more intense) and more consistent TLs than the method of adjustment. Stephens and Anderson (1971) also obtained higher TLs with a tracking method than they did with a manual method of limits when using naive subjects. The differences were minimal with experienced subjects.

Ventry et al. (1971) compared attenuation rates of 2.5 dB and 1.25 dB on MCL results obtained via a Bekesy tracking method. They found that the 2.5 dB rate produced higher MCLs than the 1.25 dB rate. The size of intensity increments used in a manual method of limits varies among investigators. Increments of 1, 2, 5, and 10 dB have all been used. Stephens and Anderson (1971) compared TLs obtained with 1 and 5 dB steps and found similar results for both size increments.

The procedural effect that seems to produce the most significant variations is that of an ascending versus a descending approach in the method of limits. As was indicated earlier, using the Ventry and Johnson (1978) study, an ascending method produces lower MCLs than a descending method. Variations with respect to this variable can be very large, as the 62.8 dB (ascending) versus 83.0 (descending) variations seen in the Ventry and Johnson study.

With respect to testing procedure, although not related to psychophysical method used, some mention should be made about sound field or free field testing and testing done under earphones. Most research investigations utilize testing done with earphones. In a clinical situation, both earphone and sound or free field testing is conducted, the latter being necessary in aided observations. Stephens and Anderson (1971) report nearly identical monaural TLs in sound field and under earphones (in dB SPL). It would appear that there is no problem in moving from one testing mode to the other as long as one is aware of the binaural sound or free field effect and as long as the sound field speakers are calibrated properly.

This section of the chapter has been a general consideration of variables that might affect TL or MCL–MCR measures. In the next sections, very specific guidelines are included.

TL

The following is offered as a suggested procedure for determining TLs. Below are instructions that should be given to the patient:

> I want to find out how loud you can tolerate speech. I am going to say some words and gradually increase their loudness. If the words should ever become so loud that you feel you could not tolerate them any louder, press the button (or raise your hand, etc.). "Okay?" or "Is that clear?"

Once the instructions have been given, the intensity dial should be set to 70 dB HL or 5 dB above the person's ST, whichever is more intense. The intensity dial should be turned up in 5 dB steps with three spondee words presented at each level. The spondee words should peak the VU meter at 0 dB on each syllable and be said relatively rapidly without long pauses between them.

The intensity at which the person responds should be noted. The intensity dial should then be turned down 15 dB and the procedure repeated. (The patient might be told: "I am going to try that again.") The highest level achieved in three trials should be recorded as the patient's TL.

Spondee words were selected as stimuli because they are readily available and audiologists usually have considerable practice at uttering spondee words at equal intensities. Live voice TL determination is thus facilitated. It is anticipated that in a clinical setting TLs will usually be obtained live voice using a method of adjustment (i.e., the clinician will vary the intensity).

The procedures could easily be adapted for use with recorded words. The clinician could prerecord spondees in groups of three. The author is in the process of preparing and standardizing recordings for the measures covered in this chapter in the event a standardized tape is wanted. If a recorded version is used, the phrase "I am going to say" might be replaced by "you are going to hear."

The procedure could also be modified to permit use of a Bekesy tracking method. Recorded spondees (not grouped in threes) would be used as stimuli and the following instructions used:

> I want to find out how loud you can tolerate speech. You are going to hear some words that will gradually increase in loudness. If the words should ever become so loud that you feel you could not tolerate them any louder, press the button and the words will start getting softer. Once the words are soft enough that you can easily tolerate them, stop pressing the button. When the words again become so loud that you feel you could not tolerate them any louder, press the button. Press the button when the words get too loud to tolerate. Do not press the button when the words can be easily tolerated.

It should be noted that while procedures and instructions are being given for speech stimuli, the same procedures and instructions could be used for tones or noise with the appropriate substitutions made for "speech" or "words" in the instructions.

MCL

The following instructions should be given to the patient:

> I want to find the loudness level where you would most like to listen to speech. I am going to say some words at two loudness levels and I want you to tell me which one you prefer, level #1 or level #2. You might find that both levels are quite comfortable, but, if possible, please tell me which of the two levels you would prefer. "Okay?" or "Is that clear?"

Start with a presentation level midway between the person's ST and TL (or midway between their ST and 100 dB HL if their TL is not known). For an example, assume a starting level of 50 dB HL. Say: "This is level no. 1: baseball, etc. (three spondee words as in TL determination). Then turn the intensity level down 5 dB (to 45 dB in the example) and say: "This is level no. 2, etc. Which do you prefer?" Based on the response obtained (assume the person preferred 50 dB), proceed to bracket the MCL (in this case 50 versus 55 dB). Alternate between presenting the more intense and the less intense level of a pair first (in the example, 50 versus 45, then 50 versus 55; if needed, it would then be 55 versus 60).

Increments of 5 dB are suggested, although many normal hearers will find it difficult to make judgments this refined and 10 dB steps may be needed. Sensorineural (cochlear) patients, particularly if the loss is pronounced, will find it easier to make judgments, and 5 dB increments should be possible.

A recorded list of spondees, in clusters of three, can be used for recorded MCL determinations (same recording as for TL). For the Bekesy tracking method, an ungrouped recording of spondee words and the following instructions can be used:

> I want to find the loudness level where you would most like to listen to speech. You are going to hear (recorded version instructions) a series of words that will change in their loudness level. When the words get at all louder than the level you would most like to listen to them, press the button. When the words get at all softer than the level you would most like to listen to them, release the button. Use the button to keep the words at the loudness level you like best. Press the button when the words get louder than what you like best; release the button when the words get softer than what you like best.

The midpoint of the Bekesy tracing would be used as the person's MCL.

MCR: LLMCR and ULMCR

To determine the LLMCR use the following instructions:

> I want to find the softest loudness level at which speech is loud enough to be comfortable to you. I am going to say some words. The words will start out very soft and gradually get louder. When the words first get loud enough to be comfortable to you, press the button (or raise your hand).

Start at the person's ST. Use three spondee words at each level. Use 5 dB steps. Once the patient first presses the button, note the intensity level and turn the intensity down 15 dB and repeat the process. Use three trials. If in three trials three different intensity levels are obtained, use the middle level as the LLMCR (as 20, 30, 35, LLMCR = 30). If only two or three intensity levels are obtained, use the most frequently occurring intensity as the LLMCR (as 20, 20, 30, LLMCR = 20).

To determine the ULMCR, use the following instructions:

> I want to determine the loudest level at which speech is still comfortable to you. I am going to say some words that will gradually get louder. When the words first get so loud that they are not comfortable for you to listen to them, press the button (or raise your hand).

Start 10 dB lower than the person's MCL (or 10 dB lower than the estimated MCL if the MCL is not known). Proceed as for LLMCR.

The person's MCR is the range between his or her LLMCR and ULMCR. Once the patient's ST, TL, MCL, and MCR (LLMCR and ULMCR) have been obtained, his or her complete DR function can be indicated as shown in Fig. 9-2.

For Bekesy determination of MCR, use the following instructions:

> I want to determine the loudness range where speech is comfortable to you. You will hear a series of words. When the words first get so loud that they are not comfortable, press the button. Keep the button pressed until the words get so soft that they are not comfortable, then release the button. Press the button when the words get too loud to be comfortable, and release the button when the words get too soft to be comfortable.

The width of the Bekesy excursions represent the person's MCR. The LLMCR is the lowest average intensity level of the Bekesy tracing, and the ULMCR is the highest average intensity level of the Bekesy tracing.

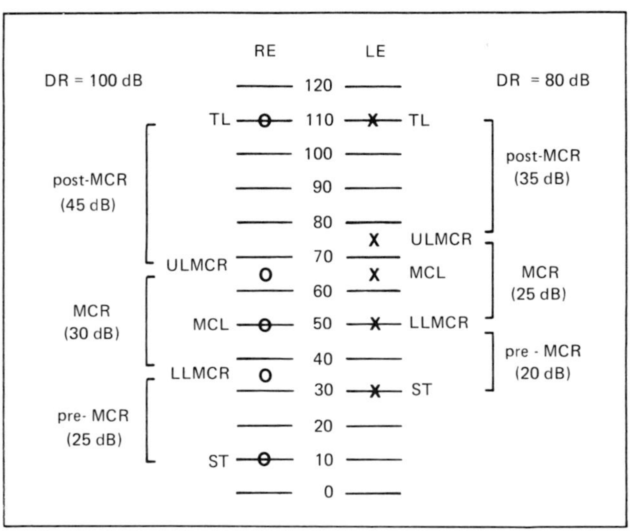

Fig. 9-2. An illustration of how DR and related concepts might be indicated. Right ear has normal hearing; left ear has a mild sensorineural loss. It may also be helpful to include acoustic reflex thresholds.

CLINICAL AND REHABILITATIVE APPLICATION

While the clinical and rehabilitative application of DR and related concepts are topics which are appropriately covered in other chapters (such as Chapter 7 with respect to site of lesion testing and Chapter 12 with respect to hearing aid fitting), a general review of the primary applications of DR and related concepts will also be included here. Applications will be considered in three areas: (1) selection of discrimination test presentation levels; (2) site of lesion implications; and (3) hearing aid selection implications. However, before specific applications are discussed some general information regarding the frequency of the use of DR measures among clinical audiologists will be considered.

Martin and Pennington's 1971 survey of clinical audiologists indicated 21.6 percent of the audiologists responding determined an MCL for most patients, 13.2 percent determined a TL for most patients, and 5.4 percent calculated a DR for most patients. For hearing aid candidates, 41.6 percent determined an MCL; 44.7 percent, TL, and 34.9 percent, DR. The percentage of audiologists who never measured MCL was 22.0 percent; TL, 25.3 percent, and DR, 48.7 percent.

While specific figures are not included for DR measures in Martin and Forbis's 1978 survey, the authors indicated that results for MCL and DR had not changed since 1971, although TL was used more often with hearing aid candidates and less with other patients than it was in 1971.

Discrimination Test Presentation Levels

Results from the two surveys cited above also indicated that 16 percent of the audiologists responding used a patient's MCL as the presentation level to obtain word discrimination scores (WDS). While the MCL has been shown to provide better WDS in some cases than a 40 dB SL presentation rule (Markle & Zaner, 1966), the bulk of research results strongly indicate that an MCL presentation will not always produce the maximum WDS. It appears that if the goal in discrimination testing is to obtain a PB maximum score, then a rule dictating that the MCL always be used as the presentation level is a poor rule.

Actually, no single rule has yet been shown to be adequate for PB max determination. A rule based on TL probably has as much merit as any (as TL minus 10 dB), but the rollover effect indicates that this approach will not work either. Clinicians should be careful, however, that no matter what rule they do use (a 32 dB SL and 40 dB SL approach seems to be gaining in popularity), they take care not to exceed the patient's TL.

TLs should be determined prior to discrimination testing, particularly when intense presentation levels are needed. If a patient has a 70 dB

HL hearing level and his or her loss is cochlear in nature, it is not possible to intelligently decide on a WDS presentation level without obtaining an indication of TL. It is not defensible to try a presentation level of 102 dB HL in this case (32 dB SL) only to find that the patient's TL is 85 dB HL.

Both MCL and TL are helpful in making a decision on WD presentation levels. Unfortunately, it appears from the Martin and Forbis (1978) survey that when MCL and TL are determined they are usually the last measures obtained.

Site of Lesion

When Watson (1944) discussed DR (his terminology was different), he indicated that the DR provided an indication of the presence or absence of recruitment. Bangs and Mullins (1953) indicated that of the four measures of recruitment they compared, the range between a patient's MCL and TL was by far the most discriminating technique.

It can be seen from the above that the use of DR as a possible site of lesion indicator is not a new idea. In spite of the early use of DR as an indicator of recruitment, its current use for that purpose appears not to be widespread in relation to site of lesion (Martin & Pennington, 1971; Martin & Forbis, 1978). Perhaps the reason for the lack of popularity in using DR as a site of lesion indicator lies in the fact that many times patients' TLs are in excess of usual maximum audiometer outputs.

In sensorineural loss patients , a TL within normal limits suggests recruitment and is a cochlear indicator. When the TL does not occur within maximum output limitations, the results are inconclusive. (It should be noted that Hood & Poole, 1966, felt otherwise; they felt that failure to find TLs within typical audiometer outputs was a strong eighth nerve indicator.)

With respect to site of lesion, the DR-related concept that appears to offer appreciable potential, and which is gaining rapidly in popularity, is the MCR rather than the DR. The most poular use appears to be a Bekesy MCR for tones, which Jerger and Jerger 1974 have called Bekesy comfortable loudness (BCL) tracings. Data from Smith and Rupp (1973) and McCarthy (1977) suggest potential for speech and tone MCRs as a site of lesion indicator.

Jerger and Jerger (1974) offer theoretical rationale as to why MCR tracings might be more sensitive to site of lesion differentiation than conventional Bekesy MCR tracings. The results of their study support their theoretical rationale. MCR tracings provided better eighth nerve versus cochlear differentiation than conventional Bekesy tracings. MCR tracings and forward and backward Bekesy threshold tracings were more comparable in their differentiation abilities but the MCR tracings proved more sensitive.

Jerger and Jerger (1974) identified six MCR tracing types, three characteristic of patients having normal hearing or peripheral hearing impairments (N*1*, N*2*, and N*3*), and three characteristic of patients having eithth nerve or brainstem problems (P*1*, P*2*, and P*3*). The reader should consult the Jerger and Jerger article for the specific classifications and the data demonstrating their site of lesion potential.

The clinical potential of Bekesy MCR tracings appears to be reflected in their very rapid adoption as a site of lesion measure. In the 1978 Martin and Forbis survey, about 225 of the audiologists surveyed used Bekesy testing. Ninety-eight of these audiologists used modifications of traditional Bekesy; about half used backward Bekesy (descending frequency) and about half used MCR tracings.

Smith and Rupp (1973) determined MCRs via a manual method of limits for speech and pure-tone stimuli in normal hearing and sensorineural loss (cochlear) patients. The MCRs for the sensorineural group were much smaller than those for the normal group. Data using their approach are needed for eighth nerve patients. It is anticipated that the manual determination of MCR also offers potential as a site of lesion indicator.

Since the AR was discussed earlier, before leaving the site of lesion topic, it should be noted that the AR and ART decay are, of course, popular and extremely useful site of lesion indicators. Specifics of this diagnostic tool are, however, outside the realm of this chapter.

Hearing Aid Fitting

It was obvious from the statistics cited earlier from the Martin and Pennington (1971) and Martin and Forbis (1978) surveys that the most extensive application of DR-related concepts is in the area of hearing aid selection. The use of DR-related concepts in hearing aid selection is both extensive and variable. A comprehensive discussion of the nature and relative merits of various DR approaches, and their relationship to other aid selection approaches, is beyond the scope of this chapter and would require a volume or more by itself. Some general comments are, however, in order.

Perhaps the most important, and probably the most widespread use of a DR concept in hearing aid fitting, is the use of TL to determine hearing aid maximum power output (MPO). If there is one most common single cause of hearing aid candidates not using their hearing aid, it appears to be excessive MPO (McCandless, 1976). Proper use of TL should minimize this occurrence.

Hearing aid selection procedures must take into account the relationship among hearing aid MPO, the patient's TL (and/or ART) and the patient's DR. The MPO of the aid, at every frequency, should be less than the patient's TL at the respective frequencies. The degree that the aid's MPO is less than the TL should be related to the user's DR. The broader the DR, the more the MPO can be reduced from the user's TL. The narrower the DR, the less the MPO can be reduced from the user's TL and the greater the likelihood that compression amplification will be helpful. Both TL and DR are essential considerations in determining MPO.

The importance of TL and DR in MPO selection is particularly important when a comparative approach is used in aid selection (i.e., the patient's scores on various measures are compared for different hearing aids to determine which aid produced the best results). An example will illustrate the point.

Assume a patient has a 50 dB HL hearing level (flat cochlear loss). His results for two aids are as follows: aid A: ST = 15dB, WDS = 84 percent, WDS in noise = 68 percent; aid B: ST = 25 dB, WDS = 72 percent, WDS in noise = 56 percent. Assume both aids were set to a volume judged most comfortably loud with a 50 dB HL sound or free field input. Aid A would be recommended.

Assume we find that the patient's aided TL with aid A is 65 dB HL and his or her tolerance level with aid B is 90+ dB HL. Now if we had to fit the patient with one of these aids, there would be no question that aid B should be the aid of choice. The patient would likely use aid B and find it quite helpful even though it would not solve all his or her communication difficulties. If the patient were fitted with aid A, he or she would not likely use it (except possibly on the "off" setting). Ideally, we would find an aid for the patient that produced the aided TL of B and WDS scores of A.

Unfortunately, while the above example is perhaps extreme, some audiologists might have obtained only the original results and have recommended aid A. No aided TL would have been determined and no careful analysis of MPO versus unaided TL and DR would have taken place. The importance of TL–DR versus MPO considerations in hearing aid selection cannot be stressed too much. Aided TLs should be a routine measure in hearing aid evaluations. Actually, with proper hearing aid fitting procedures, aided TLs need not be lower than unaided TLs and it may even be possible in some instances to allow them to be higher (because of the attenuation characteristics of the earmold and the MPO of the aid).

In the author's opinion, someone who is reasonably competent in the selection of hearing aids on the basis of unaided test results and hearing aid specifications, but who is very aware of TL–DR versus MPO relationships, is far more likely to consistently select satisfactory hearing aids for patients (without ever trying the aid on the patient) than is someone who uses a comparative evaluation procedure but who does not measure aided TLs or carefully consider TL–DR versus MPO relationships. The application of DR-related concepts to hearing aid MPO is a necessity.

With respect to gain and frequency response determination in hearing aid fitting, it appears that prescription type approaches are becoming more popular (Shapiro, 1976; Berger et al., 1977). The popularity of the in-the-ear type hearing aids has encouraged this approach and the low return rates of ITE aids seem to testify to its success. Most prescription type approaches rely heavily on DR-related concepts. The method proposed by Shapiro (1976) particularly illustrates the relationship between DR concepts and hearing aid fitting. In his approach, the gain and frequency response of an aid are based upon the patient's MCLs; the MPO of an aid is based upon the patient's TL.

As indicated at the beginning of this section of the chapter, consideration of specific hearing aid selection approaches is beyond the scope of this chapter. It should be noted, however, that regardless of the method used to select appropriate hearing aids for a patient, in comparative evaluation of hearing aids, the volume at which an aid is set is usually based on the patient's aided MCL (Walden et al., 1977). When this approach is used, the patient is asked to adjust the volume of the hearing aid until a signal presented at a normal conversational intensity level (usually 40–55 dB HL) is comfortably loud.

Walden et al. (1977) evaluated the reliability of the above approach of setting hearing aid volume. They also compared the resulting volume settings to those that patients actually used outside a clinical setting. They found the aided MCL method to be reliable and to produce settings comparable to those actually used in a nonclinical setting (when a 70 dB SPL signal was used for the clinical setting stimulus).

SUMMARY

In this chapter, DR and related concepts (TL, MCL, MCR, LLMCR, ULMCR, pre-MCR, post-MCR, recruitment, and AR) were identified, defined, and explained. The term TL was recommended as the label for the upper limit of the DR. Alternate terminology was indicated. Specific clinical procedures for manual and Bekesy determination of DR-related concepts were given.

Some areas of application of DR concepts were reviewed. It was indicated that DR concepts, particularly MCR, appear to offer potential in site of lesion differentiation. MCR Bekesy tracings appear to be gaining widespread use. It was indicated, however, that the most extensive current application of DR concepts is in the area of hearing aid selection. The importance of considering DR and TL in determining hearing aid MPO was stressed.

REFERENCES

Bangs, J., & Mullins, C. Recruitment testing in hearing and its implications. *Archives of Otolaryngology,* 1953, *58,* 582–592.

Beedle, R., & Harford, E. A comparison of acoustic reflex and loudness growth in normal and pathological ears. *Journal of Speech and Hearing Research,* 1973, *16,* 271–280.

Berger, K. The use of uncomfortable loudness in hearing aid fitting. *Maico Audiological Library Series,* 1976, *15,* Report 2.

Berger, K. Speech audiometry. In D. Rose (Ed.), *Audiological assessment.* Englewood Cliffs, New Jersey: Prentice Hall, 1971.

Berger, K., & Lowry, J. Relationships between various stimuli for MCL. *Sound,* 1971, *5,* 11–14.

Berger, K., Hagley, E., & Rane, R. *Prescription of hearing aids: rationale, procedure, and results.* Kent, Ohio: Herald Publishing House, 1977.

Berger, K., Rane, R., & Hagberg, E. Comparisons of uncomfortable loudness levels and acoustic reflex thresholds. *Audiology and Hearing Education,* 1979, *5,* 11–15; 25.

Bragg, C. Toward a more objective hearing aid fitting procedure. *Hearing Instruments,* 1977, *28,* 6–9.

Carhart, R. Tests for selection of hearing aids. *Laryngoscope,* 1946a, *56,* 780–794.

Carhart, R. Volume control adjustment in hearing aid selection. *Laryngoscope,* 1946b, *56,* 510–526.

Carver, W. Loudness balance procedures. In J. Katz (Ed.), *Handbook of clinical audiology.* Baltimore: Williams and Wilkins, 1978.

Dancer, J. *The relationship between continuous (C) and interrupted (I) tones at threshold and most comfortable loudness (MCL) in hearing-impaired ears.* Unpublished doctoral dissertation, Teachers College, Columbia University, 1976.

Davis, H., Hudgins, C., Marquis, R., Nichols, R., et al. The selection of hearing aids. *Laryngoscope,* 1946, *26,* 85–115; 135–163.

Dirks, D., & Kamm, C. Psychometric function for loudness discomfort and most comfortable loudness levels. *Journal of Speech and Hearing Research,* 1976, *19,* 613–627.

Dudich, T., Keiser, M., & Keith, R. Some relationships between loudness and the acoustic reflex. *American Electromedics Corporation Impedance Newsletters,* 1975, *4,* 12–15.

Harris, J., & Pickler, P. Compensatory and pursuit tracking of loudness. *Journal of the Acoustical Society of America,* 1960, *32,* 1129–1133.

Hemeyer, T., & Rupp, R. Loudness discomfort levels in normal and pathological ears. *Journal of the Michigan Speech and Hearing Association,* 1970, *6,* 14–20.

Hochberg, I. Most comfortable listening level for the loudness and intelligibility of speech. *Audiology,* 1975, *14,* 27–33.

Holmes, D., & Woodford, C. Acoustic reflex threshold and loudness discomfort level: Relationships in children with profound hearing losses. *Journal of the American Audiology Society,* 1977, *2,* 193–196.

Hood, J., & Poole, J. Tolerable limit of loudness: Its clinical and physiological significance. *Journal of the Acoustical Society of America,* 1966, *40,* 47–53.

Jerger, J., & Jerger, S. Diagnostic value of Bekesy comfortable loudness tracings. *Archives of Otolaryngology,* 1974, *99,* 351–360.

Kallstrom, L., & Carstensen, K. The perception of loudness. *Audiology and Hearing Education,* 1978, *4,* 36–38.

Kamm, C., Dirks, D., & Mickey, M. Effect of sensorineural hearing loss on loudness discomfort level and most comfortable loudness judgments. *Journal of Speech and Hearing Research,* 1978, *21,* 668–681.

Kavanaugh, J. *An investigation of the most comfortable listening levels for speech.* Unpublished doctoral dissertation, University of Wisconsin, 1960.

Keith, R., & Sininger, L. New ideas in hearing aid selection. *Hearing Instruments,* 1978, *29,* 6–8; 34.

Kopra, L., & Blosser, D. Effects of methods of measurement on most comfortable loudness level for speech. *Journal of Speech and Hearing Research,* 1968, *2,* 497–508.

Loftiss, C. *An evaluation of the effects of selected psychophysical methods and judgmental procedures upon comfortable loudness judgments of connected speech.* Unpublished doctoral dissertation, University of Illinois, 1964.

LeZak, R. Some aspects of comfortable loudness. *Laryngoscope,* 1963, *73,* 267–274.

Markle, D., & Zaner, A. The determination of gain requirements for hearing aids: A new method. *Journal of Auditory Research,* 1965, *6,* 371–379.

Martin, F. *Introduction to audiology.* Englewood Cliffs, New Jersey Prentice-Hall, 1975.

Martin, F., & Forbis, N. The present status of audiometric practice: A follow-up study. *ASHA,* 1978, *20,* 531–541.

Martin, F., & Pennington, C. Current trends in audiometric practices. *ASHA,* 1971, *13,* 671–677.

McCandless, G. Special considerations in evaluating children and the aging for hearing aids. In M. Rubin (Ed.) *Hearing aids: current developments and concepts.* Baltimore: University Park Press, 1976.

McCandless, G., & Miller, D. Loudness discomfort and hearing aids. *National Hearing Aid Journal,* 1972, *25,* 1; 28; 32.

McCarthy, V. *The relationship between comfortable loudness range and most comfortable loudness for pure tones and speech in sensorineural hearing loss.* Unpublished doctoral dissertation, Teachers College, Columbia University, 1977.

McElhone, M. *Loudness discomfort levels for persons aged 10–17 years with normal hearing and sensori-neural loss.* Unpublished master's thesis, Ball State University, 1971.

Melnick, W. Comfortable level and loudness matching for continuous and interrupted signals. *Journal of Speech and Hearing Research,* 1967, *10,* 99–109.

Morgan, D., & Dirks, D. Loudness discomfort level under earphone and in free field: The effects of calibration methods. *Journal of the Acoustical Society of America,* 1974, *56,* 172–178.

Morgan, D., Wilson, R., & Dirks, D. Loudness discomfort level: selected methods and stimuli. *Journal of the Acoustic Society of America,* 1974, *56,* 577–581.

Niemeyer, W. Relations between the discomfort level and the reflex thresholds of middle ear muscles. *Audiology,* 1971, *10,* 172–176.

Northern, J. Clinical measurement procedures. In J. Jerger (Ed.), *Handbook of clinical impedance audiometry.* Dobbs Ferry, New York: Morgan Press, 1975.

Olson, A., & Hipskind, N. The relation between levels of pure tones and speech which elicit the acoustic relfex and loudness discomfort. *Journal of Auditory Research,* 1973, *13,* 71–76.

Preves, D., & Orton, J. Use of acoustic impedance measures in hearing aid fitting. *Hearing Instruments,* 1978, *29,* 22–24; 34–35.

Rappoport, B., & Tait, C. Acoustic reflex measurements in hearing aid selection. *Archives of Otolaryngology,* 1976, *102,* 129–132.

Rintleman, W., & Carhart, R. Loudness tracking by normal hearers via Bekesy audiometer. *Journal of Speech and Hearing Research,* 1964, *7,* 79–93.

Schmitz, H. Loudness discomfort level modification. *Journal of Speech and Hearing Research,* 1969, *12,* 807–817.

Shapiro, J. Hearing aid fitting by prescription. *Audiology,* 1976, *15,* 163–173.

Shapiro, J. Prediction of most comfortable loudness levels in hearing aid evaluation. *Journal of Speech and Hearing Disorders,* 1975, *40,* 434–438.

Silverman, S. Tolerance for pure tones and speech in normal and defective hearing. *Annals of Otology, Rhinology, and Laryngology,* 1947, *56,* 658–677.

Smith, H., & Rupp, R. Determination of the most comfortable loudness range (MCL–R) for normal-hearing subjects and subjects with sensori-neural hearing losses. *Journal of the Michigan Speech and Hearing Association,* 1973, *9,* 65–70.

Stephens, S., & Anderson, C. Experimental studies on the uncomfortable loudness level. *Journal of Speech and Hearing Research,* 1971, *14,* 262–270.

Ventry, I. Procedural considerations in the measurement of comfortable loudness: review. *Maico Audiological Library Series,* 1977, *15,* Report 6.

Ventry, I., & Johnson, J. Evaluation of a clinical method for measuring comfortable loudness for speech. *Journal of Speech and Hearing Disorders,* 1978, *43,* 149–159.

Ventry, I., Woods, R., Rubin, M., & Hill, W. Most comfortable loudness for pure tones, noise and speech. *Journal of the Acoustical Society of America,* 1971, *49,* 1805–1813.

Watson, L. Certain fundamental principles in prescribing and fitting hearing aids. *Laryngoscope,* 1944, *54,* 531–558.

Woodford, C., & Holmes, D. Relationship between loudness discomfort level and acoustic reflex threshold in a clinical population. *Audiology and Hearing Education,* 1977, *3,* 9–12.

Walden, B., Schuman, G., & Sedge, R. The reliability and validity of the comfort level method of setting hearing aid gain. *Journal of Speech and Hearing Disorders,* 1977, *42,* 455–461.

J. C. Cooper, Jr., Ph. D.

10
Speech Protocols in the Assessment of Functional Hearing Loss

Premises

FUNCTIONALITY

There certainly exist individuals whose responses to auditory stimuli are suspect. When instructed to repeat a word, for example, they do not, although there are indications they hear well enough to do so. While they exist, there is no uniformity in labeling them. The terms functional, nonorganic, and psychogenic hearing loss, as well as malingerer, have been used. The diversity of terms undoubtedly stems from audiology's position straddling psychoacoustics and physiology while attempting to correlate the two. As audiology continues its growth it may be able to apply physiological techniques to the clinical measurement of speech discrimination. In current practice, such measures are limited to estimates of sensitivity to sound. Thus, the following approaches the above problem from the viewpoint of psychoacoustics. Since psychoacoustics is the study of input–output functions, and since the basic information which suggests less than full cooperation is the failure to discern a reasonable pattern in an individual's performance, it is appropriate that "functional hearing loss" be applied to this chapter. It is concise, descriptive, and avoids the questionable excess of meaning that might be gleaned from other terms such as malingerer (has the task to be avoided been specified?) and nonorganic (can it be said with certainty that no organic defect exists?). Even if the implied questions were answerable, the answers would most certainly not come from audiological data.

IDENTIFICATION VERSUS EVALUATION

For economy's sake it must be presumed that, in the absence of evidence to the contrary, all individuals undergoing evaluation are willing to cooperate. Thus, the audiologist is faced with two distinct tasks when considering functional hearing loss. The first is to become alert to its presence within the context of a routine evaluation. The second is to arrive at valid measures of hearing when faced with such indications. In both cases, the standard by which patient performance is gauged is the accumulated knowledge of the several patterns produced by relating acoustic input to behavioral output. For that reason, a brief summary of typical input–output functions is reviewed, the details of which can be found elsewhere is this text.

TWO ASIDES

Before beginning the review, two additional points should be made. First, this writer makes no age distinctions when dealing with the possibility of functional hearing loss. Anyone capable of deciding if and when to respond is capable of misleading the audiologist. This writer is obliged to the five-year-old who seared this truism indelibly in his memory. Second, the final "proof" of functionality in speech audiometry is obtained when the patient is induced to cooperate and "true" performance is measured. In the face of steadfast refusal to cooperate, the audiologist is stalemated. Fortunately, with the major exception of the Verterans Administration, speech measures are not critical to defining degree of hearing loss for most legal purposes. Thus, the mainstay of evaluation of functionality is the determination of valid tonal thresholds and physiologic rather than psychoacoustic techniques are likely to dominate the process. This is not to say that speech measures are unimportant. It is simply to acknowledge the more difficult task involved in obtaining valid speech measures and to acknowledge the fact that they are less than crucial to any legalistic resolution of functionality.

Parameters of Speech Discrimination

While auditory experience can be delineated along multiple dimensions, two are capitalized upon in audiologic practice: threshold sensitivity and discrimination of suprathreshold sounds. The presumably clear distinction becomes blurred when speech is presented at low levels. However, two generalizations can be made.

SENSATION LEVEL

The most fundamental generalization is that increasing sensation level (SL) should improve peformance in a discrimination task. Two obvious qualifications are that some degree of discrimination ability need be present and that the relationship between SL and performance may be complex. The factors which may complicate the relationship fall in three major categories: the acoustic composition of the signal and any concomitant noise, any defects in the anatomical system, and the nature of the cortical processing of the signal.

A discussion of the decisions which eventually result in the delivery of a particular test word with particular modifications by the delivery system are beyond the scope of this chapter, but the results can range from lists which accent the decrement in performance in high-frequency hearing loss to presentations in noise. Suffice to say that each test offered for use should be backed up by appropriate normative data specifying typical input–output functions for unimpaired listeners and the several categories of hearing loss that may be subjected to the test. In general, conductive lesions displace the performance–intensity (P–I) function to the right to a degree consistent with the magnitude of the attenuation imposed by the defect. Sensorineural losses operate to lower the level of maximum performance as well as shifting the function to the right and may alter its shape as, for instance, in the rollover noted in a variety of lesions central to the cochlea. Lastly, the nature of the patient's decisions regarding if and when to respond to the impressed signal must be taken into account. Such decisions appear to produce no consistent patterns in those with functionality. The best that can be said is that inconsistency at suprathreshold levels may be the rule.

NONAUDITORY CUES

A second generalization that can be made involves nonauditory cues. Performance can be improved by the addition of such cues which are primarily contextual and visual. While this writer knows of no formal test of functionality designed to employ context as a variable, a test employing an unusual variation of "visual" cues is discussed later.

Tonal Thresholds and Speech Measures

SPONDEE AND SPEECH DETECTION THRESHOLDS

It was stated that discrimination and threshold sensitivity are different auditory functions. It was also stated that this distinction becomes blurred in some auditory tests. The particular case alluded to involves the expectation that the spondee threshold (ST) should approximate the pure tone average (PTA). Taken at face value, it might be presumed that these two measures require equal intensity to achieve threshold. This is not the case. The equality is artificial, resulting from arbitrary calibration standards. To explain, the ANSI 1969, standards for 0 dB hearing level (HL) over the 500–2000 Hz range average 8.7 dB sound pressure level (SPL). The standard for 0 dB HL speech is 20 dB SPL. The basis for the increased level to obtain an ST is the difference in the tasks presented to the listener. In one case, simple detection of any auditory event is required. In the other case, both detection and discrimination are required. However, if normal-hearing individuals are asked simply *to detect the presence or absence* of an auditory event and if that auditory event is speech, then the speech detection threshold (SDT) averages 10 dB less than the ST.

It should also be recalled that any speech signal is spectrally complex. Deviations from the expected relationship among the PTA, SDT, and ST can be observed routinely in cases where large interoctave threshold differences occur. Such audiometric configurations act, in effect, to filter stimuli, rendering normative data suspect. In the case of either a sharply rising or falling audiogram, the effect should permit detection of speech at levels close to the best tonal threshold but may drive the ST to higher levels. However, changes in the ST require rather dramatic interoctave differences in the speech range, since there is good agreement between it and the average of the two better tonal thresholds (500–2000 Hz) in, for example, noise-induced hearing loss (Cooper & Owen, 1976). An additional factor which can distort the PTA–ST relationship is very poor discrimination ability which may raise the ST to levels higher than the PTA. When faced with an ST much poorer than the PTA, low discrimination at any SL can be expected. The SDT should be unaffected. Obviously, STs better than PTAs are illogical. (See Rupp's Chapter 4.)

SPEECH DISCRIMINATION

Because of the differences in threshold and suprathreshold tasks, there is little predictable relationship between tonal thresholds and discrimination measures. Nonetheless, increments in performance should occur with increasing SL and, while the relationship is not precise, increasing hearing loss should be accompanied by lower plateaus for the P–I function.

Strategy

IDENTIFICATION

Though difficult to reduce to quantifiable, reportable data which might stand up in a court of law, a cursory discussion with an experienced audiologist will quickly disclose that gut feeling is often used to "identify" those with functional hearing loss. While certainly not excluding himself from those using subjective reactions, this writer finds it difficult to communicate the nature of those behaviors in a clear manner. More importantly, there are concrete relationships among routinely collected data that can be examined and, when inconsistent, are indications of functionality. Prime among these is the relationship among the PTA, SDT, and ST. With less precision, inconsistencies in the pattern of suprathreshold responses as reflected in P–I functions can be valuable in alerting the audiologist to functionality.

EVALUATION

Special tests to confirm the indications of functionality and, occasionally, to estimate valid levels of performance employ several strategies. In the case of unilateral functionality, the audiologist may capitalize on the patient's lack of knowledge about crossover and the inability of the human to be aware of low SL presentations in one ear in the presence of high SL in the other. In bilateral losses, test signals are combined with other stimulation such as noise, self-hearing, and visual cues. Attempts may be made to confuse the patient by alternating the signal between ears. The assumption is that, being unable to keep the origin of information straight (better or poorer ear), the patient will repeat portions of the signal which are presented to the ear with functional hearing loss. There are also a variety of suggestions which this writer chooses to categorize as tricks. They are based upon catching the patient at the time when the artificial criteria used as a basis for responding are relaxed. An example would be instructing the patient to "take the earphones off—the test is over" at a level below the admitted ST. The problems in drawing reportable conclusions from such techniques are many although it is difficult to fault any technique which is designed to unmask functionality. Lastly, galvanic skin reponses (GSR) have been used with speech materials as stimuli.

ROUTINE PROCEDURES

Pretest Interview

Although the bulk of pretest indices of functionality will be ignored, there is one aspect of the interview that, together with a reasonable assertion, can alert the experienced audiologist to the need for assuming a skeptical posture toward certain patients. That aspect is the patient's communication efficiency in a face-to-face interview. The assertion (Davis & Silverman, 1978), simply stated, is that 50 percent discrimination at 50 dB HL will not affect communication conducted in the structured context of the typical pretest interview. Assuming that efficient communication occurs, two speech audiometry data points for the better binaural air conduction average are reasonably established. Discrimination at 50 dB HL should be no poorer than 50 percent and, reasoning backward from P–I functions, the ST should be no poorer than about 35 dB HL.

There is a piece of concrete information which must alert the audiologist to possible functionality. That is the knowledge that hearing is at issue in some claim for compensation or in some litigation. Such information is certainly not *prima facia* evidence for functionality. It is an indication that any subsequently documented hearing loss may be contested by either the injured party or by those against whom a claim is being made. The question of functionality may arise and it would be embarrassing, if nothing else, to be forced to admit that possible functionality was not considered during the evaluation.

Acoustic Reflex Thresholds

When impedance audiometry is a part of a routine evaluation, acoustic reflex thresholds and subsequent estimation of the PTA can supplement interview estimates of likely speech performance in the absence of indications of conductive loss. It is acknowledged that such estimates can be in error when a hearing loss is present, but indications of normal hearing are rarely in error (Jerger, Hayes, & Anthony, 1978).

Spondee Threshold

Presume for the moment that a patient decides to deceive the audiologist as to his or her true ST. What preparations would be made? First, an arbitrary level for responding would be nice to have, since absolute judgments of suprathreshold loudness (that sound is 30 dB SL) are more difficult to make than relative judgments (that sound is louder than the other.) A constant tinnitus or background noise would be convenient. Some knowledge of a reasonable input–output relationship would be valuable to insure that the shape of the P–I function would not alert the audiologist to the fact that something was amiss. Realizing that the P–I function for spondees is steep, the patient's task might be simplified to merely having an appropriate reference against which to compare the loudness of stimuli. The cortical decision could be reduced to responding correctly to all words at or above the level of the reference and never responding below that level, particularly if the patient were subjected to a 5-dB increment procedure.

Since some estimate of the ST is available on the basis of the interview and impedance audiometry, this writer routinely obtains STs prior to other behavioral measures. Any indication of inconsistency warrants further examination. On the basis of their P–I function, the range from 10–90 percent correct identification of spondees should not exceed 10 dB. Test–retest variability should not exceed the 6 dB range found in more than 90 percent of normals and nonfunctional hearing losses (Chaiklin & Ventry, 1963). Test–retest consistency is no assurance that valid thresholds have been obtained since Menzel (1960) noted that 60 percent of functional patients fell within those limits. It would seem reasonable, however, to accept larger differences as evidence of functionality. Presuming that the ST is consistent with face-to-face communication and the PTA estimated from acoustic reflex thresholds, the next stage in evaluating its validity is to obtain tonal thresholds and compare them to the ST. They should agree within 8–10 dB. Only 15 percent of those with functional hearing loss were reported to be able to match within 8 dB (Chaiklin & Ventry, 1963). (Although different calibration standards were used, dB SPL differences in the PTA and ST were only 1.8 dB greater than current standards.) When the ST is different from the PTA by 12 or more dB, functionality may be presumed.

The type of errors made in responding to spondees may also be used as an indicator of functionality. Half-word responses are suspect on theoretical grounds. The patient has been familiarized with the words and guessing has been encouraged whenever the word is not heard clearly. It is difficult to believe that "hot" can be repeated without realizing that the stimulus is "hotdog." Further, since the stimuli are produced with equal stress on each syllable, there is little reason to believe that "dog" has been inaudible.

Speech Detection Threshold

This writer suggests that the SDT be used as part of a triad of measures (together with the PTA and ST) which should be internally consistent. To restate the earlier discussion, the ST should approximate the PTA and the SDT should be 10 dB better than both. The establishment of a SDT takes little time and provides a reasonable transition from the patient's task in the ST (repeat the word) to the task which will be faced in generating an audiogram (indicate when any sound is heard, however faint). Since it is not a routine measure, there is no "standard" procedure for its determination. The following instructions are used by this writer.

> Now I want you to raise your hand whenever you hear my voice. It is important to respond whether or not you understand what I am saying or whether or not what you hear sounds like a word. Under no circumstances attempt to repeat or describe what you hear. Simply raise your hand whenever you hear anything.

Speech Discrimination

The decisions faced by the patient seeking to mislead the audiologist as to his or her true speech discrimination are more complex than those involved in the ST task. At least one additional reference level (ST + 30 dB, or whatever SL is used for discrimination measures) would need to be established. If full P–I functions and retesting can be expected, the task becomes seemingly impossible. Additional artificial reference levels would be helpful. Some understanding of the effects of filtering would be valuable if other than a flat audiogram will be simulated. Errors will need to be related to the spectrum of the item missed and the audiogram. Their rate will need to be made dependent upon the level of presentation so that a reasonable P–I function will be generated. The patient, one presumes, is rarely engaged in the above thought process. Nonetheless, the steps give some insight into difficulties faced by those with functional hearing loss if they chose to mask their functionality from the audiologist and if the audiologist challenges them with a thorough speech audiometry battery. Thus, three aspects of supra-ST performance can be examined in cases of possible functionality: the shape of the P–I function, the variability of scores at one level of presentation, and the nature of errors that are made.

PERFORMANCE–INTENSITY FUNCTION

The most common measure of speech discrimination is made at some level presumed to be at or above that necessary to produce maximum discrimination. This writer advocates an additional routine measure to 50 dB HL, approximately conversational level. With knowledge of interview communication efficiency, the ST, typical P–I functions for the list used, and the above two measures of discrimination, a rough estimate of the patient's P–I function can be made. It should approximate the functions typical of the lists used. Functions which are steeper than normal have not been reported to this writer's knowledge. Thus, for example, if the ST is 40 dB and discrimination at 50 dB HL is 80 percent, the only conclusion is that the offered ST is poorer than the true ST. Any indication of inconsistency renders the patient suspect and warrants the development of a complete P–I function.

RELIABILITY

An additional index of a patient's cooperation can be had by establishing repeat discrimination measures. Specific values for test–retest consistency depend upon the set of lists used. Excessive variability, with level of presentation held constant, indicates less than full cooperation. Another aspect of reliability is the consistency of errors. The expectation is that particular words in a list should be consistently identified or missed, and that errors should be consistent with the filtering effects of hearing loss. The word "cows" may be repeated as "cow" but should not be repeated as "rapt." A complication of attempts to analyze errors is that the same list must be repeated. The justifiability of reusing a specific list depends upon the evidence offered in its standardization data.

SPECIAL SPEECH TESTS

Several practical matters should be discussed before proceeding with the examination of particular tests. The first, broached earlier, involves the need to establish valid speech measures in determining hearing for legal purposes. While often desirable, they are seldom crucial to the determination of the degree of hearing loss. Second, since functional hearing loss may be complicated by organic underpinnings and since organic damage can produce a wide range of performances, it can be difficult, if not impossible, to separate the functional component from the gross performance. For these reasons, it is not surprising that the bulk of research in determining true hearing has addressed itself to the determination of tonal thresholds. There are comparatively few studies of speech measures and those that do exist address themselves to that relative of threshold sensitivity, the ST. There is virtually no research that addresses itself to determining speech discrimination measures.

The student should not be critical of the profession for these shortcomings. Aside from the reduced pressure to determine speech measures because of the emphasis in litigation on tonal thresholds, there is a second contribution to the current state of affairs. That is the fact that it is difficult to obtain experimental subjects for any investigations. First, consider the possibility that those proficient at masking their true hearing are simply not detected. Only the bunglers may ever be caught. Short of announcing a general amnesty for all functional hearing loss cases and inducing the most successful to cooperate in an extensive research effort, getting an ideal experimental group would seem to be close to impossible. It is noted that this criticism may be limited only to speech measures, depending upon the reader's definition of hearing and his or her interpretation of its relationship to physiological events such as change in skin resistance or change in averaged brainstem discharge patterns with auditory stimulation. Assume that, for most practical purposes, measures of audition reflected in physiological measures are unequivocal evidence of hearing. On the basis of such an assumption, it is relatively easy to establish experimental groups. In fact, the bulk of experimental evidence has used such measures to define those with functional hearing loss. The remaining evidence is based upon functional patients who eventually volunteered normal hearing or normals who agreed to simulate a loss. Except in the two latter cases, estimates of the speech discrimination ability have been conspicuously absent.

Two general comments about all audiological testing are particularly applicable when using special speech tests for functional hearing loss. First, when there are positive indications of functionality, it is likely to be present. Functionality may be present without indications, however. Audiological results do not rule out lesions, only indicate their site in the presence of abnormal findings. Second, it is not possible to attribute a cause for functionality when faced with positive indications. Rarely, the cause may simply be misunderstanding of instructions. Audiological results indicate site of a lesion, not its etiology.

With the reader thus warned, the following will categorize special speech tests for functional hearing loss into four groups: one test designed to confirm the existence of functional hearing loss, those that estimate the patient's level for awareness of speech stimuli but not necessarily implying speech discrimination, those that attempt to estimate a ST, and those that may estimate a level for understanding ongoing speech, a level likely to be above the ST by a degree dependent on the materials used.

Doerfler–Stewart: A Confirmatory Test

BASIS

The test is based on two principles. The first is the disruption of any internal reference used by the patient to produce artificial STs by presenting words binaurally in binaural noise. The second principle involved is a comparison of relationships among STs, noise detection thresholds (NDT), and noise interference levels (NIL). The NIL is that level at which noise masks the speech signal. Since the test is adminstered binaurally, the function of the better ear or a combination of the two ears' hearing is evaluated.

PROCEDURE

Spondaic words are used as the signal. A variety of noises have been used from sawtooth (Doerfler & Stewart, 1946) through complex noise (Ventry & Chaiklin, 1965) to speech noise (instructions for Grason-Stadler speech audiometers). The procedure involves estblishing a binaural ST using an ascending technique from 0 dB HL. This initial ST is designated SRT_1 (SRT will be used to identify those measures specified in the original studies. ST is precisely equivalent to SRT but more recent usage.) Spondaic words are then repeated 5 dB above this level while noise is introduced at 0 dB HL and increased in 10 dB steps until a level 15 dB below SRT_1 is reached. Increases are continued in 5 dB increments until the patient no longer repeats any words. The NIL is taken as the point where not more than two of six spondees is repeated. Increases in the level of the noise are continued to approximately 20 dB above the NIL. The noise level is held constant and the level of spondee presentation (spondees are continually repeated during the manipulation of noise levels) is reduced to $SRT_1 - 15$ dB in 5 dB steps, one spondee presented at each decrement. The noise is then reduced in 10 dB steps, one spondee being repeated at each decrement until the noise level is 0 dB HL or spondees are again repeated. If spondees are repeated at $SRT_1 - 15$ dB during the reduction in noise level, a new SRT_1 is established and the above procedure repeated until a stable SRT_1 is obtained. If none are repeated, or when a stable SRT_1 is obtained, the level of spondees is increased from $SRT_1 - 15$ dB until a second ST is obtained, designated SRT_2. No further spondees are presented. The patient is then instructed to indicate when the noise becomes just audible. The noise is raised from below 0 dB HL in 5 dB steps until the patient indicates that he or she hears it. This is recorded as the NDT.

INTERPRETATION

Five comparisons are made among the four measures. These are: $SRT_1 - SRT_2$, $SRT_1 - NDT$, $SRT_2 - NDT$, $SRT_1 + 5$ dB $-$ NIL, and NDT $-$ NIL. Epstein and Hopkinson (1956) and Doerfler and Epstein (1956) have reported norms for the five indices. In the order listed above, algebraic values of the subtraction process should not exceed the following ranges: -4 to $+5$, -5 to $+15$, -7 to $+15$, -18 to $+3$ and -31 to -2 dB. Ventry and Chaiklin (1965) "arbitrarily" concluded that if all results were within the above norms, there was no indication of functional hearing loss. If one of the five indices fell outside the norms, the results were considered equivocal and if two or more values fell outside the norms, the results were considered a positive indication of functional hearing loss. They found that differences between functional and nonfunctional groups on measures of $SRT_1 - SRT_2$ and NDT $-$ NIL were not significant. $SRT_1 + 5$ dB $-$ NIL, though significant, correctly identified only 18 percent of the functional group. It should be noted that the two most powerful indices in separating functional from nonfunctional groups ($p < .01$) were $SRT_1 -$ NDT and $SRT_2 -$ NDT. Such indices should be related to the ST $-$ SDT comparison discussed in a previous section, depending upon the degree to which the noise spectrum matches the average spectrum of speech. They revised the norms and established the following values for $SRT_1 - SRT_2$, $SRT_1 + 5$ dB $-$ NIL, and NDT $-$ NIL: 0 to $+10$, -24 to -12, and -40 to -20 dB. With the revision, $SRT_1 + 5$ dB $-$ NIL and NDT $-$ NIL became significant indices ($p < .01$). Reviewing the results of all five indices using the revised norms, they found that only one in 20 functional hearing loss patients had no positive indications of functionality. Six had one positive indication and 13 had two or more positive indications. In a nonfunctional group of 18, 11 had no indications of functionality, four had one indication, and three had two or more indications. They pointed out that the test is "a screening procedure rather than a threshold measuring technique." They also concluded that it is "too complex for routine screening use." Menzel (1960) also questioned the value of the test, since functionality among his cases was discovered with criteria other than the test itself. A peripheral benefit of administering the test as the first test (which he did uniformly) was the fact that while the first binaural ST (SRT_1) of functional cases was commonly inflated, the first monaural ST obtained after the test was not. The test appears to be a deterrent to functionality.

Tests of Sound Awareness

LOMBARD TEST

BASIS

The Lombard Test is based upon the fact that people tend to raise their voices in the presence of noise. Although references to the test can be found dating back to 1910, and while Hopkinson has asserted that the test was "still used regularly" in 1973, Harris (1965) implied that research was needed to develop the principle to the point where it might provide clinically useful information. In 1965, Hanley and Harvey noted that there were three major drawbacks to the test. First, it had not been standardized. Second, the sophisticated patient could control the intensity of his or her voice in noise. Third, criticism was leveled at the methods by which the increase in vocal output had been detected. Those methods were dominated by variations of simple visual monitoring of peaks produced on a VU meter which was connected to the output of a microphone placed in front of the patient. In that this writer has uncovered no research since 1965, Harris' conclusion appears to remain sound.

PROCEDURE

Administration of the test is relatively straightforward in concept. The patient is asked to read a passage aloud several times so that reading becomes relatively fluent and vocal intensity becomes relatively stable. A microphone and VU meter are used to monitor vocal intensity. The microphone is located so that its distance from the patient is held constant. When reasonably stable reading is achieved, repetitions of the reading are continued with presentation of noise to one or both ears. If vocal intensity increases, then it is presumed that the noise is audible.

INTERPRETATION

Several questions should occur to the reader. What should be the spectrum of the noise? What level of noise should be used with what levels of volunteered hearing? What criteria should be used to evaluate significant changes in vocal intensity? What conclusions about hearing can be drawn from the level at which noise produces a change in vocal intensity? Unfortunately, there is no clear answer to any of these questions. One wonders if any time at all need be spent in seeking answers since Taylor (1949) reported that seven of 12 normal-hearing individuals familiar with the effect were able to prevent any significant changes in vocal intensity in noise levels as high as 60 dB SL. Nonetheless, he presented information indicating that the naive patient will succumb. His naive, normal-hearing ad hearing-impaired subjects produced consistent average increases in vocal intensity (from .6–8 dB VU as noise was increased in 20 dB steps to 60 dB SL). Hanley and Harvey (1965) used sophisticated integrating equipment to evaluate changes in vocal intensity rather than using a VU meter. They used normal-hearing, naive subjects and found that, on the average, significant changes in vocal intensity occurred. However, 15 of 64 possible comparisons between successive noise/no-noise and no-noise/noise presentations were not different from successive no-noise/no-noise sequences.

In view of the above findings, it is difficult to commend this test to the reader for routine use. It is mentioned primarily to provide the reader with some context within which to consider other more optimistic views of the test's usefulness.

DELAYED AUDITORY FEEDBACK

BASIS

If self-hearing of speech by air conduction is delayed, then normal hearing individuals are likely to change their vocal output in several ways. Changes are primarily a function of the amount of delay and the sensation level of the delayed signal. Superficially, such changes may appear to be similar to the Lombard effect, but research provided by individuals such as Butler and Galloway (1957) and Peters (1956) clearly demonstrate that the effects are not similar to hearing noise.

PROCEDURE

A procedure is difficult to outline beyond the following brief sketch. The basics are straightforward. A patient is placed before a microphone whose output is fed to a device where it is delayed and then routed back through an amplifier and attenuator to earphones which the patient wears. One of the simplest delay devices is a three-head tape recorder. While speaking, the patient's output is recorded. The tape is then transported to a playback head where the previously recorded signal is detected, amplified and returned to the patient's earphones. The amount of delay is dependent upon the speed of the tape and the distance between the record and playback heads. On the basis of reviews such as that by Yates (1963), a .18 second delay appears to be optimum for disrupting the patient's performance by producing a significant increase in the total time necessary to complete reading a passage. Thus, a comparison of reading time with delay to reading time without delay is used as an index of whether or not the delayed speech was heard by the patient.

Part of the difficulty in specifying a procedure is that materials have not been standardized and no particular set is generally accepted. Experimental materials have ranged from such open-ended vocal output as asking a subject to repeat a proverb and explain it (Korowbow, 1955) to rapidly saying aloud a two-digit number flashed on the screen (Butler & Galloway, 1957). The more rote the materials, the less the effect. For example, a person may repeat the alphabet without demonstrating any effect, but may breakdown with rapid repetition of "sister Sally sitting on a thistle." Additionally, individuals vary in their susceptability to Delayed Auditory Feedback (DAF) and in the degree to which they adapt to the effects. While adaptation effects are not complete, some adaptation can occur with increasing exposure to DAF. Therefore, most writers suggest using ascending levels of feedback although Hanley, Tiffany, and Brungard (1958) suggest that intermittent presentations of DAF be used. While reading time to complete the passage is the most thoroughly investigated effect, other indices have been suggested. Among such measures are changes in the fundamental frequency of the speaker's voice (Fairbanks, 1955), vocal intensity (Black, 1951), the intelligibility of the speaker (Atkinson, 1954), galvanic skin responses (Hanley, Tiffany, & Brungard, 1958), as well as a variety of articulation errors summarized by Yates (1963).

INTERPRETATION

With no clear cut procedure available, generalizations regarding interpretation are impossible. Beyond that, results may be confounded by both the type and degree of organic hearing loss that may be present (Butler & Galloway, 1959; Harford & Jerger, 1959). For example, the latter authors reported higher error scores in a group of otosclerotic patients than in those in a group of normal subjects tested with earplugs simulating a conductive hearing loss. Nonetheless, when changes in vocal output occur, it can be concluded that the feedback was audible, although its SL may be in doubt.

The somewhat dismal picture generated by the above should not be taken too much to heart. A review of one experimental conclusion and a consideration of another may lend some insight into ways to improve the technique. In another context, Cherry and Sayers (1956) demonstrated that stammerers could be controlled by masking only the low-frequency components of their speech. This finding suggests that high-frequency components in feedback may not be critical to the DAF effect. If so, then DAF may simply correlate with the SDT. If effects of high-frequency feedback could be demonstrated, however, then estimates of discrimination might be possible by selective filtering of the feedback.

GALVANIC SKIN RESPONSE AUDIOMETRY

There are regulatory issues surrounding the safety of this technique when applied without medical supervision (Underwriters' Laboratories, 1976), although this writer has been unable to find either documented or anecdotal information that would lead him to believe the technique unsafe in any practical sense. The point may be moot, since the only commercial instrument designed for the test is no longer for sale. Without commending it to the reader's use, the test should be briefly discussed. Description of the technique can be found elsewhere (Hopkinson, 1978; Chaiklin & Ventry, 1963). Two points in such reviews should be mentioned. First, speech can be used as a signal to determine at least a SDT. In such a situation, any speech signal is conditioned to produce a change in skin resistance as a result of being paired with a mild electrical shock. The interpretation of such results obviously depends on he specturm of the speech signal and the shape of the true audiogram. Second, Ruhm and Carhart (1958) reported a variation in which the repsonse was conditioned to a particular word, thus indicating intelligibility rather than detection, although one would be hard pressed to call a measure based on a single spondee the ST.

Tests of Spondee Thresholds

SPEECH STENGER TEST

BASIS

If identical signals are presented to both ears of a normal-hearing individual and the SL of each is varied, conditions can be established such that the sound is perceived as coming only from the ear with the greater SL. In the case of speech stimuli, it appears that when the SL of one ear exceeds that of the other ear by approximately 10 dB or more, speech is not perceived in the ear with the lower SL. The difference necessary for the phenomenon to occur can be as high as +35 dB SL (Taylor, 1949). It is noted that the ideal case for the test's application is a unilateral functional component. However, the test may be applied to any case of asymmetrical hearing where STs are different by 20 dB or more.

PROCEDURE

Although the test can be administered with any speech materials, spondaic words are generally used to estimate true STs. The equipment must permit the introduction of identical signals to both ears with independent control of the intensity to each. After establishing monaural STs, words are presented to the ear with the better ST alone at 10 (Chaiklin & Ventry, 1963) to 15–16 dB SL (Hopkinson, 1978). The patient may be asked simply to repeat words or to repeat and point to the ear in which the word was hear (Johnson, Work & McCoy, 1956). Presentations to the poorer ear are then added (a simultaneous binaural presentation) starting at a level of no more than 20 dB *re* the ST of the better ear. Presentations are increased in 10 dB steps in the poorer ear while the level in the better ear is being held constant until the patient stops responding or it is clear that the presentation in the poorer ear is crossing over to the better ear.

INTERPRETATION

Under no circumstances should a patient without functional hearing loss in the poorer ear stop responding. If responses cease, then it is presumed that the words were heard in the poorer ear at a SL sufficient to preclude the patient being aware of the words present in the better ear and that the patient has chosen not to respond. The ST in the poorer ear is then no poorer than the level at which the patient ceased responding. If the patient has also been asked to indicate which ear heard the word, additional information can be obtained. When responses are consistently obtained and when the patient indicates having heard from the better ear at levels higher than those where crossover would have been expected, then crossover has been demonstrated. If the patient continues responding at all levels and indicates that hearing has shifted to the poorer ear, then it may be presumed that the SL in the poorer ear is higher than that in the better ear. The point at which hearing shifts from the better to the poorer ear should be higher than the monaural PTA and ST obtained from that ear in routine tests.

Menzel (1960) indicated that the test demonstrates functionality in 47 percent of applicable cases with functionality. This figure is conservative, since it included cases in which functionality was demonstrated only for pure-tone thresholds and not for speech measures. When functionality was demonstrated for speech measures, the test was a true indicator of functionality in 85 percent of the cases where it was applicable. Ventry and Chaiklin (1965) reported that it was positive in only 40 percent of applicable cases. They do note that when the test was negative, no patient had more than a 22-dB functional component for STs in the poorer ear and that the same patients had functional components as high as 25 dB in the better ear.

"LIPREADING TEST" (SPONDEE THRESHOLD INFERRED)

BASIS

Falconer's "Lipreading Test" (1966) is unique among auditory tests. In its administration, the patient's attention is explicitly drawn to visual cues which "should" supplement audition in a task requiring the repetition of words. In fact, it is the materials' inherent lack of lipreadability that is capitalized upon and the patient's "use" of such ambiguous visual cues unmasks his functionality.

PROCEDURE

The test consists of 20 monosyllabic and homophenous words, for example, "bud," "bun," or "but." Eight different test lists are available. The test is appropriate only when some degree of communication between the audiologist and the patient can be conducted in a face-to-face situation. If this had occurred and subsequent volunteered thresholds give reason to suspect functionality, the test can be applied. Falconer suggests the test be given monaurally, but adds that a binaural presentation may be used when no responses are obtained in standard audiometry or when responses are exceedingly poor bilaterally. He suggests that the increased loudness of a binaural hearing situation is an advantage. With the knowledge that binaural thresholds can be better than monaural, it is unfortunate that norms for the test were not developed for binaural presentation. Prior to the administration of the test, it is suggested that the audiologist compliment the patient's lipreading ability and present the test within the context of measuring this ability as opposed to a further measure of hearing.

The patient is seated in a darkened, sound-treated room wearing earphones. The audiologist is seated in a well-lighted adjacent room with his or her face clearly visable through a window. Test items are presented by monitored live voice while the patient is encouraged to repeat words using both visual and auditory cues. Scoring should be done in a manner which prevents the patient from determining whether or not his responses are correct. It is recommended that the first list be presented approximately 12 dB above the estimated true ST with succeeding tests presented in 6 dB decrements, one for each repetition of the test. Testing is continued until no more than three of 20 words have been correctly repeated.

If no ST estimate is available, levels near the volunteered ST are appropriate or levels in excess of 80 dB HL if a profound hearing loss has been offered. When a high initial presentation level has been used, succeeding lists are presented in decrements of 10 or 20 dB until the patient's performance falls below 15 correct repetitions for a list. Then 6 dB decrements are used.

INTERPRETATION

The lists were standardized on normal-hearing individuals by presenting them at −10, 0, and 10 dB SL *re* the ST. Normal hearers produced a linear P–I function which ranged from an average of .7 words correct at −10 dB SL to 16.1 words correct at 10 dB SL. The test was also standardized on a total of 62 hearing impaired individuals who were thought to be free from functional hearing loss and whose audiograms were relatively flat (no more than a 20 dB difference between low-frequency thresholds and those at 2000 Hz). Again, an essentially linear P–I function was obtained over the range from −6 (mean of 1.3 words correct) to 12 dB SL (mean of 13.9 words correct). It is noted that although the slopes of the normal and hearing-impaired P–I functions were practically identical, the intercepts were different. At 0 dB SL, normal hearing individuals produced a mean score of 7.0 words correct while hearing-impaired individuals produced approximately 5.3 words correct. Falconer suggests that the point at which five words are correctly repeated is the best estimate of the ST. When no list produces exactly five correct responses, the ST can still be predicted because of the linearity of the P–I function. It should be 5 dB below the point at which ten words are repeated correctly, 4 dB below nine words correct, 3 dB below eight, 2 dB below seven, or 1 dB below six words repeated correctly.

Falconer presents results from only three functional hearing loss cases. However, the three covered a wide range of functionality from no response on initial attempts to obtain a ST to one in which the initial ST was 30 dB. In the first case, the predicted ST was 5 dB and eventual volunteered responses were 10 dB. In the other case, the final volunteered ST was 18 dB and the predicted ST was 14 dB. It is unfortunate that independent verification of the test's effectiveness appears not to have been published. This writer has employed the test with success on several occasions. There are minor difficulties in getting good facial lighting for the audiologist in a standard audiometric suite where the overhead light tends to case shadows on the face. A limitation of the test, in this writer's experience, is that it is uncommon to find patients who both offer poor hearing and who appear to have reasonably efficient face to face conversation, which they attribute to lipreading ability.

Estimates of Levels for Understanding Ongoing Speech

SWINGING SPEECH TESTS

BASIS

Such tests are applicable to those presenting with asymmetrical hearing and are based on the assumption that, if the poorer ear is functional and information is presented to both ears, critical information presented to the poorer ear will be included in a later repetition of what was heard because the patient could not keep the source of the information (better or poorer ear) straight. For example, assume that a patient offers normal hearing in one ear and a functional hearing loss of 50 dB in the opposite ear. Both ears are presented a story at 30 dB HL. The material presented to the poorer ear supplements the tale. A switching device or a prepared recording is used to insure that certain words are presented to one, both, or the other ear. The following sentence will serve to illustrate a pattern of switching. The italicized words are presented only to the poorer ear. "Three men, *a boy,* and a dog took a trip in a boat with their fishing gear *and a tent.*" If the patient mentions either a boy or a tent when asked to repeat the story, he or she had heard with the poorer ear.

PROCEDURE

As can be imagined, preparation of materials, determination of appropriate presentation levels and scoring of the test could be complicated. At one extreme, one could devise an intricate story whose critical words were words of a speech discrimination test. While offering an opportunity to measure speech discrimination, the difficulties seem completely out of proportion to the information likely to be gained. At the other extreme, a relatively brief test could be devised for the purpose of estimating a level for understanding cold running speech. Although Johnson, Work, and McCoy (1956) discussed what follows within the context of the Speech Stenger, it appears to be more reasonably located in this section. They suggest that it can be used on patients with bilateral functional hearing loss. Spondaic words and short questions are presented in rapid sequence at a variety of levels to one of the two ears. The patient is pressured to respond immediately and at the same time indicate from which ear he or she is hearing, an audiometric modification of the familiar children's game, "Simon Says." The "confusion and anxiety" which may develop can lead to the patient responding at levels in either ear which are below admitted thresholds of speech.

INTERPRETATION

This writer has been unable to undercover any standardized procedure, much less any systematic study of the test scheme. Interpretation of results from any test would be dependent on such information. It is concluded, along with Chaiklin and Ventry (1963), that the test is "difficult to recommend."

SWITCHED SPEECH TESTS

A variation on the principle is offered by Calearo (1957). The variation involves switching signals between two ears on the basis of time rather than words. For exmple, the 1st second of the message would be presented to one ear while the 2nd second was presented to the opposite ear and the 3rd second once again presented to the first ear. The switching would be done without regard to whether or not words were interrupted. When the technique is applied to normal listeners, the 2nd second would be inaudible rather than shifted to the opposite ear. Under such conditions and when the on-time is equal to the off-time, a normal individual's understanding is very poor. As the interruption rate increases beyond ten per second, however, nearly normal intelligibility is achieved. At, say, 50 interruptions per second, the message would be presented for 100th of a second followed by 100th of a second with no message, etc. Over any extended period of time, the first example and the one just described would provide the listener with exactly the same amount of total information, 50 percent of the message. In the former case, however, there would be relatively long periods of time where no message would be received while in the latter case, brief, but essentially continuous, samples, of the message would be available to the listener, permitting normal understanding. Calearo contends that the test permits "unmistakable and clear-cut results" in detecting functionality. Confirmation of this assertion could not be uncovered by this writer. This is unfortunate because of the clear logic of the test. Given proper normative data with various types of materials, including P–I functions at various interruption rates, reasonably precise estimates of true speech discrimination should be possible.

SUMMARY AND CONCLUSIONS

Retrospect

THE PROBLEM

In several contexts, it has been suggested that hearing sensitivity and the discrimination of suprathreshold sound are two distinctly different categories of behavior. Current clinical technique permits the relatively easy determination of auditory sensitivity without the cooperation of the patient. This is not true in the case of speech measures. The mainstay of evaluating speech discrimination performance for possible functionality is the comparison of volunteered P–I functions to normative data describing the patterns of performance produced by normal-hearing individuals and the various categories of hearing-impaired individuals. Speech detection and spondee threshold measures fall between the extremes of sensitivity and discrimination and may be estimated by physiologic technique, their validity evaluated by comparison to other psychoacoustic measures, and reasonable estimates of their true values obtained. Fortunately, identification of those with functioal hearing loss appears to be reasonably efficient by careful examination of measures which are routinely obtained in evaluation of any hearing loss.

THE SOLUTION

Routine tests. Accepting the assumption that there is no large body of successful functional hearing loss patients in our midst, comparison of routine PTAs and STs and examination of their reliability are the best indicators of functionality when there is no pretest reason to suspect its presence. The SDT may be included in those cases where discrimination appears to be significantly impaired or when the ST is unusually variable. If, as should be the case, more than one SL is used to measure discrimination, additional information about possible functionality can be obtained. More tediously, test–retest variability of discrimination at one or more sensation levels can complete the initial picture of a patient's P–I function. To recapitulate, the ST should approximate the PTA and both should be 10 dB poorer than the SDT. The P–I function for spondaic words should be steep, with a range of no more than 10 dB from no words correct to all correct (10–90 percent). The P–I function for speech discrimination materials should be no steeper than those produced by normal and hearing-impaired individuals. They may be shallower and the plateau may be lower. For those individuals who appear to communicate reasonably well in a face-to-face situation, the 50 percent performance level for speech discrimination materials should occur at presentation levels of no more than approximately 50 dB HL. Beyond these routine measures, the experienced audiologist may develop an ability to use other indices of a patient's behavior to detect functionality. Because of this writer's inability to describe such indices with the clarity necessary to insure that the naive reader will understand, no discussion of the indices was provided. It was noted that any case presenting within the context of possible or certain litigation should alert the audiologist to the possibility of functional hearing loss.

Special tests. A description of special tests for evaluating functionality was prefaced by pointing out that such tests are seldom critical for legal purposes and that present physiological techniques preclude precise evaluation of speech discrimination. Tests were categorized into four groups, graded in ascending degrees of approximations to speech discrimination from one which confirms impressions of functionality through estimates of SDTs to levels for understanding ongoing speech.

The Doerfler–Stewart Test is a variation on measures that are obtained in a routine evaluation (ST and an approximation of SDT, NDT, plus NIL). Aside from comparing NDT to NIL, the remaining four indices for the detection of functionality are variations of SDT–ST comparisons and test–retest reliability. The assumption behind the test is that noise will disrupt whatever internal standard the patient has established for responding. For a test almost universally cited as a special test for functionality, it is curious that one writer (Menzel, 1960) has suggested that its major value may be in discouraging functionality rather than unmasking it. This writer concludes with Menzel that, if used routinely enough so that the complexity of the test administered is overcome, the test has its greatest potential value in being routinely applied as the first measure whenever functionality is suspected. The reader should bear in mind that the test serves merely to unmask functionality.

A second group of tests (DAF, the Lombard, and GSR audiometry using speech stimuli) form a transition from confirming the presence of functionality to estimating levels of sound awareness. The phrase "sound awareness" is used advisedly in this context, and only to the extent that the noise or speech involved in a test must have been heard to see any change in performance. It is noted that although the DAF may be presumed to be a function of the intelligibility of the delayed signal, one study reviewed suggests it may be based predominantly on low-frequency hearing. As such, it may be expected that it would correlate best with SDTs. Of the three measures, GSR appears to be the most clearly defined procedure. The technique has been refined to the point where a true intelligibility, as opposed to detection, can be inferred from the results. The limitation, of course, is that conditioning is achieved to only a single word. Of the three tests, GSR audiometry would seem to be the test of choice where possible safety hazards are overcome and when appropriate medical supervision is available. Those conditions are rare, particularly since no commercially available instrument is currently available.

The Speech Stenger appears to be a valid test for obtaining an ST in unilateral functionality so long as the ST arrived at is qualified by the phrase "no poorer than." Because of the variability in the relationship between better and poorer ear SLs to achieve the effect, the true ST *may be better than* the estimated. The "Lipreading Test" appears to be a valuable test for establishing STs. It has three limitations. The patient must have decided to use the facade of lipreading as part of his or her overall functionality to buttress a claim against those situations in which he or she inadvertently responds more appropriately than he or she would have with a true hearing loss. The patient must be willing to undergo examination of this presumed modality of communication and, lastly, must be unaware of the true nature of the test.

The swinging speech test (alternate words between ears) and the switched speech test (switching on the basis of a time schedule) have a distinct capability when compared to the other tests. That capability is that responses which include the full message clearly indicate that hearing has occurred at some suprathreshold level. There is no standard test so that use of any test must be categorized as experimental in nature.

THE REPORT

At some point in time, collection of data is complete and the audiologist faces the task of reporting results. The first matter to be addressed is the consistency between tonal and speech thresholds by either routine or special tests. The best of these measures is the best estimate of sensitivity. While statements may be made about a patient's sensitivity to either tonal or speech stimuli with a reasonable degree of confidence, there is nothing in the way of formal testing that can demonstrate a person's ability to discriminate speech at suprathreshold levels without his cooperation. Inferences can be made, of course. The most fundamental can be developed when a patient offers reasonable communication efficiency in a face-to-face situation. Such performance allows the audiologist to backtrack known P–I functions to a conclusion that the ST is no poorer than about 35 dB. If there is a flaw in such reasoning, it is that P–I functions steeper than normal are conceivable if improbable.

A completely different tack may also be taken in the interpretation of results. It is of particular value in the case of children where functionality may be seen as a transient problem arising out of attempts to cope with stress. It may be wise to ignore all indications of functionality and focus upon communication effeciency at conversational levels. If within the range of normal, it would seem reasonable to emphasize that normality in both the posttest interview with parents and in any reports to school officials or the like. This emphasis on communication ability at conversational level may bring to mind visions of Davis' Social Adequacy Index (1978) and possible revisions proposed in Chapter 2. It is also noted that the position from which communication efficiency (as opposed to auditory sensitivity) is evaluated in compensation cases is receiving some attention. For example, the Department of Labor has shifted away from a classic PTA for estimating hearing loss to the use of hearing thresholds at

1000, 2000, and 3000 Hz in, presumably, an effort to arrive at measures which more accurately reflect the difficulty a person is encountering in day-to-day communication (Telcom, Hearing Loss Task Force, Department of Labor, Washington, D.C., July 28, 1978).

Prospect

There appears to be no significant future for speech protocols in the evaluation of functional hearing loss, as long as sensitivity measures remain the bulwark of evaluating the degree of hearing loss. Should society ever find it necessary to estimate speech discrimination, and should it be willing to pay for the development of measures to do so, then audiology would seem to have two alternatives available.

The first would be to develop physiological measures to the point where speech materials might be used as stimuli. In principle, the anticipatory response or the contingent negative variation response of electrical response audiometry might be applied to speech discrimination. However, a paradigm for their application might be exceedingly cumbersome as suggested by the complexities one might expect in raising GSR audiometry to a level where responses among several spondaic words could be separated.

Of the currently available techniques, switched speech tests have the greatest promise of measuring discrimination in spite of the complexities that would be encountered in matching critical portions of the acoustic signal to the "off" times. In the final analysis, some compromise between the principle of the story tests and the principle of the switched speech tests might be arrived at. The DAF, while figuring predominantly in recent reviews of tests for functional hearing loss, would seem to require a great deal of further experimentation to arrive at anything approaching a standard test.

Unfortunately, such speculation is pie-in-the-sky. Realistically, there is little in the way of currently standardized procedures that might permit an audiologist to make confident statements about the ST or discrimination score of patients with bilateral functional hearing loss who adamantly refuses to cooperate or to give up their mask of functionality.

REFERENCES

Atkinson, C. J. Some effects on intelligibility as the sidetone level and the amount of sidetone delay are changed. *Proceedings of the Iowa Academy of Science,* 1954, *61,* 334–340.

Black, J. W. The effect of delayed sidetone upon vocal rate and intensity. *Journal of Speech and Hearing Disorders,* 1951, *16,* 56–60.

Butler, R. A., & Galloway, F. T. Performance of normal-hearing and hard-of-hearing persons on the delayed auditory feedback test. *Journal of Speech and Hearing Research,* 1959, 2, 84–90.

Butler, R. A., & Galloway, F. T. Factorial analysis of the delayed speech feedback phenomenon. *Journal of the Acoustical Society of America,* 1957, *29,* 632–635.

Calearo, C. Detection of malingering by periodically switched speech. *Laryngoscope,* 1957, *67,* 130–136.

Chaiklin, J. B., & Ventry, I. M. Functional hearing loss. In J. Jerger (Ed.), *Modern developments in audiology,* New York: Academic Press, 1963, pp. 76–125.

Cherry, C., & Sayers, B. Experiments upon the tonal inhibition of stammering by external control and some clinical results. *Journal of Psychosomatic Research,* 1956, *1,* 233–246.

Cooper, J. C., Jr., & Owen, J. H. Audiologic profile of noise-induced hearing loss. *Archives of Otolaryngology,* 1976, *102,* 148–150.

Davis, H., & Silverman, S. R. *Hearing and deafness,* (4th ed.) New York: Holt, Rinehart & Winston, 1978.

Doerfler, L. G., & Stewart, K. Malingering and psychogenic deafness. *Journal of Speech and Hearing Disorders,* 1946, *11,* 181–186.

Fairbanks, G. Selective vocal effects of delayed auditory feedback. *Journal of Speech and Hearing Disorders,* 1955, *20,* 333–345.

Falconer, G. A. A "lipreading test" for nonorganic deafness. *Journal of Speech and Hearing Disorders,* 1966, *31,* 241–247.

Hanley, C. N., & Harvey, D. G. Quantifying the Lombard effect. *Journal of Speech and Hearing Disorders,* 1965, *30,* 274–277.

Hanley, C. N., Tiffany, W. R., & Brungard, J. M. Skin resistance changes accompanying the sidetone test for auditory malingering. *Journal of Speech and Hearing Research,* 1958, *1,* 286–293.

Harford, E. R., & Jerger, J. F. Effect of loudness recruitment on delayed speech feedback. *Journal of Speech and Hearing Research,* 1959, *2,* 361–368.

Harris, J. D. Speech audiometry. In A. Glorig (Ed.), *Audiometry: principles and practices,* Baltimore: Williams & Wilkins, 1965, pp. 151–170.

Hopkinson, N. T. Speech tests for nonorganic loss. In J. Katz (Ed.), *Handbook of clinical audiology,* Baltimore: Williams & Wilkins, 1973, 374–394.

Hopkinson, N. T. Speech tests for pseudohypacousis. In J. Katz (Ed.), *Handbook of clinical audiology,* Baltimore: Williams & Wilkins, 1978, pp. 291–303.

Jerger, J., Hayes, D., Anthony, L. Effect of age on prediction of sensorineural hearing level from the acoustic reflex. *Archives of Orolaryngology,* 1978, *104,* 393–394.

Johnson, K. O., Work, W. P., & McCoy, G. Functional deafness. *Annals of Otology, Rhinology, and Laryngology,* 1956, *65,* 154–170.

Korowbow, N. Reactions to stress: a reflection of personality trait organization. *Journal of Abnormal Social Psychology,* 1955, *51,* 464–468.

Menzel, O. J. Clinical efficiency in compensation audiometry. *Journal of Speech and Hearing Disorders,* 1960, *25,* 49–54.

Peters, R. W. The effect of acoustic environment upon speaker intelligibility. *Journal of Speech and Hearing Disorders,* 1956, *21,* 88–93.

Ruhm, H. B., & Carhart, R. Objective speech audiometry; a new method based on electrodermal response. *Journal of Speech and Hearing Research,* 1958, *1,* 169–178.

Taylor, G. J. An experimental study of tests for the detection of auditory malingering. *Journal of Speech and Hearing Disorders,* 1949, *14,* 119–130.

Underwriters' Laboratories Standard for medical and dental equipment. UL 544: July 7, 1976.

Ventry, I. M., & Chaiklin, J. B. Multi-discipline study of functional hearing loss. *Journal of Auditory Research,* 1965, *5,* 179–272.

Yates, A. J. Delayed audiotory feedback. *Psychological Bulletin,* 1963, *60,* 213–232.

Robert M. McLauchlin, Ph.D.

11

Speech Protocols for Assessment of Persons With Limited Language Abilities

In this chapter, the protocols employed to obtain speech audiometric results with language-limited individuals are reviewed. Language limited is defined for purposes of this chapter to mean verbal language skills are insufficient to permit the use of conventional adult speech audiometric procedures with English materials. Therefore, infants and young children who are acquiring verbal language on time are considered language limited. Non-English-speaking persons are viewed as language limited even though they may possess very high verbal skills in their own language. Moreover, hearing-impaired persons with reduced verbal language skills, despite the possible presence of exceptionally good written and manual language abilities, are considered language limited. Two other populations reviewed under this definition include persons who are mentally retarded or aphasic. These latter two populations probably are more traditionally thought of as language limited.

Some general considerations related to modified conventional speech protocols are discussed including masking, monitored live-voice presentation, calibration, auditory-visual presentation, probing language limitations, familiarization and selecting familiar materials, response reinforcers, and documentation. Modified speech protocols are discussed including speech detection threshold (SDT), speech reception threshold (SRT), speech discrimination (SD), as well as most comfortable loudness (MCL) and uncomfortable loudness (UCL) level tests. Finally, the specific language-limited populations of infants, young children, severely and profoundly hearing-impaired, mentally retarded, aphasic, and non-English-speaking persons are reviewed. Far too often, an audiometric report indicates speech audiometry or one of the speech protocols, such as SRT or SD, could not be tested because the client was too young, too retarded, or simply had limited verbal language abilities. Unfortunately, the limitation sometimes exists because the clinician and researcher have not modified routine speech protocols or devised new ones to accommodate the verbal language abilities of specific populations and individuals.

GENERAL CONSIDERATIONS

In modifying speech audiometric procedures to accommodate language-limited individuals, there are several general considerations. Most of the considerations are discussed in greater detail elsewhere in this book. Therefore, the purpose of this section is merely to reinforce that good clinical procedures are equally important when testing language-limited clients and to emphasize some special considerations when working with these persons.

Masking

Whenever speech stimuli possibly can cross over to the nontest ear—whether testing for SDT, SRT, SD, or MCL—masking obviously is essential. Clinicians should not assume masking will disrupt or confuse the aphasic, mentally retarded individual, or a young child to the extent that they will be unable to respond. In this clinician's experience, if language-limited clients can be instructed, shown, or conditioned to respond appropriately on speech audiometric tests without masking, then masked speech measures also can be obtained following additional verbal or gestural instruction or reconditioning to respond selectively to the speech stimuli. If masking cannot be used when it is essential, the fact should be indicated on the audiometric record. Moreover, the uncertainty of the audiometric results should be explained in order to preclude any misinterpretation of reported speech audiometric data. A reasonably good general rule is to mask whenever the speech stimuli are being presented to the test ear 40 dB above the established or possible bone conduction thresholds in the nontest ear. In the absence of bone conduction threshold measurements, masking should be used in the nontest ear whenever speech materials are being presented at or above 40 dB HL in the test ear.

Monitored Live-Voice Presentation

At least for clinical speech audiometry, monitored live-voice (MLV) usually is preferred over the use of recorded materials in evaluating most language limited persons. One exception, however, is the non-English-speaking individual being evaluated in a clinic where no clinician or resource individual is available who speaks the client's language. An MLV procedure increases the flexibility to eliminate the words not familiar to the listener, to vary the rate of presentation to match the quickness or slowness of the listener's response, to allow for extraneous interruptions, and to provide reinforcement at intervals based on the examiner's determination of need. When MLV is used, clinicians should adhere to acceptable techniques for using microphones and VU meters. Clinicians also should be aware when they may be using a dialect which is substantially different than the listener's. In the case of a very young child or infant, it may be helpful to train a parent to administer the MLV speech audiometry. Similarly, a person who speaks the language of a non-English-speaking client can be trained to present the speech materials by MLV. Finally, clinicians should be aware that an MLV procedure can yield differences in speech audiometric results, particularly in speech discrimination findings, when different speakers are used. Speech discrimination differences do occur with different speakers (Harris, Haines, Kelsey, & Clack, 1961). The author of this chapter often finds speaker differences to be dramatic in cases of moderate-to-marked high frequency hearing loss, having observed as much as 20–25 percent better speech discrimination scores for male versus female voices with such cases even when the materials are presented in quiet.

Calibration

Although speech protocols have to be modified and sometimes less formal for assessing language limited clients, clinicians should strive to attain and maintain accurate calibration of stimulus and environmental conditions. Without appropriate calibration protocols, findings are of little or no value. MLV and recorded speech materials should be presented at a VU meter level consistent with the level intended for the materials and instrumentation. Moreover, the listerner should be seated at the appropriate location in the sound-treated room to maintain calibration when testing in the soundfield. When client placement becomes impossible as sometimes is the case with a "terrible-two" child, this fact should be noted on the audiometric record.

Auditory-Visual Presentation

For individualized habilitation or rehabilitation planning, it is important to assess speech perception with the hearing-impaired client using his or her visual as well as auditory modality. Therefore, clinicians are encouraged to assess auditory-visual as well as auditory performance as an integral part of speech audiometric protocols with the hearing impaired.

The interaction between and relative reliance on the visual and auditory modalities for speech perception are crucial to most habilitative and rehabilitative decisions, particularly for moderately to profoundly hearing-impaired clients.

Probing Language Limitations

For purposes of performing speech audiometry, the clinician is most interested in any limitation in the client's verbal receptive vocabulary or general responsiveness to speech stimuli. Any possible limitations can be pursued in a variety of ways. First, a careful case history can reveal valuable information. For example, if the parents report that their three-year-old son is unable to follow any verbal instructions, the clinician has reason to suspect that an SRT cannot be obtained even using a protocol appropriate for most normal two-year-old children. On the other hand, the clinician should not rule out the possibility of the parents' observations being erroneous or of the child being unable to hear the instructions because of impaired hearing. Second, other diagnostic tests such as the Peabody Picture Vocabulary, subtests of childrens intelligence tests, and the Illinois Test of Psycholinguistic Abilities are useful in obtaining an auditory receptive vocabulary age which can assist in knowing whether the PBK-50 (Haskins, 1949) or Word Intelligibility by Picture Identification test (Ross & Lerman, 1970) is appropriate and possible to administer. See the discussion in this chapter under the section on speech discrimination about the appropriate vocabulary ages at which to administer these tests. Third, speech protocols known to be appropriate for normal clients of a given chronological age may be attempted. If they cannot be administered, this fact may serve to demonstrate language limitations. If scores on speech discrimination tests are below normal, then it should be determined if the items were missed because of a discrimination problem or a limitation in recognition vocabulary. When this author and others write about speech protocols being appropriate for specific aged infants and children, reference is being made to the chronological age of "normal" listeners. Therefore, probing the language limitations of individual listeners is essential to knowing which speech protocols can be or are being used appropriately.

Familiarization and Selecting Familiar Materials

Familiarizing the language-limited client with the speech stimuli intended for use and selecting alternate familiar materials are essential if valid, and sometimes if any, speech audiometric results are to be obtained. Even with adults, spondee thresholds (STs) are improved 4–5 dB by familiarizing them with the spondees when the CID W-1 (Hirsh et al., 1952) words and a 2-dB step procedure are used (Tillman & Jerger, 1959). Conn, Dancer, and Ventry (1975) devised a list of 15 spondees taken from the CID W-1 list which yielded unfamiliarized STs comparable to the familiarized STs using the entire list of 36 spondees. These 15 spondees fell within a 4 dB range of audibility as recommended by Curry and Cox (1966). Unfortunately, since these spondees were derived from the CID W-1 list, few of the 15 will meet concomitant criteria of being able to be illustrated pictorially and be within the recognition vocabulary of young children. Perhaps three to seven of these items might meet these two criteria including: baseball, airplane, armchair, stairway, birthday, railroad, and sidewalk.

With the language-limited, the task often is to select some speech items that are familiar to the listeners rather than familiarizing them with a preselected set of speech materials. Parents, spouses, friends, speech-language pathologists, special education teachers, and others who are in frequent contact with the clients may provide the clinician with speech materials that are within their auditory or auditory-visual recognition vocabulary. Clinicians may not be familiar with the common vocabulary of a very young child or with such television programs as "Sesame Street" and "The Electric Company." Additionally, they may not be familiar with the daily routine and language abilities of an institutionalized mentally retarded adult, may not know the residual language abilities of a young woman suffering from aphasia, or may not know the current colloquial vocabulary of a severely or profoundly hearing-impaired high school student. For example, "Big Bird" might be a better spondee than "wristwatch," "snowman," or "sandbox" to use in a picture-pointing ST test with a young child.

The number of items found to be within the recognition vocabulary of some language-limited persons may be extremely small and insufficient for any but the crudest of speech protocols. Under these circumstances, the clinician may engage in a familiarization process involving the training of clients to recognize a sufficient number of words to permit more elaborate, reliable, and valid speech protocols. This concomitant treatment and assessment protocol may be essential with mentally retarded, aphasic, profoundly hearing impaired, and very young clients. Parenthetically, training also may be necessary to familiarize these clients with the listening and response task as well as the materials. With a group of severely and profoundly hearing-impaired children five to nine years old, it took four to ten sessions on consecutive days before recognition scores stabilized using ten selected spondees (Cramer & Erber, 1974).

Whereas many clinicians familiarize adults with spondees before determining an ST, this author is unaware of any clinicians who routinely familiarize adults with lists of monosyllabic words or provide any practice in listening to these materials before assessing speech discrimination ability. This routine clinical practice continues despite cautions by Egan as early as 1957. The author of this chapter believes familiarization with the speech discrimination materials and listening task is equally important as it is with SRT testing, regardless of whether the listener is or is not language limited. When the client's receptive vocabulary is limited, familiarization with the SD materials, listening, and response task is paramount. To derive meaningful conclusions from WIPI scores when a listener does not recognize seven pictures from one list and three from a second list is impossible if the clinician is unaware that these items are unknown to the listener. Among many other possible erroneous conclusions, the clinician might believe there is a 16 percent difference in speech discrimination between the ears or hearing aids when making comparisons with these two WIPI lists. At a minimum, if prior familiarization is not done, the clinician should review all missed items with the client to determine if the errors are due to a discrimination, recognition vocabulary, or some other problem. An example of another problem includes pictures illustrated inappropriately on picture pointing tests. Familiarization encompasses many considerations when performing speech audiometry with the language-limited listener.

Response Reinforcers

Maintaining the attention of language-limited clients to the listening task often poses a problem. Therefore, clinicians and researchers routinely use various forms of reinforcers to establish and sustain appropriate responses to the presentation of speech stimuli. For non-English-speaking and aphasic clients as well as for severely and profoundly hearing-impaired children and adults, social reinforcement such as an appropriately timed smile, gesture, or verbal comment may suffice. With infants beginning at about six and 12 months, activating toy animals to flash on and off or mechanically move helps to obtain and maintain responses to speech as well as other auditory stimuli. Tangible reinforcers such as candy, trinkets, and other objects determined to be of interest to individual listeners are useful with mentally retarded clients and sometimes are used with young children. When planning to use tangible reinforcers, it is important to inquire of parents what might be most successful and what should not be used. For example, candy would be inappropriate if parents have their child on a sugarfree diet for health or personal reasons. This author finds enthusiastically presented social reinforcement to be satisfactory for most young children.

Documentation

In order to preclude misinterpretation of speech audiometric results obtained on language-limited listeners, documentation of most protocols is essential. The speech materials, type and levels of presentation, any modification in standardized procedures or calibration references, the listening and response task, the reliability and validity of responses, and opinion why specific speech protocols were modified or could not be performed should be specified clearly on the audiometric record. Extensive documentation also is important so that the same protocol may be used in subsequent testing or that it may serve as a basis for understanding obtained differences between sessions. Much of this documentation should be provided routinely for all speech audiometry. However, documentation tends to become more important with language-limited individuals because speech protocols seldom are routine with these clients. It is important: (1) to know if speech discrimination scores were derived using the WIPI; (2) to know which and how many words were not within a three-year-old child's recognition vocabulary for the lists employed; (3) to explain why an SRT was not obtained and why an SDT test was administered only in the soundfield; (4) to know the instructions given for measuring MCL and UCL; (5) to know the five of 18 spondees found to be within the recognition vocabulary of an aphasic or mentally retarded person. Clinicians are encouraged to provide this type of detailed documentation on all clients, but particularly on those persons with limited language.

These are some of the more important general considerations in performing speech audiometry with language-limited persons. Most of them are essential for routine speech protocols with all clients; although other considerations such as response reinforcers, documentation, and probing language limitations take on additional importance when testing language-limited individuals.

MODIFIED SPEECH PROTOCOLS

Speech protocols for language-limited persons are modified in a variety of ways to accommodate the language abilities of these individuals. In some instances, new rather than modified protocols are needed. The speech protocols reviewed in this section include SDT, SRT, SD, MCL, and UCL measurements.

Speech Detection Threshold

Speech detection threshold may be defined as the lowest intensity level at which a person can auditorily detect the presence of speech. An SDT is usually obtained when a clinician is unable to derive an SRT because of the listener's limited language abilities. According to Martin (1978), the listener, in addition to detecting the presence of speech, must identify the stimulus as speech. Giolas, (1975) recommends that a child make a repeated play response to verbal instruction. If the child is able to follow the verbal instruction, the intensity is lowered until the child ceases to respond. The author of this chapter believes these procedures (1) vary substantially from the traditional definition of SDT; (2) would result in poorer test–retest reliability with thresholds somewhere between SDT and SRT; and (3) would be difficult or impossible to follow by language-limited subjects on whom SDTs were being attempted because SRTs can not be obtained.

At least in the case of very young children, SDTs may yield a more accurate indication of threshold sensitivity than pure tones. Studies and reports indicate better responsiveness to speech and speech-like stimuli than to pure tones (Hardy & Bordley, 1951; Eisenberg, 1976; Northern & Downs, 1979). However, clinicians should understand that SDTs will be lower than the best pure-tone thresholds for a relatively flat audiometric configuration if the pure-tone and speech circuitry are calibrated to ANSI –1969. One of the purposes of this calibration is to achieve good agreement between the pure-tone average for 500, 1000, 2000 Hz and the speech reception threshold. But in achieving this end, speech detection thresholds are then going to be better than the pure-tone thresholds by about 8–10 dB, approximately the same difference found between the SDT and SRT (Beattie, Svihovec, & Edgerton, 1975; Hodgson, 1978). Thus, the SDT is not better than pure-tone thresholds, but appears to be because of an artifact related to the way audiometers are calibrated. Stated another way, if both pure-tone and speech audiometric testing was done with a single reference of 0 dB SPL, SDTs should agree closely with the best pure-tone thresholds obtained.

An SDT may be obtained on any specific language-limited person employing the same procedures used, or to be used, in measuring pure-tone thresholds. Depending upon the listener's capabilities, a hand raising, conditioned play, or visually reinforced orienting response might be employed. Depending also on the client's attentiveness and the clinician's professional philosophy, a five or two decibel step procedure might be used. For clinical purposes, a 5-dB step procedure is usually adequate and frequently desirable with a language-limited person whose attention span may be limited. This author recommends documenting on the audiometric record whether two or five decibel steps were used because current practices vary on which procedure is used throughout the United States.

Many different speech signals are used to determine SDTs including spondees, nonsense syllables, cold running speech, or the listener's name. Martin (1977) believes that cold running speech is inappropriate for children. According to Hodgson (1978), [bʌ-bʌ-bʌ] appears to have become conventional as a speech stimulus for determining SDT. Whatever speech stimuli are used to obtain SDTs, they should be noted on the audiometric record.

Clinicians should not attempt to predict the pure-tone audiogram or SRT based on an SDT. An SDT will relate to the best pure-tone threshold on the audiogram. Consequently, flat, rising, precipitously falling, and trough-shaped audiograms can all yield identical SDTs. Moreover, the SRT can be influenced by the audiometric configuration, thus making its accurate prediction based on the SDT impossible. Although the SDT can be predicted from the pure-tone audiogram, it is of little benefit other than to confirm agreement between SDT and the best pure-tone thresholds. As indicated earlier, agreement, may mean SDTs which are 8–10 dB better than the best pure-tone thresholds if the pure-tone and speech instrumentation is calibrated to ANSI-1969. Because of the limited value of the SDT, this author recommends its use only when an SRT cannot be obtained. Investigation of filtered speech and the Ling (1978) Five-Sound Test might prove useful in deriving some information about the shape of the audiogram from an SDT measurement.

Speech Reception Threshold

Speech reception threshold might be defined broadly as the lowest intensity level where 50 percent recognition of speech occurs. Whereas adults and children with normal language routinely are asked to repeat spondaic words from a fairly lengthy list, many alternate procedures are used with language-limited individuals. These procedures may include (1) presenting simple verbal instructions; (2) using a picture-pointing closed response format; or (3) selecting spondees which are found to be within the recognition vocabulary of individuals.

Early in the profession of audiology, Keaster (1947) developed a test of 25 simple directions with key nouns to be used for assessing speech reception in children as young as three years old. Pictures representing 25 nouns were placed on an easel in front of the child, and he or she was asked to name each picture. The reported purpose of this preliminary procedure was to insure that none of the pictures confused the child. Then the child was given several sample directions such as "put the baby on the floor," and told that this voice gradually would become very soft. Speech reception threshold was defined as the lowest level where at least three directions were followed correctly. Other than requesting the child to name the pictures which restricts the test to those with an intelligible expressive vocabulary, this speech reception threshold test would be as effective as many such tests in use today with young children. The thresholds of intelligibility for connected discourse and spondees are in close agreement (Falconer & Davis, 1947; Chaiklin, 1959). Therefore, simple commands may be used effectively as an alternate means for determining SRT with language-limited individuals. A 50 percent response criterion should still be used to define threshold.

Because young children learn about their body at an early age, asking them to "point to your . . .," "show me your . . .," or "touch your . . ." nose, arm, ear, and other body parts is usually an effective technique with two-year-old chidren. The clinician also can ask the child to "touch my . . ." or "touch Mommy's . . ." followed by the name of a body part. A more elaborate version of this procedure was investigated by Martin and Coombes (1976). They used a multicolored clown and candy reinforcing dispenser to assess speech reception thresholds of 40 normal-hearing preschoolers ranging in age from 17–56 months. Each child was instructed or shown how to push buttons on the appropriate part of the clown upon hearing "put your hand on the . . ." and one of the following words: hair, hat, hand, eye, nose, ear, foot, arm, leg, tummy, mouth, or ball (held in the clown's hand). All 20 children ranging in age from 30–56 months were tested successfully. SRTs were obtained on nine of ten children between the ages of 27 and 33 months. None of the ten 17–20 month old children could be tested with this technique. Simple instructions to stand up, sit down, bring me the ball, open the door, raise your hand, give mommy a kiss, and so forth can be used to establish an SRT.

A point-to-the-picture or -object technique is used extensively with language-limited individuals. It requires only a recognition vocabulary for the test items. Some clinicians apparently prefer the actual objects to pictures (Sortini & Flake, 1953; Northern & Downs, 1978). Objects are easier to obtain, less abstract, and do not have to be illustrated so as to realistically represent the object. However, this author prefers pictures when working with young children because he has found children more inclined to pick up objects than pictures and begin playing with them in a way not intended by the clinician.

To increase the reliability of spondee thresholds, various attempts have been made to select and record spondees which are close in intelligibility across intensity. As one attempts to accomplish this goal while simultaneously selecting spondees that can be represented pictorially and which are within the recognition vocabulary of very young children, the task becomes complicated. Although several studies have identified more homogeneously audible spondees from the CID W-1 pool of 36 words (Bowling & Elpern 1962; Curry & Cox, 1966; Beattie, Svihovic & Edgerton, 1975), less than six of these spondees, in this author's opinion, could be represented pictorially and be within the recognition vocabulary of young children.

McLauchlin, Rosenblatt, and Rupp (1971) developed a recorded list of 84 spondaic words including the CID 36 words and other spondees considered appropriate for use with young children. The range of the mean SLs for the 84 spondaic words was 9.6 dB, 66 of these spondees were recognized correctly within a 4 dB range of SLs, and 38 fell within a more stringent 2 dB range for a group of 10 normal-bearing young adults. Within the 4 dB range, at least 12 and possibly as many as 30 spondees could be illustrated pictorially and appear to be within the recognition vocabulary of young children. Even within the very homogeneous range of 2 dB, seven to 14 spondees appear to be appropriate for use in a picture-pointing test with young children. Hurley and McLauchlin (1972) expanded the investigation using 35 audiologically unsophisticated normal-hearing listeners. Recognition of the 84 spondees ranged over mean SLs of 13.7 dB. Forty-seven and 31 spondees fell respectively within a 4-dB and 2-dB range of mean SLs. Fifteen to 24 of the 47 spondees and 10 to 16 of the 31 spondees can be represented pictorially and appear to be suitable for use with very young children.

Wilson and McLauchlin (1973) presented water color paintings of the 24 spondees that fell within a 4-dB range of mean SLs in the Hurley and McLauchlin study to 44 young normal-hearing children ranging in age from 2.6 to 6.3 years old. The purpose was to determine whether these words were within the recognition vocabulary of young children and appropriately illustrated. Because each child was faced with 24 pictures from which to choose, the stimulus word was presented twice when there was no response or an error was made on the first presentation. Based on the summed scores, all spondees were eliminated where more than 4 (10 percent) of the 44 children were unable to select the correct picture. Six spondees were eliminated in this procedure, leaving 18 that were highly recognizable across a wide range of young children. All 24 spondees were correctly identified by the children 6.0–6.5 years old, but increasing numbers of spondees were not identified as the age of the children decreased. Most children above the age of 4.6 years were able to recognize 18 of the spondees. Table 11-1 illustrates the 18 spondees found to be highly homogeneous in audibility and within the recognition vocabulary of most normal-hearing children ranging in age from 4.6–6.5 years old. Twelve items were recognized nearly 100 percent of the time by even the younger aged children and have been asterisked.

Of the 18 spondees found to be within the recognition vocabulary of most normal-hearing young children and pictorially illustratable, only three (airplane, hotdog, toothbrush) appeared in the homogeneous grouping by Bowling and Elpern (1961), two (airplane, toothbrush) in the Curry and Cox study (1966), and none in th Beattie et al. investigation (1975).

The ASHA "Guidelines for Determining the Threshold Level for

Table 11-1
Spondees Selected for Use With Language Limit Populations

Wilson & McLauchlin, 1973	Griffing et al., 1967	Lloyd et al., 1967	Erber, 1974	Cramer & Erber, 1974
*snowman	snowman		snowman	snowman
*shotgun				
*toothbrush	toothbrush	toothbrush		
*wristwatch	wristwatch	wristwatch		
*hairbrush				
*bandaid				
*sandbox	sandbox			
*hotdog			hotdog	
*doghouse				doghouse
*airplane	airplane	airplane	airplane	airplane
*cupcake	cupcake			
*ice cream	ice cream		ice cream	ice cream
sailboat	sailboat		sailboat	
jumprope		jumprope		
baseball			baseball	
shoelace				
sidewalk				
highchair	highchair			
	bathtub		bathrub	bathtub
	firetruck			firetruck
	cowboy	cowboy	cowboy	
		blackboard	blackboard	
			birthday	
			cubscout	
			doughnut	
			earphone	
			eyebrow	
			haircut	
			lunchroom	
			mailbox	
			notebook	
			paintbrush	
			playground	
			popcorn	popcorn
			schoolbus	
			sidewalk	
			stopsign	
			toothpaste	toothpaste
				lunchbox
				raincoat

*Words found to be highly homogeneous in audibility, within the recognition vocabulary of very young children, and pictorially illustrable.

Speech'' (1979) recommend spondaic words as the standard test material and use of the term "Spondee Threshold" (ST) to denote the materials used. Although two half lists of the CID W-1 spondees separated according to the criteria of dissimilarity and homogeneity of audibility are presented, the guidelines recognize that different lists of spondees may be necessary for children, neurologically impaired clients, and other special populations. Clearly, the problem with the W-1 list of 36 spondees is that only a few of the items are able to be represented pictorially and are concomitantly within the recognition vocabulary of young children.

Although the Verbal Auditory Screening for Children (VASC) was developed as a screening test (Griffing, Simonton & Hedgecock, 1967), the twelve spondee pictures are sometimes used by clinicians to establish spondee thresholds. This author recommends separating the 12 VASC pictures mounted on a single sheet so the spondees can be eliminated which are found not to be within the recognition vocabulary of the person being tested. Table 11-1 shows that seven of the 12 VASC spondees appear in the Wilson and McLauchlin (1973) list of 12 spondees found to be highly homogeneous in audibility and within the recognition vocabulary of very young children. Lloyd, Reid, and McManis (1967) used six spondee pictures to establish STs with mentally retarded children. Table 11-1 illustrates that three of these six spondees were identical to three of the 12 Wilson and McLauchlin spondees. Erber (1974) as well as Cramer and Erber (1974) used 25 and 10 spondees, respectively, for obtaining recognition scores with severely and profoundly hearing-impaired older children. As illustrated in Table 11-1, only three of the Erber and four of the Cramer and Erber spondees were identical to the 12 homogeneous Wilson and McLauchlin spondees. Further studies are necessary to determine which spondaic words are within the recognition vocabulary of different language-limited populations. For young children, this author recommends the 12 spondees asterisked in Table 11-1.

A variety of ST procedures are used clinically. Chaiklin and Ventry (1964) recommended a descending 5-dB step procedure, but indicated another study by them suggested an ascending procedure might be faster. Lloyd and Reid (1966) used a descending 2-dB step procedure with a group of mentally retarded children. Tillman and Olsen (1973) recommended a descending 2-dB step procedure which was subsequently supported by Wilson, Morgan, and Dirks (1973). Martin and Stauffer (1975) developed a modification in the Tillman and Olsen procedure for use when testing the ST before pure-tone thresholds or when examiner bias based on prior knowledge of the pure-tone average needs to be minimized. Martin and Stauffer indicated that the modification might be useful in testing small children. The ASHA "Guidelines for Determining the Threshold Level for Speech" (1979) recommended an ascending 5-dB step procedure. Threshold was defined as the lowest level at which at least half (two or more) of the spondees were repeated correctly with a minimum of two ascending sampling series. According to Martin (1978), a 5-dB and even 10-dB step procedure frequently yields rapid and acceptable STs with children.

In the interest of standardization and efficiency in clinical testing of language-limited clients, this author recommends the ascending 5-dB step procedure suggested in the ASHA "Guidelines." However, clinicians are cautioned against allowing too much time to elapse while presumably in the range of inaudibility with some language-limited clients. A listener may tire of the task before an ST can be established. Given the current variation in techniques used to determine the ST, this author also recommends documenting on the audiometric record the dB unit of measurement and whether a descending or ascending approach were used to obtain the ST.

Due to the additional time involved in using a carrier phrase, which may be at a premium with some language-limited cases, this author does not recommend its use with these clients unless the clinician determines a carrier phrase is essential as an alerting signal for specific cases. Martin (1978) suggests using a carrier phrase for a few initial presentations and then deleting it if the child understands the task. Northern and Downs (1978) recommend using a carrier phrase 10–15 dB above the presentation level of the spondee to hold the child's attention while searching for the threshold. A final recommendation concerning procedures is to use a monitored live-voice presentation for accommodating the reduced recognition vocabularies, slower responses, interferences, and other problems often encountered with language-limited clients.

There have been several studies to develop formuli for calculating the SRT from pure-tone thresholds (Carhart, 1946; Fletcher, 1950; Harris, Haines, & Meyers, 1956; Quiggle, Glorig, Delk, & Summerfield, 1957; Graham, 1950; Carhart, 1971). Carhart's more recent formula (1971) predicts the SRT by adding the pure-tone thresholds at 500 and 1000 Hz, dividing by two, and then subtracting 2 dB. He believes this is a reasonably good formula when specific audiometric configurations are not taken into account and audiometric equipment is calibrated to ANSI-1969. Unfortunately, these generalized formuli are accurate for individuals only with relatively flat audiometric configurations. Therefore, Carhart and Porter (1971) provide some guidelines for selective use and weighting of the pure-tone frequencies 500, 1000, 2000, and 4000 Hz to predict SRTs depending on the audiometric configuration. To predict SRTs based on pure-tone data for clients with audiometric contours other than relatively flat ones, further reseach is needed to clarify the relative contributions of pure-tone thresholds by frequency for different audiometric patterns.

There predictive formuli would be beneficial for language-limited clients on whom SRTs cannot be obtained but pure-tone measurements are possible.

Since occasionally an SRT can be obtained when pure-tone thresholds are unobtainable, it conversely would be beneficial to predict pure-tone audiometric thresholds from an SRT. However, too many different audiometric configurations are associated with an identical SRT. Selective high, mid, or low frequency hearing impairment can be missed if predictions about hearing sensitivity for 125 through 8000 Hz are attempted solely on the basis of SRT measurements.

Speech Discrimination

The conventional monosyllabic speech discrimination materials such as the PB-50 and CID W-22 lists, combined with a verbal response, are inappropriate for use with language-limited clients. These materials were developed for adults with reasonably good language skills. Therefore, many of the words are not within the recognition vocabulary of young children and other language-limited persons. Articulation and voice problems associated with hearing impairment, mental retardation, and other disorders frequently preclude accurate scoring of verbal responses given by these persons. Often, writing skills ae insufficiently developed or are sufficiently disordered, thus preventing a written response. Even the multiple-choice tests by Fairbanks (1958), Black (1968), and Kreul et al. (1968) are usually inadequate because they depend on the person being able to read word choices.

Haskins (1949) developed a modification of the PB-50 lists for use with children or adults with limited language. Although these materials gained wide acceptance throughout the United States during the 1950s and 1960s, they still required a verbal or written response and a receptive vocabulary of about 5–6 years of age. Matkin (1977) recommends use of the PBK-50 lists for children with receptive vocabulary ages between six and 12 years.

One of the earliest available picture-pointing tests of speech discrimination ability was the Boston University Speech Sound Discrimination Test (Pronvost & Dumbleton, 1954). There are 36 sets of three similar-sounding word pairs pictured on each set. Vowel as well as consonant discrimination ability is assessed. The clinician names one of the word pairs, and the listener is to point to the appropriate picture representing the verbal stimulus. A sample of the three word pairs would be *cat–bat, bat–bat,* and *cat–bat*. Two of the three pairs are used as test items, thus allowing a total possible score of 72. Thirty-six items can be used for a shortened version. In 1957, Templin reported on the development of a picture-pointing test, which is referred to as the Templin Picture Sound Discrimination Test. Upon hearing the stimulus word, the listener is to point to one of two pictures on a card. The paired stimulus words are like-sounding, and the total possible score is 59.

This author's interest in a test of speech discrimination for language-limited persons dates back to 1963–64 while working on the predecessor to the Word Intelligibility by Picture Identification (WIPI) test at the University of Connecticutt. In 1963, Myatt and Landes reported on the standardization of a speech discrimination test used with groups of normal, speech defective, and mentally retarded trainable as well as educable children. The ages of the children in this study ranged from three years, seven months to six years, ten months for the intellectually normal children and from five years, two months to 15 years, six months for the mentally retarded children. Each child's task was to point to one of four pictures on a page upon hearing a monosyllabic noun word. There were twenty pages with a total of 80 items, which were all used to form four lists of 20 items per list. After reviewing a large number of pictures from magazines, children's books, and speech audiometric cards, these investigators ultimately selected the final 80 test items which were "recognized by virtually all of the children" (p. 361) in this study. These authors concluded that this test was applicable for children whose IQs were about or exceeded 50. In addition, the possibility of using this test with hearing-impaired children was implied.

Consequently, Lerman, Ross, and McLauchlin (1965) explored this implied possibility. Following a discouraging attempt to find existing realistically colored pictures of uniform size and background for the 80 words selected by Myatt and Landes, a commercial artist was employed to paint these pictures to specification. The four lists were found to be comparable and reliable for assessing speech discrimination with hearing-impaired children ranging in age from four years, eight months to ten years, 11 months. These children had varying degrees and types of hearing impairment. However, (1) some words such as "gate," "belt," and "vase" did not appear to be within the recognition vocabulary of the young hearing-impaired children sampled; (2) some pictures were inadequate representations of the words; and (3) chance scores were too high with only four choices.

Therefore, the author of this chapter reviewed preschool and kindergarten reading materials and word-count lists to select additional monosyllabic nouns judged to be within the recognition vocabulary of young children and capable of being represented pictorially. Nursery school and kindergarten teachers then judged whether these words would be familiar to the children they taught. Although an attempt was made to select rhyming words with variations only in the initial and final consonants, this goal was not achieved entirely because of the limited number of known noun words suitable to illustrate pictorially for this population. Given these limitations, 26 sets of six words each were assembled. It was considered desirable to add at least five more words per list so the unit value could be reduced from five to four percent.

This author moved to Detroit in 1966 to begin a doctoral program, and Ross and Lerman (1970) completed the final standardization study with the assistance of James Peck. In a preliminary evaluation, 15 hearing-impaired children ranging in age from six to 12 years old were used to select four of the six words in each set which were within the recognition vocabulary of these young children and to screen out any pictures which were poor representations of the test words. Four lists of 25 words each were chosen, leaving two additional pictures on each plate as foils. These additional pictures reduce the probability of high scores based on chance or recall of what pictures were identified on precedingly presented lists.

This final version of the WIPI was standardized on 61 hearing-impaired children. Ross and Lerman found the four lists to be comparable and to yield good test–retest reliability. The WIPI, they concluded, was suitable for moderately hearing-impaired children five to six years old and for severely hearing-impaired children seven to eight years old. The authors further concluded that: (1) additional data were needed on the use of the WIPI with children under five years old, (2) WIPI scores, based on theoretical and limited research considerations, should exceed conventional open ended response speech discrimination scores by 25 percent; (3) speech discrimination functions should be derived for the four lists; and (4) norms should be established for presenting the WIPI in the presence of noise.

Although Ross and Lerman predicted that WIPI scores should exceed conventional speech discrimination scores by 25 percent, Hodgson (1973) found only ten percent better scores with normal hearing children between the ages of five and nine years of age on an open response versus closed response presentation of the WIPI test items. In cases of hearing-impaired children with substantially reduced speech discrimination ability, possibly differences between tests of as much as 25 percent may occur.

Schwartz (1971) found Lists 1 and 2 of the WIPI test applicable for use with preschool normal-hearing children down to the age of two years, six months. Lists 3 and 4 were not evaluated. The mean scores were 83 percent for the two year, six month to three year-old-group and 93 percent for the five year to five year, six-month-old-group. The mean score even for the three year to three year, six-month-old children was 89 percent, which suggests the WIPI test is relatively acceptable for use with three-year-old children. Because even some five-year-old children were missing items, the author of this chapter recommends that all missed words be checked to determine if they are within the recognition vocabulary of each person being tested. An analysis of errors according to age conducted by Schwartz provides some indication of what words may not be appropriate for very young children.

Sanderson-Leepa and Rintelmann (1976) compared the results of the WIPI, PBK-50, and Northwestern University Auditory Test No. 6 (NU–6) lists on 60 normal hearing children ranging in age from 3½–11½ years old. As might be suspected, scores on the WIPI test were highest; scores on the PBK-50 test were intermediate; and those on the NU–6 test were poorest. Moreover, the WIPI test appeared to be most appropriate for preschool children as young as 3½ years. The mean score for the 3½ year old children was 92 percent at a 32 dB SL with a standard deviation of 6.26. This finding is in close agreement with the 89–94 percent mean scores and 4.5–6.4 standard deviations obtained on three- to four-year-old normal-hearing children by Schwartz (1971). The PBK-50 or WIPI test seemed to be adequate for the normal hearing children of about 5½ years. According to these researchers, however, the WIPI test might be preferred because it can be administered faster, is not as limited by differences in speech and language abilities among children, and is intrinsically a more interesting task for young children. These investigators also provide an error analysis, which should be helpful in predicting words that are unfamiliar to young children.

Weber and Reddell (1976) devised 100 sentences using the WIPI test words. Seventy-five normal hearing and hearing-impaired children were given both the word and sentence forms of the test. Scores were similar for 50 of the children who had either very good or poor speech discrimination ability. Twenty-one children with moderate speech discrimination problems demonstrated an average improvement of 20 percent on the sentence test with a range from 12–40 percent. These investigators were surprised to find four children who yielded an average decrement of 19 percent on the sentence version of the WIPI test, with a range from 12–44 percent. They hypothesized that if these four children were found to have language disorders, the sentence form of the WIPI test might provide diagnostic usefulness in identifying otherwise unsuspected language problems. The sentences appear in Weber and Reddell's article.

A speech discrimination test entitled Picture Identification for Children—A Standardized Index (PICSI) was developed by Seidel (1963). Three lists of 58 monosyllabic noun words were selected based on the familiarity of these words by three- to five-year-old children and on whether the word could be represented pictorially. Each of the 58 cards contained three pictures of nouns which varied only in an initial or final consonant. Although the test was administered to 60 preschool children, the test was never made available commercially.

Siegenthaler and Haspiel (1966) devised a picture-pointing speech discrimination test for children called the Discrimination by Identifcation of Pictures (DIP) test. It consists of three lists and 48 cards with two pictures on each card. To obtain three lists, words are reused in a different order of presentation. Because there are only two pictures on each card, a 50 percent score is possible by change selection.

Several speech discrimination tests involve paired stimuli and a response indicating whether the pairs are the same or different. Wepman (1960) devised the Wepman Auditory Discrimination Test which requires such a response. The listener hears ten pairs of identical and 30 pairs of dissimilar words for a possible score of 40. Upon hearing each pair of words, the listener is to state whether the words were the same or different. Schlanger and Galanowsky (1966) developed a similar test using nonsense syllables. They found the results to be almost identical to those on the Wepman Test for groups of mentally retarded and normal children with mental ages of seven years, seven months, and seven years, three months respectively. Using paired nonsense syllables, Kelly and Pillow (1979) developed a same-different test with nonsense syllables for use with young children. If the verbally presented paired stimuli are the same, the child is to point to a picture of two Charlie Browns. If they are different, the child is to point to a picture of Charlie Brown and Snoopy. This test consists of five lists of ten paired nonsense syllables. Four of each ten syllable pairs are the same and the remaining six pairs are different. The test was administered to 12 normal hearing children between the ages of 4.6 and 6.0 years. A mean score of 84 percent (ranging from 72–92 percent) was obtained, which the authors thought supported the contention that nonsense syllables are too abstract for young children. In an earlier study using the same test with normal hearing adults, Kelly (1968) had obtained a mean percentage correct score of 98 percent.

Only a mean score of 81 percent, however, was obtained on a same-different task with the Wepman word pairs for children with a mental age of seven years, three months. Thus, the reduced percentage correct scores obtained by Kelly and Pillow with young children may be related more to factors such as discrimination ability, attentiveness or short-term memory associated with the same-different response task rather than to the abstractness of nonsense syllables.

Schwartz and Goldman (1974) have expressed concerns about the use of the same–different type of auditory discrimination test. According to these authors, this type of test may contain unfamiliar vocabulary, the response task may be unfamiliar, and paired stimuli may require memory which can adversely affect the response score. This author believes the first concern is relevant to all tests of speech discrimination, not just same–different tests, but this author would add another concern. Scores can be influenced by the chance probability of obtaining a 50 percent score with a two-alternative choice. Despite these concerns, there may be instances where a same–different speech discrimination test would be more appropriate than a multiple-choice picture pointing test for specific language limited individuals. This type of test traditionally has been used with clients exhibiting articulation and language rather than hearing disorders.

Most Comfortable Loudness and Uncomfortable Loudness Levels

The MCL and UCL level measurements for speech are useful in selecting appropriate amplification for hearing-impaired persons. Even for clients without language problems, these measurements sometimes are difficult to establish and vary substantially depending upon instructions and psychophysical procedure. Despite these difficulties, clinicians are encouraged to modify their existing procedures whenever and however necessary to measure the MCL and UCL of language limited persons. The UCL measurement is particularly important in determining what a hearing aid's saturation sound pressure level (SSPL) should be set at to preclude extreme discomfort and possible additional hearing loss due to noise exposure. With infants as well as some mentally retarded and aphasic patients, UCL may have to be estimated from reflex measurements or by observing nonverbal signs of discomfort as the intensity of sound stimuli is increased. The MCL can be determined in a more leisurely time frame during an extended hearing aid orientation program.

LANGUAGE LIMITED POPULATIONS

Five specific types of language-limited clients are discussed in this section, including: (1) infants; (2) young children; (3) mentally retarded; (4) severely and profoundly hearing impaired; (5) aphasic; and (6) non-English-speaking persons.

Infants: Zero–Two Years

With the extreme importance of early intervention and habilitation for hearing-impaired infants, clinicians need new and improved speech audiometric procedures to use with this population. Treatment decisions have to be made such as how much emphasis to place on audition; which hearing aid to select; whether the aid is to be monaural, binaural, or a CROS-type; and whether previous habilitation has been successful. The accuracy and appropriateness of these decisions will improve correspondingly with the development of new speech protocols for infants. Clinicians typically rely on any consistent reflexive or volitional responses to the presentation of a variety of speech stimuli as the only speech audiometric procedure to use with infants. Visual reinforcement usually is presented following appropriate responses from infants six to 24 months.

Northern and Downs (1978) review the responses of normal-hearing infants to speech stimuli. A startle response is obtained from most infants, including newborns, to a speech signal suddenly introduced into a quiet environment at 65 dB HL (ANSI-1969). Between four and seven months, infants begin to turn their heads toward the source of sounds and respond on the average to speech stimuli presented at 21 dB HL (ANSI-1969). Infants of this age may be more responsive to the name they are called at home, other words frequently used with them, and the voices of the persons who have spent the most time with them during the first few months of life. Between seven and nine months of age, infants on the average turn their head consistently in the correct lateral direction toward the source of speech presented at about 15 dB HL (ANSI-1969). By 13 months, infants usually localize the source of speech stimuli in both a vertical and horizontal plane presented at only 5 dB HL (ANSI-1969). Between 18 and 20 months, infants begin to recognize the names of a few objects and body parts, thus permitting the estimate of SRT. Clinicians can give instructions to infants of this age such as "pick up the ball" or "bring me the cup." This author usually asks infants of this age to "show me . . ." or "point to your . . ." nose, mouth, hand, and other body parts.

Simmons-Martin (1978) states that "Regrettably, infants' speech discrimination cannot be tested but must be observed" (p. 373). Fortunately, because of extensive research being conducted on normal language acquisition with some emphasis on early speech discrimination ability (Moffitt, 1968; Friedlander, 1970; Eimas et al., 1972; Condon & Sander, 1974; Ling & Ling, 1974; Miller & Morse, 1976; Spring & Dale, 1977; and Davis, 1978), the potential exists for developing new and more formal clinical tests of speech discrimination ability for use with infants. These research findings indicate the ability of the infant to discriminate between fairly subtle speech differences even during the first few months of life and delineate some conditioning protocols for possible clinical adaptation. Hopefully, the applied research necessary to develop these clinical tests is currently in process. In the meantime, clinicians should continue to assess informally the speech discrimination abilities of infants by observing the rate or lack of speech development. Specifically, clinicians can assess the ability to imitate, differentiate between and spontaneously produce phonemes, syllables, and words.

Young Children: Two–Four Years

Speech protocols are possible with young children, but many modifications are necessary. Valid SDTs can be obtained by using a visual reinforcer for appropriate orienting responses with most infants down to about 13 months and is a technique sometimes necessary with some two-year-olds. A conditioned play response such as dropping a block in a box can be used to determine the SDT with many two-year-olds, and is the protocol of choice with most three-year-old children. This play technique can be used with four-year-old children, although a simple hand or arm raising response is possible with many children of this age. Some indication of audiometric frequency pattern may be obtained by using filtered speech of the Ling (1978) Five-Sound Test.

Generally, speech reception threshold measurements can be obtained using simple instructions for two-year-old children and a picture-pointing protocol for three- and four-year-old children. Two- to three-year-old children should be able to follow many simple auditory directions, including pointing to many pictures or objects. The major problems usually are trying to retain the attention of these children during their "terrible twos" and finding those nouns which are within their recognition vocabulary. Three- and four-year-old children usually have sufficient receptive vocabulary to permit the routine use of selected spondee picture cards and a pointing response. This author recommends the use of the 12 asterisked spondees appearing in Table 11-1 and a familiarization procedure to eliminate any items not within the recognition vocabulary of individual children.

Speech discrimination testing with the two-year-old is easier than with the infant, but currently still involves some informal procedures. By asking the parents for a list of words the child understands and by reviewing a collection of simple pictures or objects with the child, some selected items can be obtained for measuring speech discrimination ability. The WIPI test can be used as a source for these pictures. Although some clinicians use environmental sounds to assess auditory discrimination of two-year-old children and infants, they should be cautious in generalizing their findings to speech discrimination ability (Ling, 1976).

With three-year-old children, clinicians can use the WIPI to test speech discrimination ability; but it must either be predetermined or determined after the fact which words are not within the recognition vocabulary of each child. The error analysis data reported by Schwartz (1971) and Sanderson-Leepa and Rintelmann (1976) provide some information on those words which may be appropriate with this age child. With four-year-old children, the WIPI can be used routinely. However, the author still recommends a posttest check of those items missed to determine if they are within the recognition vocabulary of individual children being tested.

Mentally Retarded

Several investigators have used modified speech protocols with mentally retarded persons. Studies by Lloyd (1965), Lloyd and Melrose (1966), and Lloyd, Reid, and McManis (1967) all showed that "point-to-the-picture" and "say-the-word" spondee thresholds were virtually identical for clinical purposes with mentally retarded normal-hearing subjects. Mean differences between the two procedures were less than 3 dB for all three studies and less than 1 dB in the 1967 study. Test–retest reliability also was found to be good in all three of these studies for either response method used with mentally retarded subjects. The selected six spondees used by Lloyd and his associates appear in Table 11-1. The test–retest reliability was slightly better for speech than pure-tone thresholds with retarded persons (Fulton & Graham, 1964; Lloyd & Melrose, 1966; and Lloyd & Reid, 1966).

Schlanger and Galanowsky (1966) administered four tests of auditory discrimination to 85 institutionalized mentally retarded children and 86 normal children matched according to mental age on the Peabody Picture Vocabulary Test. The mean mental ages were seven years, three months and seven years, seven months for the normal and retarded groups, respectively. All of the children had normal hearing. The four tests included the Templin Picture Sound Discrimination Test (Templin, 1957); Boston University Speech Sound Discrimination Test (Pronovost and Dumbleton, 1954); Wepman Auditory Discrimination Test (Wepman, 1960); and a Nonsense Syllable Discrimination Test patterned by the authors of this study after the Wepman Test. The retarded group scored poorer on all four tests by the mean differences in percent correct scores of six percent for the Templin, 12 percent for the Boston, 12 percent for the Wepmen, and 13 percent for the authors' Nonsense Syllable Test. These reduced scores for the retarded group were attributed by these investigators possibly to adverse factors associated with institutionalized living. When the children were asked to point to the appropriate picture, 94 percent and 93 percent scores were achieved on the Templin and Boston tests, respectively. But when asked to indicate verbally whether what they heard was the same or different, only an 81 percent score was obtained on both the Wepman and Nonsense Syllable Test. Apparently, the discrimination or response task or combination of these two factors are easier with the Templin and Boston than with the Wepman and Nonsense Syllable Tests.

Wilson and McLauchlin (1972) administered the WIPI lists to 40 normal hearing institutionalized mentally retarded children ranging in age from nine years, one month, to 19 years, one month with a mean age of 15 years. List equivalency remained high, despite progressively reduced scores associated with decreasing intelligence. Many of the WIPI items were taken from the Myatt and Landes (1963) test, which was standardized on a group of mentally retarded children. The mean scores by degreee of mental retardation were 95.4 percent for the mild, 72.5 percent for the moderate, 60.4 percent for the severe, and 31.8 percent for the profound groups. As can be seen by these scores, the WIPI test was found suitable in its present form for use with the mildly retarded, but would require modification for use with the more severely retarded. An item analysis was performed to determine which words were missed most frequently and what were the error responses.

This author recommends the use of selected spondees for determining SRTs, and the WIPI for determining SD scores with mentally retarded children and adults when they exhibit sufficient capability to perform these tests. Error analysis data can help in preselecting words which are unlikely to be within the recognition vocabulary of persons with greater than a mild degree of retardation. Familiarization and usually reinforcement procedures are essential with this population.

Severely and Profoundly Hearing Impaired

Conventional speech audiometric procedures designed for adults occasionally are appropriate for persons with severe hearing impairments, but are virtually useless with the profoundly hearing impaired. Therefore, numerous procedures and materials have been devised for conducting speech audiometry with severely and profoundly hearing-impaired clients.

Watson (1957) constructed a picture vocabulary test consisting of twenty cards with six pictures on each card for use with deaf children. The words were printed beneath each picture for the benefit of children who could read. Although he administered the test to deaf children between the ages of ten and 15 years, he found the test useful with only some of the children and did not standardize these materials.

Jones and Studebaker (1974) found the Oklahoma University Closed-Response Test (OUCRT) more beneficial than the open-response W-22 test for measuring speech discrimination of severely and profoundly hearing-impaired children who ranged in age from nine to 16 years. Using conventional speech audiometric procedures and materials, SRTs could not be obtained on 11 of 23 children; and zero percent speech discrimination scores were obtained for nine of 23 children with an open-ended response to presentation of a W-22 word list. In contrast, all 23 subjects achieved greater success in choosing the appropriate items on a closed-response task. Speech discrimination scores for the 23 children ranged from 11–94 percent on the OUCRT compared to zero to 34 percent of the W-22 test. Moreover, according to Jones and Studebaker, the closed-response paradigm permitted an analysis of phonemic errors.

Erber and his associates at the Central Institute for the Deaf have published extensively on procedures for assessing speech discrimination among the severely and profoundly hearing impaired. Cramer and Erber (1974) used ten spondaic words recorded on Language Master Cards and a picture-pointing response to assess speech "recognition" (discrimination) in 58 severely and profoundly hearing-impaired children ranging in age from five to nine years. Average pure-tone thresholds for 500, 1000, and 2000 Hz ranged from 52–123 dB HL (ANSI-1969). The ten spondees determined to be familiar to these children are shown in Table 11-1. Special precautions were taken to insure that the words were recorded at a similar duration and intensity. Use of the Language Master allowed for easier randomization of the ten spondees, and the children also were very familiar with this device. The spondees then were presented at "maximum tolerable levels—at least 15 dB above each child's threshold for detection of speech" (p. 306), and verbal reinforcement was used to maintain attentive behavior. Generally, children with pure-tone averages between 52 and 92 dB HL obtained recognition scores of 66–100 percent, and those with averages exceeding 103 dB HL scored between zero and 65 percent. Children with pure-tone averages from 93–103 dB HL were less predictable based on their audiometric thresholds, yielding recognition scores from 8–100 percent. Moreover, in contrast to consistently high or low scores with the other two groups, the 93–103 dB HL group showed steadily improving or inconsistent performance for repeated measures on consecutive days. Cramer and Erber hypothesized that the children scoring 0–65 percent may have perceived speech based primarily on a time—intensity envelope, whereas those scoring 66–100 percent may have perceived speech by also using spectral characteristics. This speech recognition task should be beneficial in making decisions about hearing aid selection as well as determining auditory training goals and procedures according to these researchers.

Erber and Alencewicz (1976) found high word recognition scores on a closed-response picture-pointing test with children having average hearing threshold levels better than 95 dB at 500, 1000, and 2000 Hz. The test words included four monosyllabic, four trochaic, and four spondaic noun words. The performance of children with average thresholds between 95 and 110 dB on this test varied extensively, and the performance of children with average thresholds exceeding 110 dB was poor. These results, like those by Cramer and Erber (1974), indicated that predicting speech discrimination ability of children with average thresholds between about 93 and 110 dB HL was nearly impossible. These investigators reported successful use of this simple test with most children over five years old, regardless of their loss in hearing sensitivity. Erber (1972, 1977) also has described a closed-set videotaped syllable recognition test to be used with hearing-impaired children in assessing visual and auditory-visual as well as auditory recognition. Auditory-visual and visual recognition have been explored further by Erber (1971) and Erber and McMahan (1976).

Finally, Erber and Witt (1977) described the use of ten monosyllabic, ten trochaic, and ten spondaic words for determining speech detection, preferred and speech discomfort levels, as well as for assessing word categorization by stress pattern and word recognition with ten severely and ten profoundly hearing-impaired children. The materials were recorded on Language Master cards. Children responded in the recognition and categorization portion of the test by repeating the word and pointing to it on a list. Word recognition and categorization scores reached maximum levels at 24–36 dB SL (105–129 dB SPL) for the severely impaired group. In contrast, word recognition scores remained low regardless of SL for the profoundly impaired, but categorization of words according to three stress patterns improved with increasing intensity to maximum levels of 12–30 dB SL (117–129 dB SPL). Best performance occurred within 6 dB of preferred listening levels for both groups. This procedure, concluded Erber and Witt, should be beneficial in selecting optimal hearing aid volume settings for young hearing-impaired children.

Johnson (1975) described the procedures for assessing speech discrimination of students at the National Technical Institute for the Deaf (NTID). Of 1345 students enrolled at NTID during the early 1970s, the average hearing level in the better ear was about 95 dB HL (ANSI-1969), necessitating the use of a variety of speech audiometric materials and procedures. The CID every day sentences with 50 keywords and ten selected spondees were used for materials. Recognition responses were required for the 50 keyword and selected spondees. If students were unable to perform this recognition task, or recognition scores were less than 50 percent for the ten selected spondees, then a same–different response was required on a test using the ten selected spondees. All materials were presented at a predetermined most comfortable loudness level for each student. Depending upon performance on these tests of speech discrimination, students were rated on a five-point scale with one indicating a score of less than 15 correct responses in identifying whether 20 paired spondees were the same or different. A five denoted the ability to identify correctly 90–100 percent of 50 keywords in the CID Everyday Sentences.

The highest percentage (33–36 percent) of NTID students obtained a rating of two, indicating a score of 15 or more correct responses on a same–different task with 20 paired spondees. Receptive verbal communicative skills also were assessed for speech reading with and without sound. Simms (1975) reported on the validation of the CID Everyday Sentences for use with severely hearing-impaired NTID students.

Aphasic Patients

It is important to assess the hearing sensitivity and speech discrimination ability of persons with aphasia because of the possibility of a concomitant peripheral hearing impairment. Many aphasic patients are older and thus may have such an impairment due to aging, noise, ototoxic drugs, and several other etiologies. At least 30 percent of Americans 65 years of age and older have some degree of hearing impairment (U.S. Public Health Service, 1975). Moreover, persons having aphasia as a result of head trauma also may have incurred damage to the peripheral auditory system from the insult. Regardless of whether the person with aphasia is elderly or acquired the disorder from a head trauma, good rehabilitative management would imply the need for a comprehensive audiological assessment because of the mere existance of a communicative disorder.

Winchester and Hartman (1955) found aphasic patients were able to perform satisfactorily on standard speech discrimination tests when recordings of phonetically balanced words were presented in quiet, but performed significantly poorer than a normal control group when noise was introduced. In an attempt to determine SRTs, Miller (1960) was able to test only six of 18 aphasic patients. Even then, the mean result was 11.4 dB poorer than the mean pure-tone average for 500, 1000, and 2000 Hz. This discrepancy, however, could have been a calibration artifact, because reference levels were not reported, discrepancies in the same direction occurred for nonaphasic patients, and a calibration problem existed in the early 1960s for those who used the less stringent 1951 ASA reference levels for pure-tone testing and the more stringent 1953 ASA reference level for speech threshold testing. Only four of the 18 aphasic patients could be given a speech discrimination test, presumably by a conventional procedure. Left ear and binaural speech discrimination scores dropped more for aphasics than for nonaphasic hemiplegics when noise was introduced.

Because of the importance in assessing speech discrimination among aphasic patients, Soffin and McLauchlin (1972) explored the use of the WIPI and PBK-50 List #1 with ten aphasic patients. With the exception of one 73-year-old subject, the remaining nine ranged in age from 22–50 years with a mean age of 35 years. Eight subjects were aphasic as a result of CVA and the other two because of head trauma. Most of the subjects had normal or near normal hearing bilaterally. One trauma victim yielded a unilateral mixed high-frequency loss. The materials were presented in quiet at a most comfortable loudness level. The mean percentage correct scores were: 95.6 for WIPI List #1, 95.2 for WIPI List #2, 92 for WIPI List #3, 95 for WIPI List #4, and 85.6 for PBK-50 List #1. The lower score on the PBK-50 list was, at least partially, the result of the examiner's inability to discriminate the verbal responses of one aphasic with apraxic speech. Subjectively, it appeared that the aphasics (1) exhibited less frustration with the picture-pointing task of the WIPI than with the verbal response required on the PBK-50 test; (2) were not insulted by the WIPI task and use of simple pictures; and (3) were attentive for longer periods of time with the WIPI than with the PBK-50 test.

Clearly, there is a need for clinicians to report their experiences in assessing the peripheral hearing of aphasic patients and for audiologic research to be conducted on this population. For aphasics with concomitant peripheral hearing impairment, it is important rehabilitatively to know whether misunderstood speech is a result of central or peripheral processing.

Non-English-Speaking Persons

American audiologists sometimes are confronted with performing speech audiometry on non-English-speaking individuals. Using non-English speech materials poses a problem for most American audiologists because relatively few of them are multilingual. If an audiologist's professional practice is in the southwest United States, however, he or she is likely to encounter clients who may speak and understand only Spanish. Similarly, clients who know only French may be encountered in the far northeast United States. Particularly in large cities, a clinician may be confronted with a variety of clients from ethnic communities who do not know the English language. Although non-English-speaking persons may have sufficient proficiency with their own native language, they pose problems for a clinician who does not know the client's language. The three major problems include: (1) where are foreign speech materials available; (2) how are the materials to be presented; and (3) what type of listener response is appropriate.

As for the availability of such materials, Martin and Hart (1978) devised a recorded 12-item Spanish spondee picture-pointing test that can be administered to Spanish children or adults by non-Spanish-speaking examiners. Clinicians practicing in states other than Texas who want to obtain this test are cautioned that the spondees are recorded by a person with Spanish dialect common to Texas. Tosi (1969) devised a multiple-choice rhyme test in Spanish which Cooper and Langly (1978) video recorded for use in determining audiovisual as well as auditory speech discrimination abilities of Spanish-speaking clients. Cooper and Langly also reported expected auditory and auditory-visual scores under several signal-to-noise ratios for normal hearing subjects. Barr (1969) reported on 20 German spondees and a list of 50 German monosyllabic words. Keydar and Katz (1978) selected and recorded 40 two-syllable Hebrew words for a Staggard Spondaic Word Test and 50 monosyllabic words for assessing speech discrimination of Hebrew speaking persons. Sometimes non-English speech materials and even recordings of those materials can be obtained by contacting professional colleagues who practice audiology in geographic regions of the United States having high concentrations of particular ethnic groups. Another alternative is to obtain speech audiometric materials from members of the International Society of Audiology who practice in non-English-speaking countries of the world.

The simplest solution for presenting speech materials in many clinics would be to have these materials recorded in the foreign languages frequently encountered among the population being served. Caution must be taken to select speakers with the most widely used dialect within a foreign language or at least to specify the geographic regions in which the dialect is used. Recorded materials will, as is always true, limit the versatility of their use for individual clinical needs. Another solution includes locating people in the community or employment setting who are multilingual and occasionally will assist in conducting speech audiometry using a monitored live-voice procedure. Sometimes, a family member or friend who speaks both English and the client's language will accompany the client to the clinic and assist the clinician in performing speech audiometry. With these last two solutions, time must be spent in training the speaker to use appropriately a monitored live-voice procedure.

The response obviously can be verbal only if the examiner, assistant, friend, or family member understands the client's native language. This problem can be circumvented by having the listener write the recorded words he or she hears. By using a recording of non-English words and a written response, the examiner can check the listener's responses against a list of the test items spelled in the listener's native language. If spelling or other expressive language problems exist, a closed set of spelled words or pictures may be employed. To further minimize the language barrier between the English speaking clinician and non-English client, a closed set visual display can contain both pictures and respective written noun words. The examiner can have a list of the test stimuli with both the non-English and English spellings.

Even for adults who have learned English within four years of the evaluation as a second language, significantly poorer word discrimination is expected in noise than would occur with native speakers of English (Gat & Keith, 1978). Thus, non-English speech materials also are appropriate for these clients.

SUMMARY

Language limited for purposes of this chapter refers to those persons whose verbal language skills are insufficient to permit the use of conventional adult speech audiometric protocols and English materials. Eight general considerations in performing speech protocols with language limited listeners are reviewed, including: (1) masking; (2) monitored live-voice; (3) calibration; (4) auditory-visual presentation; (5) probing language limitations; (6) familiarization and selecting familiar material; (7) response reinforcers; and (8) documentation. Moreover, speech protocols modified to accomodate limited language clients are discussed including: SDT, SRT, SD, MCL, and UCL measurements. Finally, the problems involved in administering speech audiometry to six different language limited populations are presented. These populations are infants, young children, severely and profoundly hearing impaired, mentally retarded, aphasic, and non-English speaking clients. Hopefully, this chapter provides some guidelines and knowledge about the administration of speech audiometric protocols for language-limited listeners as well as some directions for future research.

REFERENCES

American Speech-Language-Hearing Association. Guidelines for determining the threshold level for speech. *ASHA,* 1979, *21,* 353–356.

American Standard Specification for Audiometers for General Diagnostic Purposes, Z 24.5. New York: American Standards Association, 1951.

American Standard Specification for Speech Audiometers, Z 24.13. New York: American Standards Association, 1953.

Barr, D. F. Speech audiometry materials. *Audecibel,* 1969, *18,* 115–117.

Beattie, R. C., Svihovec, D. V., & Edgerton, B. J. Relative intelligibility of the CID spondees as presented via monitored live voice. *Journal of Speech and Hearing Disorders,* 1975, *40,* 84–91.

Black, J. W. Responses to multiple-choice intelligibility tests, Forms A and B. *Journal of Speech and Hearing Disorders,* 1968, *28,* 77–86.

Bowling, L. S., & Elpern, B. S. Relative intelligibility of items on CID Auditory Test W-1. *Journal of Auditory Research,* 1961, *2,* 152–157.

Carhart, R. Speech reception in relation to pattern of puretone loss. *Journal of Speech and Hearing Disorders,* 1946, *11,* 97–108.

Carhart, R. Observations on the relations between thresholds for puretones and for speech. *Journal of Speech and Hearing Disorders,* 1971, *36,* 476–483.

Carhart, R., & Porter, L. S. Audiometric configuration and prediction of threshold for spondees. *Journal of Speech and Hearing Research,* 1971, *14,* 486–495.

Chaiklin, J. B. The relation among three selected auditory speech thresholds. *Journal of Speech and Hearing Research,* 1959, *2,* 237–243.

Chaiklin, J. B. & Ventry, I. M. Spondee threshold measurement: a comparison of 2- and 5-dB methods. *Journal of Speech and Hearing Disorders,* 1964, *29,* 47–59.

Condon, W. S., & Sander, L. W. Neonate movement is synchronized with adult speech: Interactional participation and language structure. *Science,* 1974, *183,* 99–101.

Conn, M., Dancer, J., & Ventry, I. M. A spondee list for determining speech reception threshold without prior familiarization. *Journal of Speech and Hearing Disorders,* 1975, *40,* 388–396.

Cooper, J., & Langley, L. R. Multiple-choice speech discrimination tests for both diagnostic and rehabilitative evaluation: English and Spanish. *Journal of the Academy of Rehabilitative Audiology,* 1978, *11,* 132–141.

Cramer, K. D., & Erber, N. P. A spondee recognition test for young hearing-impaired children. *Journal of Speech and Hearing Disorders,* 1974, *39,* 304–311.

Curry, E. T., & Cox, B. P. The relative intelligibility of spondees. *Journal of Auditory Research,* 1966, *6,* 419–424.

Davis, S. M. Auditory speech perception. In R. L. Schiefelbush (Ed.), *Basis of language intervention.* Baltimore: University Park Press, 1978, pp. 43–66.

Egan, J. P. Remarks on rare PB words. *Journal of the Acoustical Society of America,* 1957, *29,* 751.

Eimas, P. D., Siqueland, E. R., Juscyzk, P., & Vigarit, J. Speech perception in infants. *Science,* 1972, *171,* 303–306.

Eisenberg, R. B. *Auditory competence in early life.* Baltimore: University Park Press, 1975.

Erber, N. Auditory and audiovisual reception of words in low-frequency noise by children with normal hearing and by children with impaired hearing. *Journal of Speech and Hearing Research,* 1971, *14,* 496–512.

Erber, N. P. Auditory, visual, and auditory-visual recognition of consonants by children with normal and impaired hearing. *Journal of Speech and Hearing Research,* 1972, *15,* 413–422.

Erber, N. P. Pure-tone thresholds and word-recognition abilities of hearing-impaired children. *Journal of Speech and Hearing Research,* 1974, *17,* 194–202.

Erber, N. P. Evaluating speech-perception ability in hearing-impaired children. In F. H. Bess (Ed.), *Childhood deafness: causation, assessment, and management.* New York: Grune and Stratton, 1977, pp. 173–181.

Erber, N. P. & Alencewicz, C. M. Audiologic evaluation of deaf children. *Journal of Speech and Hearing Disorders,* 1976, *41,* 256–267.

Erber, N., & McMahon, D. A. Effects of sentence context on recognition of words through lipreading by deaf children. *Journal of Speech and Hearing Research,* 1976, *19,* 112–119.

Erber, N. P., & Witt, L. H. Effects of stimulus intensity on speech perception by deaf children. *Journal of Speech and Hearing Disorders,* 1977, *42,* 271–278.

Fairbanks, G. A test of phonemic differentiation: the Rhyme Test. *Journal of the Acoustical Society of America,* 1958, *30,* 596–600.

Falconer, G. A., & Davis, H. The intelligibility of connected discourse as a test for the threshold of speech. *Laryngoscope,* 1947, *57,* 531–595.

Fletcher, H. A method of calculating hearing loss for speech from an audiogram. *Acta Oto-Laryngologica Supplement,* 1950, *90,* 26–37.

Friedlander, B. Z. Receptive language development in infancy. *Merrill-Palmer Quarterly of Behavior and Development,* 1970, *16,* 7–51.

Fulton, R. T., & Graham, J. T. Pure-tone reliability with the mentally retarded. *American Journal of Mental Deficiency,* 1964, *69,* 265–268.

Gat, I. B., & Keith, R. W. An effect of linguistic experience: auditory word discrimination by native and non-native speakers of English. *Audiology Journal of Auditory Communication,* 1978, *17,* 339–345.

Giolas, T. G. Speech audiometry. In R. T. Fulton and L. L. Lloyd (Eds.), *Auditory assessment of the difficult-to-test.* Baltimore: Williams and Wilkins Co., 1975, pp. 37–70.

Graham, J. T. Evaluation of methods for predicting speech reception threshold. *Archives of Otolaryngology,* 1960, *72,* 347–350.

Griffing, T. S., Simonton, K. M., & Hedgecock, L. D. Verbal auditory screening for preschool children. *Transactions; American Academy of Opthamology and Otolaryngology,* 1967, *71, 105*–110.

Hardy, W. G., & Bordley, J. E. Special techniques in testing the hearing of children. *Journal of Speech and Hearing Disorders,* 1951, *16,* 122–131.

Harris, J. D., Haines, H. D., Kelsey, P. A., & Clack, T. D. The relation between speech intelligibility and the electroacoustic characteristics of low fidelity circuitry. *Journal of Auditory Research,* 1961, *1,* 357–381.

Harris, J. D., Haines, H. L., & Meyers, C. K. A new formula for using the audiogram to predict speech hearing loss. *Archives of Otolaryngology,* 1956, *63,* 158–176 (and correction, 1956, *64,* 477).

Haskins, H. *A phonetically balanced test of speech discrimination for children.* Unpublished master's thesis, Northwestern University, Chicago, Illinois, 1949.

Hirsh, I. J., Davis, H., Silverman, S. R., Reynolds, E. G., et al. Development of materials for speech audiometry. *Journal of Speech and Hearing Disorders,* 1952, *17,* 321–337.

Hodgson, W. *A comparison of WIPI and PB-K discrimination test scores.* Paper presented at the meeting of the American Speech and Hearing Association, Detroit, October, 1973.

Hodgson, W. R. Testing infants and young children. In J. Katz (Ed.), *Handbook of clinical audiology.* Baltimore: Williams and Wilkins, 1978, pp. 397–409.

Hurley, R., & McLauchlin, R. *The relative intelligibility of an expanded list of spondaic words, with implications for children.* Unpublished research. The University of Michigan, Ann Arbor, Michigan, 1972.

Johnson, D. J. Communication characteristics of NTID Students. *Journal of the Academy of Rehabilitative Audiology,* 1975, *8,* 17–32.

Jones, K. O., & Studebaker, G. A. Performance of severly hearing-impaired children on a closed-response auditory speech discrimination test. *Journal of Speech and Hearing Research,* 1974, *17,* 531–540.

Keaster, J. A quantitative method of testing the hearing of young children. *Journal of Speech and Hearing Disorders,* 1947, *12:* 159–160.

Kelly, B. R. An analysis of the discrimination ability of four discrimination tests. Unpublished master's thesis, Florida State University, Tallahassee, Florida, 1968.

Kelly, B. R., & Pillow, G. Nonsense syllable discrimination by picture identification with young children. *Journal of the American Audiologic Society,* 1979, *4,* 170–172.

Keydar, B., & Katz, J. The Hebrew version of the Staggered Sponaic Word (SSW) Test. *Journal of Auditory Research,* 1976, *16,* 135–142.

Kreul, E. J., Nixon, J. D., Kryter, K. D., Bell, D. W., et al. A proposed clinical test of speech discrimination. *Journal of Speech and Hearing Research,* 1968, *11,* 536–552.

Lerman, J. W., Ross, M., & McLauchlin, R. M. A picture identificaiton test for hearing-impaired children. *Journal of Auditory Research,* 1965, *5,* 273–278.

Ling, A. H. The training of auditory memory in hearing-impaired children: some problems of generalization. *Journal of the American Audiologic Society,* 1976, *1,* 150–157.

Ling, D. Auditory coding and recoding. In M. Ross and T. G. Giolas (Eds.), *Auditory management of hearing-impaired children: prerequisites for intervention.* Baltimore: University Park Press, 1978, pp. 181–218.

Ling, D., & Ling, A. H. Communication development in the first three years of life. *Journal of Speech and Hearing Research,* 1974, *17,* 146–159.

Lloyd, L. L. *A comparison of selected auditory measures on normal hearing mentally retarded children.* Unpublished doctoral thesis, University of Iowa, Iowa City, Iowa, 1965.

Lloyd, L. L., & Melrose, J. Inter-method comparison of selected auditory measures used with normal hearing mentally retarded children. *Journal of Auditory Research,* 1966, *6,* 205–217.

Lloyd, L. L., & Reid, M. J. The reliability of speech audiometry with institutionalized retarded children. *Journal of Speech and Hearing Research,* 1966, *9,* 450–455.

Lloyd, L. L., Reid, M. J., & McManis, D. L. The effect of response mode on the SRTs obtained from retarded children. *Journal of Auditory Research,* 1967, *7,* 219–222.

Martin, F. N. Speech tests of hearing—age one year through five years. In F. N. Martin (Ed.), *Pediatric audiology.* Englewood Cliffs, New Jersey: Prentice-Hall, 1978, pp. 236–264.

Martin, F. N., & Coombes, S. A tangibly reinforced speech reception threshold procedure for use with small children. *Journal of Speech and Hearing Disorders,* 1976, *41,* 333–338.

Martin, F. N., & Hart, D. B. Measurement of speech thresholds of Spanish-speaking children by non-Spanish speaking clinicians. *Journal of Speech and Hearing Disorders,* 1978, *43,* 255–262.

Martin, F. N., & Stauffer, M. L. A modification of the Tillman-Olsen method for obtaining the speech reception threshold. *Journal of Speech and Hearing Disorders,* 1975, *40,* 25–28.

Matkin, N. D. Hearing aids for children. In W. R. Hodgson and P. H. Skinner (Eds.), *Hearing aid assessment and use in audiological rehabilatation.* Baltimore: Williams and Wilkins, 1977, pp. 145–169.

McLauchlin, R., Rosenblatt, T., & Rupp, R. R. The relative intelligibility of an expanded list of spondaic words. *Journal of the Michigan Speech and Hearing Association,* 1971, *7,* 43–49.

Miller, C. L., & Morse, P. A. The "heart" of categorical speech perception in young infants. *Journal of Speech and Hearing Research,* 1976, *19,* 578–589.

Miller, M. H. Audiologic evaluation of aphasic patients. *Journal of Speech and Hearing Disorders,* 1960, *24,* 369–379.

Moffitt, A. B. *Speech perception in infants.* Unpublished doctoral dissertation, University of Minnesota, Minneapolis, Minnesota, 1968.

Myatt, B. D., & Landes, B. A. Assessing discrimination loss in children. *Archives of Otolaryngology,* 1963, *77,* 359–362.

Northern, J. L., & Downs, M. P. *Hearing in children.* Second Ed. Baltimore: Williams and Wilkins, 1978.

Pronovost, W., & Dumbleton, C. A picture type of speech sound discrimination test. *Journal of Speech and Hearing Disorders,* 1954, *19,* 258–266.

Quiggle, R. R., Glorig, A., Delk, J. H., & Summerfield, A. B. Predicting hearing loss for speech from puretone audiograms. *Laryngoscope,* 1957, *67,* 1–15.

Ross, M., & Lerman, J. A picture identification test for hearing-impaired children. *Journal of Speech and Hearing Research,* 1970, *13,* 44–53.

Sanderson–Leepa, M. E., & Rintelmann, W. Articulation functions and test–retest performance of normal hearing children on three speech discrimination tests: WIPI, PB-50, and N. U. Auditory Test No. 6. *Journal of Speech and Hearing Disorders,* 1976, *41,* 503–519.

Schlanger, B. B., & Galanowsky, G. I. Auditory discrimination tasks performed by mentally retarded and normal children. *Journal of Speech and Hearing Research,* 1966, *9,* 434–440.

Schwartz, D. *The usefulness of the WIPI—A speech discrimination test for preschool children.* Unpublished master's thesis, Central Michigan University, Mount Pleasant, Michigan, 1971.

Schwartz, A. H., & Goldman, R. Variables influencing performance on speech-sound discrimination tests. *Journal of Speech and Hearing Research,* 1974 *17,* 25–32.

Seidel, S. *The PICSI test: Picture Identification for Children, a Standardized Index.* Unpublished master's thesis, Indiana University, Bloomington, Indiana, 1963.

Siegenthaler, B., & Haspiel, G. *Development of two standardized measures of hearing for speech by children.* U.S. Department of Health, Education, and Welfare, Project No. 2372, Contract No. OE 5-10-003, 1966.

Sims, D. C. The validation of the CID everyday sentence test for use with the severely hearing impaired. *Journal of the Academy of Rehabilitative Audiology,* 1975, *8,* 70–79.

Simmons–Martin, A. Early management procedures for the hearing-impaired child. In F. Martin (Ed.), *Pediatric audiology.* Englewood Cliffs, New Jersey: Prentice-Hall, 1978, pp. 356–385.

Soffin, B., & McLauchlin, R. *Performance of aphasic patients on the WIPI.* Unpublished study. The University of Michigan, Ann Arbor, Michigan, 1972.

Sortini, A., & Flake, C. Speech audiometry testing for preschool children. *Laryngoscope,* 1953, *63,* 991–997.

Spring, D. R., & Dale, P. A. Discrimination of linguistic stress in early infancy. *Journal of Speech and Hearing Research,* 1977, *20,* 224–232.

Templin, M. *Certain Language Skills in Children: Their Development and Interrelationships.* Minneapolis: University of Minnesota Press, 1957.

Tillman, T. W., & Jerger, J. F. Some factors affecting spondee threshold in normal-hearing subjects. *Journal of Speech and Hearing Research,* 1959, *2,* 141–145.

Tillman, T. W., & Olsen, W. O. Speech audiometry. In J. Jerger (Ed.), *Modern developments in audiology* (2nd ed.). New York: Academic Press, 1973.

Tosi, O. E. Estudio experimental sobra la inteligibilidad de un test de multiple eleccion en idioma espanol. *Fonoaudiologia,* 1969, *15,* 28–35.

U.S. Public Health Service. Prevalence of Selected Impairments United States, 1971. Series 10, No. 99. Rockville, Maryland: National Center for Health Statistics, 1975.

Watson, T. J. Speech audiometry for children. In A. W. G. Ewing (Ed.), *Educational guidance and the deaf child.* Manchester, England: University Press, 1957, pp. 278–296.

Weber, S., & Reddell, R. C. A sentence test for measuring speech discrimination ability in children. *Audiology and Hearing Education,* 1976, *2,* 25–27; 30; 49.

Wepman, J. M. Audiotry discrimination, speech and reading. *Elementary School Journal,* 1960, *60,* 325–333.

Wilson, K., & McLauchlin, R. M. *Assessment of speech intelligibility of mentally retarded with the Word Intelligibility by Picture Identification (WIPI) Test.* Unpublished study, University of Michigan, Ann Arbor, Michigan, 1972.

Wilson, S., & McLauchlin, R. M. *Standardization of a picture pointing speech reception threshold test for use with children.* Unpublished study, University of Michigan, Ann Arbor, Michigan, 1973.

Wilson, R. H., Morgan, D. E., & Dirks, D. D. Proposed SRT procedure and its statistical precident. *Journal of Speech and Hearing Disorders,* 1973, *38,* 184–191.

Winchester, R. A., & Hartman, B. T. Auditory de-differentiation in the dysphasic. *Journal of Speech and Hearing Disorders,* 1955, *20,* 178–182.

Roger N. Kasten, Ph.D.

12
Speech Protocols for Hearing Aid Evaluations

Hearing aid evaluation procedures utilizing speech materials are as old as hearing aids themselves. Prior to the development of hearing aids (of any kind), individuals experiencing difficulty with the reception of speech had to acquire the art of speech reading by whatever means possible. With the advent of useable amplification devices, however, a means was at hand to amplify speech and to make communication easier for those who suffer from a hearing impairment.

There is always a tendency when the words *hearing aid evaluation* are used to think only of approaches utilized by audiologists. Indeed, the words *hearing aid evaluation* tend to be equated with the selection and fitting of amplification performed by college-trained audiologists. Unfortunately, this term has proven to be one of great controversy. Proponents of the *hearing aid evaluation* procedures contend that this is a truly objective and worthwhile manner of selecting appropriate amplification for hearing-impaired individuals, while opponents contend that hearing aid evaluations are neither valid nor reliable.

Prior to a discussion of speech protocols for hearing aid evaluation procedures, it might be worthwhile to reflect upon the meaning and significance of the words hearing aid evaluation. Carhart is generally considered to be the originator and chief proponent of techniques for accomplishing a hearing aid evaluation. He has described these procedures in numerous publications and presented a philosophical justification for the total hearing aid evaluation procedure in 1950. In this publication entitled, "Hearing Aid Selection By University Clinics," he stated, "The clinic probably should not seek to find the 'best hearing aid fitting.'" Rather, the task is to assess an individual's needs and difficulties with wearable amplification. The goal is to select a hearing aid which meets these combined requirements as satisfactorily as one can reasonably expect for any given patient (Carhart, 1950). In short, Carhart stated that the hearing aid evaluation procedure is not designed to select the one and only hearing aid that will provide the ultimate of performance for a given patient, but the procedure should sort out a selected number of instruments that might be appropriate for a given individual and permit one of that group to be chosen.

With this in mind, it is altogether possible for an individual to be evaluated in more than one audiology center and receive more than one appropriate recommendation. This philosophical statement needs to be recalled as a basis for the entire discussion of speech protocols for hearing aid evaluation procedures. This writer knows of no audiologist who claims that the evaluation procedure selects the one and only instrument that is ultimately most appropriate for a given hearing-impaired individual. Rather, the procedure selects from among a family of aids an instrument that provides significant improvement and whose performance capabilities, for the given hearing-impaired individual, may be equalled but probably not exceeded.

PREAUDIOLOGY EVALUATIONS

There is a tendency today on the part of many to think of hearing aid work prior to World War II as being in the Dark Ages. Lybarger (1979) has pointed out that many hearing aid fitters in the 1930s utilized very informal but realistic speech evaluations. Speech testing tended to consist of questions and conversation that would provide a rough approximation of the user's ability with an average voice, across a typical room, or in a noisy environment. He also stated that systematic work had been initiated regarding speech testing. Fletcher (1926, 1932, and 1933) described the development of speech materials for the evaluation of hearing aid performance. Knudsen and Jones (1936) discussed the use of speech testing as a means of evaluating an individual's efficiency with the hearing aid. Steinberg (1936) also described speech materials appropriate for the evaluation of hearing aid performance. Lybarger (1979) further points out that pre-World War II hearing aids did not have as much versatility and had considerably more harmonic distortion and frequency distortion, but the hearing aids were of great benefit to a sizeable number of people. Lybarger also stated that the real impetus for formalized speech testing came from Carhart. He indicated that the materials and procedures for formal evaluations were present prior to World War II, but Carhart initiated the systematic work that resulted in a formalized evaluation procedure.

WORLD WAR II EVALUATIONS

Formalized hearing aid evaluation procedures were established in the aural rehabilitation centers (Borden General Hospital, Chickashee, Oklahoma; Deshon General Hospital, Butler, Pennsylvania; Hoff General Hospital, Santa Barbara, California; U.S. Naval Hospital, Philadelphia, Pennsylvania) during World War II. The best known and most widely accepted of these procedures were those established by Carhart at Deshon Hospital (Carhart, 1946a; Carhart, 1946b). In these publications, Carhart described a detailed and time-consuming procedure for the evaluation of hearing aid performance using a variety of speech materials. Indeed, it was not unheard of for a full hearing aid evaluation to take anywhere from two weeks to one month to complete. Carhart described the procedures employed in minute detail and it is easy to believe that these same procedures, if time constraints were no objection, would be tremendously successful today. Unfortunately, it is difficult to find individuals today who will devote two to four weeks to the evaluation of a set of prosthetic devices.

Interestingly, the original Deshon procedure was highly weighted toward the reception of speech. The "listening hour" that was employed in each hearing aid evaluation included the reception of familiar songs, unfamiliar songs, musical comedy, reading of prose in quiet, reading of prose with background music, and recorded continuous speech. In addition, these evaluations included the use of semiformalized speech tests to evaluate the potential user's ability to understand speech materials.

In 1947, Carhart presented a further description of the hearing aid evaluation procedure and, for the first time, discussed the use of formalized speech test materials. He advocated the measurement of aided speech thresholds, aided speech discrimination and aided tolerance levels for speech. It is at this point in time that what we refer to today as the formal hearing aid evaluation procedure had its beginning in the literature.

PRESENT-DAY SPEECH MATERIALS

One of the first problems that must be dealt with relates to the question of whether or not speech materials can actually be used to demonstrate differences in individual performance that can be brought about as a result of differently performing hearing aid systems. Probably the first systematic investigation of this type was carried out by Carhart (1946c) when he evaluated the ability of patients to employ a "comfort setting" for volume control adjustment during the evaluation procedure. For these measurements, Carhart utilized spondaic words and pointed out that new hearing aid users were quite capable of making very consistent adjustments of the volume control as reflected by test–retest threshold measurements. He further pointed out that patients were able to demonstrate differences in performance between and among different instruments on the basis of threshold measurements at the comfort setting.

Davis et al. (1946), in a detailed manuscript, questioned the clinical significance of Carhart's findings. The fact remains, however, that Carhart was able to demonstrate consistency in performance with one aid and differences in performance with more than one aid on the basis of the results of measurements made using spondaic words as speech stimuli.

By far the greatest emphasis, however, has been placed upon the measurement of speech discrimination. It has long been articulated that clarity of speech may be the most important single factor to consider when examining an individual's performance with a hearing aid. Obviously, this may not be totally appropriate for every single hearing aid user, but clarity of speech appears to be one factor of prime importance for the vast majority of hearing aid users.

Monosyllabic Word Tests

Considerable controversy has arisen over the question of whether monosyllabic speech materials are sufficiently sensitive to detect differences in hearing aid performance on the basis of differences in user performance. Shore et al. (1960) pointed out that speech discrimination measurements, either in quiet or in the presence of noise, were not able to demonstrate differences in user performance with different hearing aids. They used as their stimulus materials the Rush Hughes recordings of PAL phonetically balanced words (Egan, 1948). Their 25-word lists were presented to a variety of experimental subjects under conditions approximating those of a typical hearing aid evaluation, and they were not able to demonstrate clear-cut differences in performance achieved with different hearing aid systems. They also reported that they were unable to achieve good test–retest reliability with monosyllabic words presented either in quiet or in the presence of noise.

Interestingly, McConnell et al. (1960), at approximately the same time, investigated test–retest reliability for discrimination performance by hearing aid users in a clinical evaluation setting. They utilized the PAL materials, the CID W-22 monosyllabic words (Hirsh et al., 1952) and the PBK monosyllabic words. McConnell and his coworkers were able to demonstrate a high degree of test–retest reliability for aided speech discrimination performance even though a total of five different clinicians were involved in the live-voice presentation of the materials. Not only did these authors demonstrate high test–retest reliability in the immediate testing environment, but they were also able to achieve a high degree of clinical consistency in a remote test–retest situation.

These types of controversial findings continued for a number of years. No attempt will be made in this brief coverage to describe in detail the various contributors to the controversy, but some of the more pertinent materials will be cited. Zerlin (1962) discussed what he referred to as a new method of evaluating hearing aid performance that involved quality judgments of hearing aid processed continuous discourse in the presence of cafeteria noise. At the same time, he also recorded through each of his experimental aids 25-word lists of W-22 monosyllabic words in quiet. Zerlin was able to demonstrate that sensorineural subjects could rank order the performance of the various aids on the basis of the quality judgments made using continuous discourse in the presence of cafeteria noise. His subjects were not able to demonstrate a meaningful difference in performance for five of the six experimental aids on the basis of intelligibility scores achieved with the half-lists of W-22 monosyllabic words recorded in quiet. On the basis of these results, Zerlin concluded that quality judgments were more efficient predictors of hearing aid performance than were intelligibility scores achieved with monosyllabic words (in quiet).

Jerger et al. (1966) evaluated the performance of a group of hearing impaired subjects utilizing four different types of speech materials that had been processed through three different hearing aid systems and stored on magnetic tape. The speech materials included the PAL monosyllabic words in quiet and low-pass filtered at 500 Hz, CID W-22 monosyllabic words recorded in quiet, CNC monosyllabic words (Lehiste & Peterson, 1959) recorded in quiet, and the PAL Auditory Test no. 8 (a sentence intelligibility test) recorded in the presence of competing speech at a primary-to-secondary ration of -6 dB. The findings of Jerger and his coworkers are presented in Fig. 12-1.

Careful note should be taken of the information presented in this figure. Casual examination would lead one to conclude, as had Zerlin earlier, that differences between hearing aids could not be detected through the use of monosyllabic test stimuli. In this instance the conclusion would be that differences among hearing aids could be detected only through the use of a sentence-type test material. It is important, however, to carefully consider the method in which the various speech materials were utilized. Recall that all three monosyllabic word lists were presented in quiet and

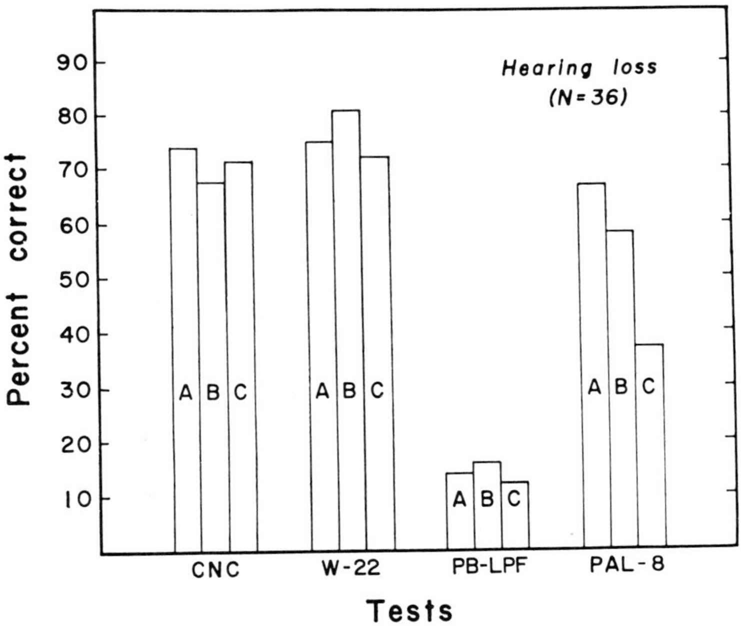

Fig. 12-1. Average intelligibility scores for four tests through three aids on 36 hearing-impaired listeners. [From Jerger, J., Malmquist, C., & Speaks, C. Comparison of some speech intelligibility tests in the evaluation of hearing aid performance. *Journal of Speech and Hearing Research,* 1966, *9,* 253–258. Reproduced with permission.].

also represented performance from a single presentation of the materials. The PAL-8 word lists were presented with a speech competition and the scores shown represent a mathematical calculation of the composite obtained from six presentations. Thus, it is questionable at best to make a realistic comparison between and among these different types of test materials. In their discussion of the results, the authors stated that:

> . . . although it is possible to devise a behavioral measure that will, in fact, differentiate among hearing aids, one is not justified in assuming that such performance differences will necessarily be reflected by monosyllabic word lists as they are currently used in conventional hearing aid selection procedures. (p. 257)

Jerger and his coworkers presented a strong condemnation of the use of the monosyllabic words for hearing aid evaluation procedures, even though the monosyllables had been presented in quiet and the sentence material presented in competition. Indeed, at that time, Jerger's attitude toward the use of monosyllabic words for the purpose of discrimination measurements can best be summarized by a question he posed at the conclusion of the 1966 Summer Institute of the Academy of Rehabilitative

Audiology. To the best of this writer's knowledge, this statement does not appear in print in any journal and this writer quotes from memory the statement of Jerger as he summarized the Summer Institute on Hearing Aid Evaluation Procedures. Jerger closed his presentation with the question, "How long must the ship of Audiology float aimlessly on a sea of monosyllables?"

Not all researchers in the area of hearing aid performance were reaching the same conclusion regarding the efficiency of monosyllabic words as Jerger or Zerlin. Kasten et al. (1967) evaluated user performance with four different hearing aid systems obtained through gain control manipulation of a single hearing aid. The four systems represented, among measured characteristics, different frequency responses and different distortion levels. CNC words were processed through each aid and stored on magnetic tape. These materials were then presented to individuals with normal hearing, conductive hearing losses, mixed hearing losses and sensorineural hearing losses. Their results are shown in Fig. 12-2.

Hearing aid conditions varied according to the levels of harmonic and total nonlinear distortion present in the hearing aid system with condition D representing the most favorable condition and condition A representing the least favorable condition. The monosyllabic words had been recorded in the presence of cafeteria-type noise (the same type of noise as that used by Jerger in the previously discussed investigation) at a fixed primary-to-secondary ratio of +10 dB. Clearly, according to this experimental design, not only did the subjects rank order their performance according to the integrity of their auditory systems, but also according to the distortion levels or frequency characteristics inherent in the amplification systems. Without belaboring the point, this monosyllabic word test in the presence of a competing auditory signal did appear to be sufficiently sensitive to indicate differences, not only in subject ability, but in system ability.

Through that same period of time, Olsen and Wilber (1967, 1968) clearly demonstrated that Northwestern Auditory Test no. 6 (a monosyllabic word test) could be used to rank order subject performance with varying amplification systems. In each instance, Olsen and Wilber utilized a competing message and did not present the monosyllabic stimuli in quiet for other than a comparison condition. Thus, the results of the last two investigations demonstrated that monosyllabic word tests can be used to measure performance differences as a function of amplification system differences.

Jirsa and Hodgsen (1970) utilized monosyllabic words and sentence-type materials to evaluate subject performance with three different hearing aid systems. The speech materials included Northwestern University Auditory Test no. 6 (Tillman & Carhart, 1966) in both quiet and noise, CID W-22 monosyllabic words, and PAL Auditory Test no. 8 sentence

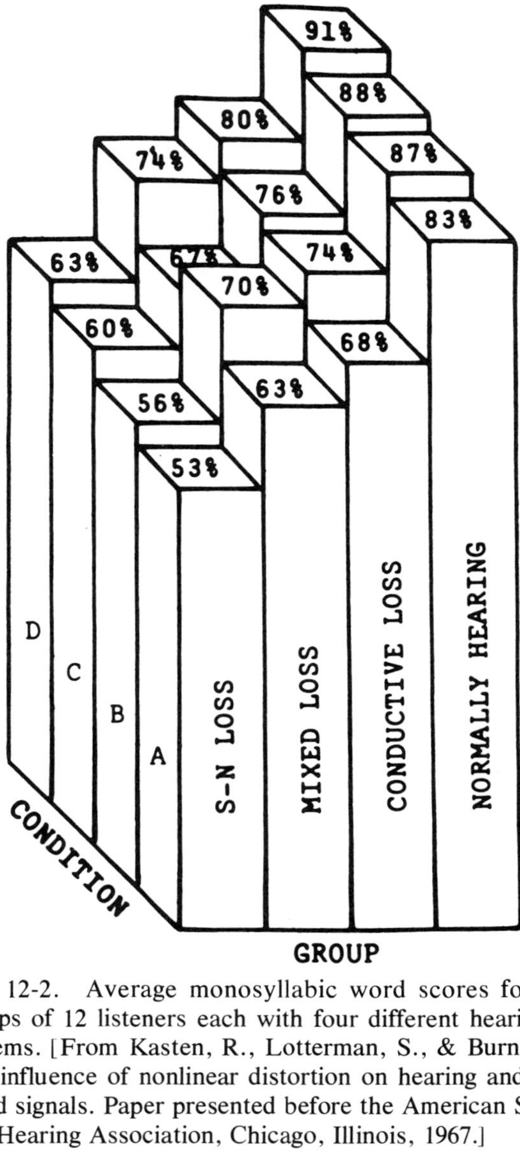

Fig. 12-2. Average monosyllabic word scores for four groups of 12 listeners each with four different hearing aid systems. [From Kasten, R., Lotterman, S., & Burnett, E. The influence of nonlinear distortion on hearing and processed signals. Paper presented before the American Speech and Hearing Association, Chicago, Illinois, 1967.]

materials. These materials were recorded through three different hearing aid systems. Each of the speech materials, whether monosyllabic words or sentence constructions, were presented in combination with speech spectrum noise as a competing signal. Their results are shown in Fig. 12-3.

It is immediately apparent that each of the speech materials, both in quiet and competition, clearly differentiated among the three hearing aid

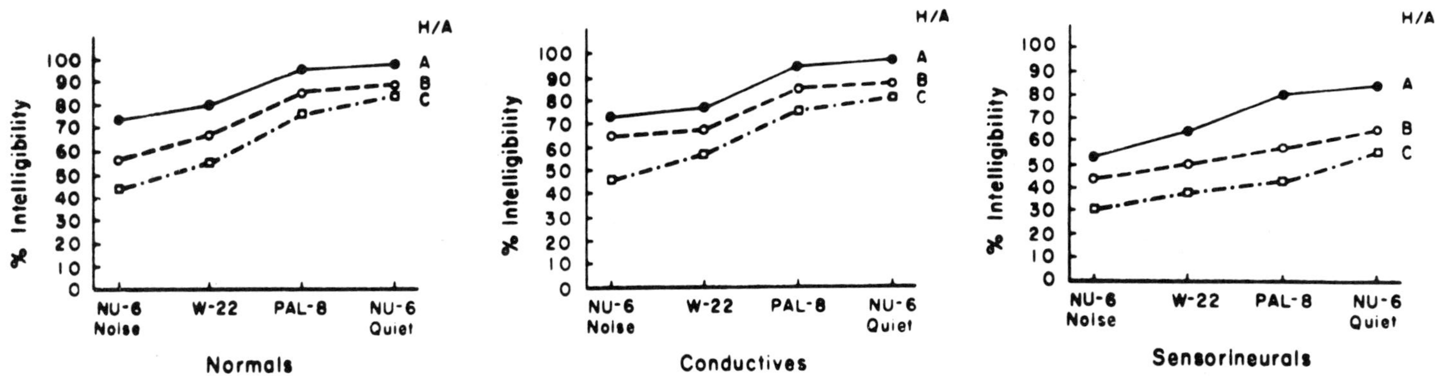

Fig. 12-3. Mean word scores for each discrimination test under each hearing aid condition for three groups of subjects. [From Jirsa, R., & Hodgsen, W. Effect of harmonic distortion in hearing aids on speech intelligibility for normals and hypacusics. *Journal of Auditory Research,* 1970, *10,* 213–217. Reproduced with permission.]

systems. The authors point out that the differences among the three aids were statistically significant for each of the test materials. It should be noted that the largest numerical difference was seen when the sentence material was utilized with the sensorineural subjects, but the magnitude of that numerical difference was not materially greater than that observed with the monosyllabic words with any of the subject groups.

In terms of actual clinical application, Haug et al. (1971) reported on the clinical results for 298 patients being seen in an otologic–audiologic treatment facility. Each patient had been seen for a complete hearing aid evaluation and discrimination performance in the aided setting was measured for each patient via live-voice presentation using PAL monosyllabic word lists. Table 12-1 provides the range in discrimination scores between the aids providing the highest performance levels and those providing the lowest performance levels.

It can be noted that the range in performance for the 298 patients was rather high between the best performing hearing aid and the poorest performing hearing aid. Indeed, in only 13.5 percent of the evaluations was the range in discrimination scores 9 percent or less. Of significance is the fact that 76 percent of the patients achieved ranges in discrimination performance of between 10 percent and 39 percent. It should be remembered that these wide performance ranges were achieved as a result of evaluations carried out utilizing monosyllabic word tests. This represents a rather significant departure from the clinical assertions presented earlier by Zerlin and Jerger. In fact, it would appear that monosyllabic words, utilized appropriately, are fully capable, in either the clinical or research setting, of detecting differences in performance among varying amplification systems.

Table 12-1
Differences in Speech Discrimination Between Hearing Aids With Highest and Lowest Scores

Discrimination Score Range, %	No. of Evaluations	Percentage
2–9	41	13.5
10–19	119	40.0
20–29	76	26.0
30–39	29	10.0
40–49	21	7.0
50–59	8	2.5
60–69	2	0.5
70–79	2	0.5
Total	298	100

From Haug, O., Baccaro, P., & Guilford, F. Differences in hearing aid performance. *Archives of Otolaryngology,* 1971, *93,* 183–185. Reproduced with permission, copyright 1971, American Medical Association.

Other monosyllabic word type tests have been advocated in recent years. Among these are the Modified Rhyme Test (House et al., 1965), the High-Frequency Consonant Discrimination Test (Gardner, 1971) and the California Consonant Test (Owens & Schubert, 1977). Although clinical experience with each of these materials indicates a potential value in each case, extensive systematic evaluations regarding material efficiency in the hearing aid evaluation setting are lacking. It would seem reasonable to assume that these materials, like other monosyllabic word materials, could be used in a meaningful manner in specific evaluation procedures designed to elicit specific types of test results.

One note of caution should be raised regarding the use of monosyllabic word tests for the evaluation of hearing aid performance. While it is reasonably clear that monosyllabic word tests, particularly in the presence of competition, are able to detect differences in hearing aid performance, none of the advocates or users of these types of tests have indicated that the test results provide a valid or meaningful measure of an individual's ability to communicate in everyday situations. Indeed, those who have utilized monosyllabic word tests seem to have implied that the prime benefit of these tests is that they will allow a rank ordering of the relative performance of different hearing aid systems. When the intent of the hearing aid evaluation procedure is viewed as originally articulated by Carhart, it would appear that monosyllabic word tests have accomplished his originally stated purpose of indicating the amplification systems that tend to provide maximum benefit for each individual user. It is sincerely hoped that those practitioners making use of monosyllabic word tests for hearing aid evaluation procedures go no further in the interpretation of the results than the results would tend to indicate for safe prediction.

Multi-Word Tests

A variety of sentence type materials have been utilized for the evaluation of hearing aid performance. This brief section will attempt to review some of the more traditional, more popular and more promising types of materials.

Jerger et al. (1966) presented an investigation in which they utilized PAL-8 sentence materials in evaluating the performance characteristics of three different hearing aids with varying degrees of harmonic distortion. This writer does not wish at this time to enter into the controversy as to whether harmonic distortion is good or bad, but rather desires only to discuss the results obtained by Jerger and his coworkers utilizing sentence-type speech materials. They recorded the sentence tests through three hearing aids with differing physical characteristics and presented these materials to a variety of experimental subjects. Their results, classified according to configuration of hearing loss, are presented in Fig. 12-4.

It should be noted that their hearing-impaired population is divided according to flat hearing loss, gradually sloping hearing loss, and severely sloping hearing loss. Further, the results are presented for six successive trials with the sentence materials under each of the aided conditions. It should also be realized that the results are plotted on a logrithmic progression which allows for the presentation of a straight line performance function.

Of significance is the fact that the results reveal a systematic rank ordering of the three aids under investigation. Regardless of the type of hearing loss or the order in the trial sequence, the aid designated "A" was superior to aid "B" which was generally markedly superior to aid "C". As a result, it is relatively easy to conclude that these sentence-type materials, presented with a speech competition, were sufficiently sensitive to detect differences among the three different hearing aid systems. Indeed, Jerger and his coworkers point out that 34 of the 36 subjects rank ordered the three instruments in this same general pattern. They concluded, "Analysis of individual performance data showed that most listeners ranked the three conditions in the same order. . . ."

One of the more widely used sentence materials for the measurement of speech intelligibility has been synthetic sentences (Jerger et al., 1968). These materials consist of third order approximations of real sentences and have been used in some extensive studies of speech discrimination performance for differential diagnosis, for the identification of individuals with central auditory processing problems and for the identification of individuals with central auditory nervous system disorders.

The use of synthetic sentences for the purpose of hearing aid evaluation procedures has not been extensive, but has yielded some very promising new approaches. Undoubtedly the most innovative use of synthetic sentences for hearing aid evaluation procedures has been presented by Jerger and Hayes (1976). The synthetic sentences emanated from a loudspeaker located directly in front of the aided patient while a competing continuous discourse was presented from a loudspeaker immediately behind the aided patient. The synthetic sentence materials were always presented at an intensity of 60 dB SPL while the competition was varied in 10 dB steps between 40 and 80 dB SPL. This arrangement provided message-to-competition ratios for the evaluation that ranged from +20 dB (very easy) to −20 dB (very difficult). An example of their findings is presented in Fig. 12-5.

Note that the individual in Figure 12-5 has a mixed loss in the right ear and normal speech discrimination ability as measured by monosyllabic words. The dashed line on the hearing aid evaluation form is a representation of the performance ability of a normal hearing population at the various message-to-competition ratios. The distance between the dashed

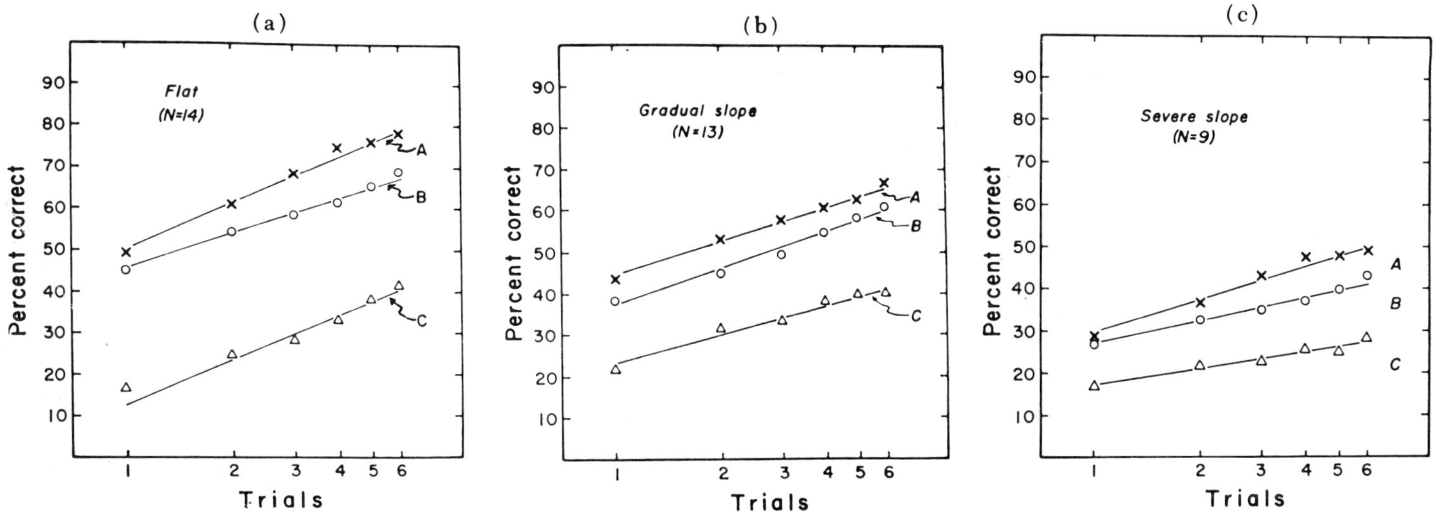

Fig. 12-4. Comparison of PAL–8 performance functions. Subjects categorized according to shape of loss: (a) flat, (b) gradual slope, (c) severe slope. [From Jerger, J., Speaks, C., & Malmquist, C. Hearing-aid performance and hearing-aid selection. *Journal of Speech and Hearing Research,* 1966, *9,* 136–149. Reproduced by permission.]

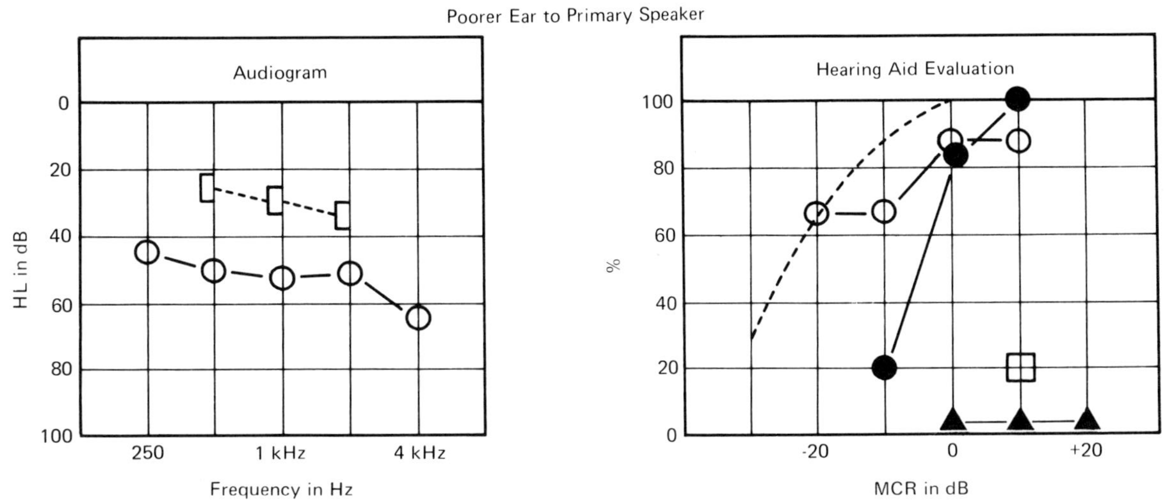

	PTA	PB Max
Right Ear	53	96%
Left Ear	NR	CNE

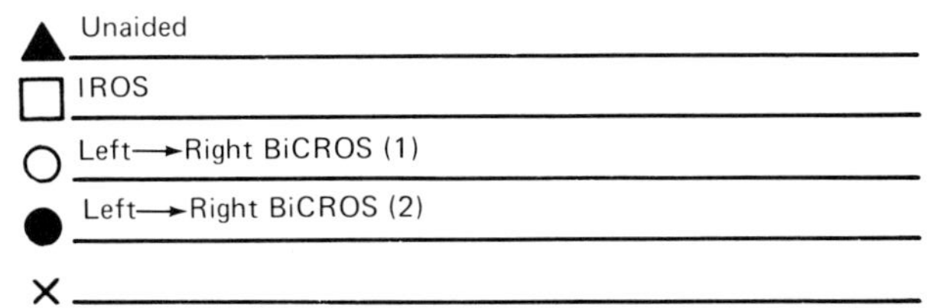

Fig. 12-5. Audiogram and hearing aid evaluation summary form for 56-year-old man with moderate mised loss in right ear and profound loss in left ear. [From Jerger, J., & Hayes, D. Hearing aid evaluation. *Archives of Otolaryngology,* 1976, *102,* 214–225. Reproduced with permission, copyright 1976, American Medical Association.]

line and the solid lines, which display performance ability with a given hearing aid system, would be an indication of the residual auditory deficit that still exists even after the aid is in place. In this illustration, the patient was unable to perform in the unaided situation, even at the easiest signal-to-noise ratios. Thus, any aided score greater than "no response" would be an indication of the amount of improvement offered at the various message-to-competition ratios for each hearing aid system.

The IROS aid, even at the easy message-to-competition ratio, was able to provide only a 20 percent discrimination score. The aid identified as "BiCROS-(1)" provided near normal performance levels in the easier listening conditions and allowed reception equivalent to normal ability at the most difficult message-to-competition ratio. The aid identified as "BiCROS-(2)" provided normal reception at the easiest listening condition, but performance with this system decreased markedly and a discrimination score of only 20 percent was achieved at the difficult message-to-competition ratio.

This approach to the evaluation of hearing aid performance with synthetic sentences allows a relatively comprehensive view of overall hearing aid performance. It is quite obvious that the aid identified as "BiCROS-(1)" provided excellent improvement in performance at all message-to-competition ratios. In the more difficult listening situations particularly, this aid was markedly superior to the other two systems under evaluation. However, had the evaluation been conducted only at the single message-to-competition ratios of either 0 dB or +10 dB, the performance of the two BiCROS systems would have appeared very similar.

Jerger and Hayes presented a series of examples to illustrate the usefulness of their procedure utilizing the synthetic sentence materials. It would appear that this type of approach provides a far more comprehensive picture of an individual's ability to perform in the aided situation than that achieved with the traditional evaluation procedure utilizing a single list of speech materials presented at one fixed message-to-competition ratio. Also, Jerger and Hayes point out that each list consists of only ten synthetic sentences; therefore, the overall time for the total evaluation procedure using the proposed method is not any greater than that required for a traditional hearing aid evaluation.

One final sentence-type speech material that should be considered, primarily because of its careful development, is the Kent State University Speech Discrimination Test (Berger, 1977). Berger has described a sentence test which consists of thirteen items in each list and one key word, embedded within each sentence, is scored for each item. These materials have been meticulously prepared and they can be presented either by live voice or by means of a commercially available tape recording. The KSU

Test has been demonstrated to have excellent test–retest reliability, both in terms of immediate and remote retest. The performance of hearing impaired individuals with the Kent State sentences and the W-22 monosyllables has been compared and Berger concluded,

> . . . the W-22 lists are more sensitive for testing auditory impairment, while the KSU test may more accurately predict how efficiently one can utilize hearing for daily communication. (p. 12)

One unique feature of the Kent State test is that the thirteen sentence items in each list have been graded according to difficulty. Each test list begins with the easiest sentence and ends with the most difficult sentence. Subject performance is graded as being correct or incorrect and a score is obtained by subtracting the sentence numbers (1 through 13) of the *incorrect* responses from 100 percent. Thus, if an individual missed sentence #10 and sentence #13, his or her score for the list would be 77 percent. This type of presentation does have one major advantage in that it allows most subjects to experience some degree of success during the early part of each presentation.

The Kent State Sentence Test has not been reported extensively in the literature as a tool for hearing aid evaluation procedures. This writer, however, is highly enthused over the potential of this type of material and would encourage the use of these sentences in the clinical setting. These materials provide an innovative approach and increased use of materials of this type will allow a more detailed description of the performance abilities of hearing impaired individuals in both unaided and aided listening situations.

CURRENT PRACTICES

While it is apparent that a variety of materials do exist for the measurement of aided performance in the evaluation setting, it is only fair that we concern ourselves with the types of materials and procedures that are in common clinical usage today. The Zenith Professional and Educational Services (1972) published a compilation of 177 individual responses to the statement, "In steps, briefly describe your clinical procedure for administering hearing aid evaluations." Since each respondent was free to make any manner of response, it is extremely difficult to provide summary statements from these data. A careful examination of the 177 responses, however, does give the impression that a majority of those who replied utilzed a measurement of aided speech threshold, aided speech discrimination (usually both in quiet and in noise), most comfortable loudness level obtained with speech stimuli, and uncomfortable loudness level obtained with speech stimuli. In general, it appeared as though the "Carhart procedure" was still the method of choice.

A much more structured and data specific vehicle was constructed by Smaldino (1979) for the Academy of Rehabilitative Audiology in an attempt to gather information regarding hearing aid evaluation procedures. This discussion of Smaldino's findings is presented with permission of the Academy of Rehabilitative Audiology. Responses were received from 83 individuals who consider themselves to be primarily rehabilitationists.

The following information is only a partial summary of the data supplied by Smaldino on behalf of the Academy of Rehabilitative Audiology. Eighty-one percent of the respondents measured speech reception threshold by means of a live-voice technique and 93 percent utilized spondaic words for these measurements. For speech discrimination testing, 63 percent of the respondents utilized live-voice testing and 37 percent made use of recorded materials. Since there was no breakdown in Smaldino's preliminary data regarding the type of facility in which testing was done, it may be assumed that many of the responses came from university training facilities where live-voice testing is frequently chosen as a teaching technique. Of those facilities that utilized monosyllabic words for the measurement of aided speech discrimination, 39 percent employed the CID W-22 words, 23 percent used Northwestern Auditory Test no. 6, and 21 percent made use of the PAL PB-50 lists.

Fifty-three percent of the respondents utilized 25-word lists for aided testing, and only 30 percent made use of 50-word lists. This is a particularly interesting finding in view of the work of Edgerton et al. (1978) regarding the use of 25-word monosyllabic lists in hearing aid evaluations. They pointed out that the use of half-list materials reduced the consistency by which hearing aids were rank ordered, and also that half-lists were not equivalent to full lists with respect to intelligibility scores. It would appear that greater attention will need to be paid to this aspect of the evaluation procedure in order to ensure maximum efficiency from the use of monosyllabic speech material.

Smaldino's findings also indicated that approximately 12 percent of the respondents did utilize synthetic sentences in the hearing aid evaluation procedure and 12 percent utilized the CID sentence materials. Fully 94 percent of those individuals responding measured speech discrimination in quiet as a routine part of the evaluation procedure, while 80 percent measured speech discrimination in the presence of competition. Of those indicating that they measured aided speech discrimination in the presence of noise, 38 percent utilized a signal-to-noise ratio of +10 dB, 23 percent use a signal-to-noise ratio of +5 dB, while 29 percent accomplished their measurements at a 0 dB signal-to-noise ratio. Finally, 72 percent of those responding stated that they measured the aided threshold of discomfort or uncomfortable loudness level using cold running speech. In contrast, only 7 percent indicated the use of pure-tones for these tolerance measures and 9 percent made use of narrow band noise. Thus, it would appear that the ''Carhart procedure'' was still the dominent method among this sample of audiologists.

SUMMARY

The purpose of this brief chapter is to discuss the procedures and the materials that are in common use in evaluating the interactions between auditory systems and amplification systems. Other esoteric materials were not included since they are not in general or popular usage.

There appears to be little doubt that either monosyllabic word or sentence materials can be used to demonstrate individual performance differences with different amplification systems. When speech materials are used in quiet for the evaluation procedure they have the tendency to provide only an indication of the maximum performance an individual can achieve under optimum conditions. Frequently, the materials in quiet do not have enough sensitivity to be able to reflect subtle performance differences in amplification systems. When these same materials are presented with a competing signal, however, performance differences have been readily elicited.

An important task of the audiologist appears to be one of determining how the resultant scores from a hearing aid evaluation are to be used. If the purpose of the evaluation is primarily to provide a rank ordering of instrument efficiency on the basis of the clarity of speech, monosyllabic words appear to be capable of meeting that task. On the other hand, if the audiologist wishes to be able to make some meaningful inferences regarding performance in more real life settings, the use of some form of sentence material appears to be appropriate. It is hoped that rigorous investigations will continue to examine the use and clinical efficiency of a variety of speech stimuli in the hope of providing even more sensitive measures of evaluating hearing aid performance.

REFERENCES

Anon. *A Collection of Shared Letters*. Chicago: Zenith Hearing Instrument Corporation, 1972.

Berger, K. *The K.S.U. Speech Discrimination Test*. Kent, Ohio: Herald Publishing House, 1977.

Carhart, R. Selection of hearing aids. *Archives of Otolaryngology,* 1946a, *44*, 1–18.

Carhart, R. Tests for selection of hearing aids. *Laryngoscope,* 1946b, *56*, 780–794.
Carhart, R. Volume control adjustment in hearing aid selection. *Laryngoscope*, 1946c, *56,* 510–526.
Carhart, R., & Thompson, E. The fitting of hearing aids. *Transactions: American Academy of Opthamology and Otolaryngology,* 1947, *51,* 354–361.
Carhart, R. Hearing aid selection by university clinics. *Journal of Speech and Hearing Disorders,* 1950, *15*, 106–113.
Davis, H., Hudgins, C., Marquis, R., Nichols, R., et al. The selection of hearing aids. *Laryngoscope,* 1946, *56,* 85–115; 135–163.
Edgerton, B., Klodd, D., & Beattie, R. Half-list speech discrimination measures in hearing aid evaluations. *Archives of Otolaryngology,* 1978, *104,* 669–672.
Egan, J. Articulation testing methods. *Laryngoscope,* 1948, *58,* 955–991.
Fletcher, H. *Hopeful trends in the testing of hearing aids and in the prescription of hearing aids.* Paper given before the 50th annual meeting of the American Federation of Organizations for the Hard of Hearing, 1926.
Fletcher, H. Can we scientifically advise patients as to the effectiveness of hearing aids? *Annals of Otology, Rhinology, and Laryngology,* 1932, *41,* 727–739.
Fletcher, H. Evaluating hearing aids. *Bell Lab. Record,* 1933, January, 1–3.
Gardner, H. Application of a high-frequency consonant discrimination word list in hearing-aid evaluation. *Journal of Speech and Hearing Disorders,* 1971, *36,* 354–355.
Haug, O., Baccaro, P., & Guilford, F. Differences in hearing aid performance. *Archives of Otolaryngology,* 1971, *93,* 183–185.
Hirsh, I., Davis, H. Silverman, S., Reynolds, E., Eldert, E., & Benson, R. Development of materials for speech audiometry. *Journal of Speech and Hearing Disorders,* 1952, *17,* 321–337.
House, A., Williams, C., Hecker, M., & Kryter, K. Articulation testing methods; consonantal differentiation with a closed-response set. *Journal of the Acoustical Society of America,* 1965, *37,* 158–166.
Jerger, J. *Summary presentation.* Presented before the annual meeting of the Academy of Rehabilitative Audiology, Denver, Colorado, 1966.
Jerger, J., & Hayes, D. Hearing aid evaluation. *Archives of Otolaryngology,* 1976, *102,* 214–225.
Jerger, J., Malmquist, C., & Speaks, C. Comparison of some speech intelligibility tests in the evaluation of hearing aid performance. *Journal of Speech and Hearing Research,* 1966, *9,* 253–258.
Jerger, J., Speaks, C. & Malmquist, C. Hearing-aid performance and hearing-aid selection. *Journal of Speech and Hearing Research,* 1966, *9,* 136–149.
Jerger, J., Speaks, C., & Trammel, J. A new approach to speech audiometry. *Journal of Speech and Hearing Disorders,* 1968, *33,* 318–328.
Jirsa, R., & Hodgsen, W. Effect of harmonic distortion in hearing aids on speech intelligibility for normals and hypacusics. *Journal of Auditory Research,* 1970, *10*, 213–217.
Kasten, R., Lotterman, S., & Burnett, E. *The influence of non-linear distortion on hearing aid processed signals.* Paper presented before the American Speech and Hearing Association, Chicago, Illinois, 1967.
Knudsen, V., & Jones, I. Audiometry and the prescribing of hearing aids. *Laryngoscope,* 1936, *46*, 523–536.
Lehiste, I., & Peterson, G. Linguistic considerations in the study of speech intelligibility. *Journal of the Acoustical Society of America,* 1959, *31,* 280–286.
Lybarger, S. Personal communication, 1979.
McConnell, F., Silber, E., & McDonald, D. Test–retest consistency of clinical hearing aid tests. *Journal of Speech and Hearing Disorders,* 1960, *25,* 273–280.

Olsen, W., & Wilber, S. *Physical performance characteristics of different hearing aids and speech discrimination scores achieved with them by hearing-impaired persons.* Paper given before the American Speech and Hearing Association, Chicago, Illinois, 1967.

Olsen, W., & Wilber, S. *Hearing aid distortion and speech intelligibility.* Paper given before the American Speech and Hearing Association, Denver, Colorado, 1968.

Owens, E., & Schubert, E. Development of the California Consonant Test. *Journal of Speech and Hearing Research,* 1977, *20*, 463–474.

Smaldino, J. Personal communication, 1979.

Steinberg, J. Telephone research and problems of the deafened. *Bell Telephone Quarterly,* 1936, *15, 3* – 12.

Tillman, T., & Carhart, R. An expanded test for speech discrimination utilizing CNC monosyllabic words. Technical Report, SAM-TR-66-55, USAF School of Aerospace Medicine, 1966.

Zerlin, S. A new approach to hearing-aid selection. *Journal of Speech and Hearing Research,* 1962, *5,* 370–376.

Harold L. Bate, Ph. D.

13

Speech Protocols in Aural Rehabilitation With Adults

AURAL REHABILITATION

Aural rehabilitation, as viewed by this writer, is the rehabilitation of the hearing-impaired individual through the procedures, separate or variously combined, of speechreading training, auditory/listening training, related skills training, speech training, manual communication training, hearing aid orientation and guidance, informational and personal adjustment counseling, and family/significant-other counseling, so as to enable the individual to function meaningfully with *a minimum of handicap*. The latter part of this definition relates to realistic expectations, wherein the intention is not to say ". . . to function as a normal hearing individual." Some individuals will, to be sure, come close to such a goal, but there always will be some situations where the imposition of the hearing loss, with or without a hearing aid, will preclude it. It is more realistic, and attainable, to aim toward helping the individual to function with as minimal a handicap as is reasonable to expect for that individual. This writer has found that hearing-impaired clients, though surprised at first by such an orientation, come to appreciate such realism and find it conducive to more relaxed functioning, enabling them to deal more realistically with their own specific limitations. It should be noted that, as used in this chapter, the term *rehabilitation* is contrasted with *habilitation* and refers to a restorative process, returning the person to as near as possible to the level of communication ability that existed prior to the loss of hearing. This writer concurs with Alpiner (1978) that ". . . habilitation should be defined as the process of developing the communication function, a skill not previously possessed by the individual . . ." and should not be used synonymously with rehabilitation.

It is the purpose of this chapter to provide guidelines and hints for rendering rehabilitative services to adults who have acquired a hearing loss. The intent, therefore, is to be succinctly pragmatic. The reader will be referred to other sources for relevant theory and research and other additional information. The main focus of this chapter is on materials and methods which are or may be used for assessment and improvement of communication skills per se, especially as have been incorporated into the aural rehabilitative services provided at Western Michigan University during the past several years. This chapter is basically the personal orientation of the writer and does not include an effort to review or relate to all the pertinent literature. Throughout the chapter an assumption is made that *any* degree, shape, or type of loss of hearing sensitivity, or other type of deviation from normal hearing, may be handicapping, depending on the given individual and the daily living demands on that individual. Any interpretation of audiometric/audiologic data which does not consider the person's complaints and daily living demands and needs and which concludes that the person has no handicap or problem is professionally naive, if not unforgivable. An assumption is also made that the best rehabilitation relates specifically to the individual seeking service, and that the best materials and activities are tailor-made for the given hearing-impaired client. It is this writer's bias that rehabilitation implies a highly individualized focus and, while group *lipreading lessons* and similar broadly designed activities may have rehabilitative value, without tailoring the therapeutic activities and materials to the individual problems and needs of a given client, the process might more accurately be described as *educative* rather than *rehabilitative*. It is realized that the two are reciprocally beneficial and intertwined and that various constraints in terms of time, personnel, and money may preclude heavy emphasis on individual attention. This is not to say that there are not commercially available materials that have value for given individuals. Indeed there are, as this chapter will identify and describe. It is in the application and use of those materials, and tailor-made materials, that the difference can arise between group education, with its more general opportunity for remedial or rehabilitative benefit, and individual therapy, with its more specific focus on rehabilitation. This writer advocates a combination of individual and group activities with as many clinicians as there are clients. This arrangement is, of course, ideal and typically possible only in situations such as university training programs where student clinicians can be used. However, it is quite possible in other settings to make use of student clinicians or paraprofessionals, aides, or volunteers under the supervision of qualified personnel.

As is evident in the definition given earlier, aural rehabilitation is a multifaceted process. It may or may not include all of the various components listed in the definition depending on individual needs. The main goal—more effective communication—is a broad one. This is a point many people, professional and lay, seem to miss. It is comparable to saying that the goal of speech therapy is more effective communication, which it certainly is. However, that broad goal does not mean the clinician is always going to employ all forms of speech therapy. The therapy will be designed to concentrate on that aspect of the person's speech or language production which interferes most with effective communication. Articulation skills, or language skills, are not likely to be worked on when the person is manifesting a vocal disorder; likewise with aural rehabilitation. Aural rehabilitation is an umbrella term to refer to a variety of possible procedures for dealing with a breakdown in free and easy communication arising from a loss of hearing. While aural rehabilitation so defined is broad, the focus of this chapter will be intentionally narrow. The chapter will deal primarily with materials and activities used in specific work on speechreading skills, auditory/listening skills, and the combination of these various skills in the bisensory mode. The chapter will not detail the various other aspects of the rehabilitative process, some of which may, in any given instance, be far more critical to effective rehabilitation than drill and practice on specific communication skills. Indeed, in some instances, it is feasible to effect rehabilitation successfully without any designed activities or emphasis upon specific communication skills, e.g., speechreading and/or hearing. An example of such rehabilitation would be that of changes in attitude and orientation brought about through informational and/or personal adjustment counseling, or through counseling the family or other significant persons in the daily life of the hearing-impaired client. This approach is what Alpiner (1978) describes as the progressive rather than the traditional approach. In any given situation, one must consider the total needs of the individual and not feel compelled to focus only on basic visual and auditory skills when other factors may well be primarily responsible for impeding meaningful communication and interaction with others. It is the simple admonition to work with the person, not just the hearing loss.

This chapter will relate primarily to those instances, however, when one is attempting to improve specific communication skills through more effective use of vision and hearing in interpreting spoken language. The reader should recognize the absolute importance of the other components of aural rehabilitation which are listed in the definition and should consult such resources as Alpiner (1978), Garstecki (1974), Oyer and Frankmann (1975), Ross (1972), and Sanders (1971; 1975) for discussions and guidance pertaining to those components. Likewise, for special considerations concerning aural rehabilitation efforts with the geriatric population the reader should consult Alpiner (1978), Hull (1977), and Maurer and Rupp (1979).

Again, this chapter is a personal orientation to aural rehabilitation based upon specific experiences with hearing-impaired adults. It deals strictly with that portion of the rehabilitative process which seeks to improve the relative contributions of vision and hearing to the understanding of speech. It is hoped that the discussions will result in some new insights, ideas, and directions for the reader.

ASSESSMENT OF COMMUNICATION PROBLEMS AND ABILITIES

There is a variety of ways to assess the hearing-impaired person's problems and needs, both quantitatively and qualitatively. These various techniques may be of value before, during, and after rehabilitative intervention.

Case History Information

Considerable guidance for determining the kinds of aural rehabilitative services to provide can come from what typically is referred to as the case history. The reference here is not limited to the usual audiological/otological case history which seeks to determine, through questioning the client, information pertaining to onset of the hearing loss, presence of tinnitus and vertigo, earaches, and so on, but one which goes beyond that important information to elicit from the hearing-impaired client highly specific information relevant to the problems and experiences the individual encounters in daily living. While this may often be done in a very general way, the intent here is to obtain highly specific information. In the interview situation, the elicitation of such information requires careful and creative listening combined with a knowledge of the various implications and nuances of hearing loss and reactions to hearing loss in order to recognize pieces of information that serve as signals to pursue certain lines of questioning. Such information can and should serve as a basis for the eventual selection and design of rehabilitative materials and activities. One should pursue the presenting complaints, seeking greater detail regarding frustrating situations; difficult communication encounters with others; communication demands and needs at work and/or at home; social demands, desires, and settings typical for the individual; special vocabulary needs, if any; typical acoustical environments; typical situations with respect to distance, lighting, and angle; existence of, and problems with, background noise and/or competing messages; need for good localization skills; frequency of business/social lunches and dinners; difficulty in small groups; need/desire to attend concerts, plays, large meetings; needs and problems related to church services, lodge meetings, club meetings; typical recreational and leisure time activities; problems at home in terms of the arrangement of the house, or the idiosyncrasies of family members; need for using the telephone; the list can go on. Such information can and should set the stage for the direction of the therapy and help determine what types of materials and activities will be used in the rehabilitative effort. Every one of the foregoing categories can be simulated or in some way incorporated into the rehabilitative program. This compilation will be referred to later in the discussions of materials and activities for working on specific communication skills. Such information, if the clinician will take the time to ferret it out, can help focus on the most needed experiences, materials, and methods, and consequently allow more effective rehabilitation by avoiding time spent on general material and situations with which the person has no difficulty. Granted, there are many commonalities in terms of problems of hearing impaired adults which can be dealt with in a general way and at the group level. For many clients, however, the most effective rehabilitation will be achieved only when highly specific needs are met, which usually can be done only on an individual basis. One of the reasons hearing-impaired adults will become disillusioned with aural rehabilitation services is that the clinicians seem to expect the client to fit the service rather than fit the service to the client. As a consequence, valuable time is spent practicing what the person can already do and ignoring areas of great suffering and need. This disillusionment is especially likely to occur for adults between the approximate ages of 20–55 years who are in their busiest and perhaps most productive periods of life in terms of families, careers, and social interactions. People who suffer from the breakdown in free and easy communication attributable to hearing impairment need and deserve highly relevant and innovative assistance. In such situations, the rehabilitation program should be open ended rather than eight lessons, or 30 lessons, or however many lessons are already prepared and inflexible before the client even arrives. The burden can be on the client to decide when therapy has accomplished its purpose. The clinician should make every effort to enable the individual to return to the mainstream as quickly as possible. Rehabilitation materials and activities can and should be designed for any given individual to simulate their problem areas and meet their specific needs. Such an approach is what makes it a rehabilitative effort. Certainly, general vocabulary and colloquial speech material also have a place in the aural rehabilitation program and are common to all, as will be described later. However, one must always relate to the unique situations and needs of each individual if meaningful rehabilitation is to occur and if the handicap is to be minimized as much and as quickly as is reasonable to expect. Careful elicitation of case history information in the manner described can identify such problems and needs.

Communication Scales and Questionnaires

In addition to helpful information obtained in the case history interview, considerable valuable information can be obtained from a variety of communication scales and questionnaires such as the Hearing Handicap Scale, the Test of Actual Performance, the Hearing Measurement Scale, the Denver Scale of Communication Function, and the Profile Questionnaire for Rating Communicative Performance (in various environments). These particular assessment tools are designed mainly to assess attitudes and problem areas. They are described and discussed by Alpiner (1978). Another similar tool is the Hearing Performance Inventory developed by Giolas et al. (1979). The HPI was developed to provide an assessment of hearing performance in various problem areas experienced by the hard-of-hearing person in certain everyday listening situations and to yield a profile of that performance. Such tools can be of considerable value in aural rehabilitation, not only in terms of giving direction regarding counseling needs and the design of specific rehabilitative experiences, but also in the pre-and postservice assessments which enable one to evaluate progress. These tools have an important place in the provision of aural rehabilitation services, and should be incorporated in order to assist the clinician in better identifying specific areas of need for a given hearing-impaired client. Indeed, these tools may be used as an excellent basis for the case history interview referred to earlier.

Audiologic Test Battery

Additional useful information of an evaluative nature can be obtained, of course, from the typical audiologic test battery. The results of pure tone audiometry certainly provide some basis for anticipating the types of problems the person is likely experiencing. The degree, type, and pattern of loss all have fairly characteristic implications for daily communication problems of the person affected. One should be cautious, however, in interpreting the implications of pure tone audiograms because of the variety of additional potential influential factors, such as the nature of the damage in the auditory system, the unique personality and intellectual characteristics of the person in question, and the daily life demands on that individual. The results of speech audiometry also can provide information of rehabilitative value depending upon what information is collected. Unfortunately, the possibility for the collection of some very useful information is too often ignored. If, for example, the examiner only marks responses on a speech discrimination test as right or wrong, the only information obtained is a score. In such a case, information useful for counseling or suggesting rehabilitative need and/or direction is lost. If, on the other hand, the examiner records the specific response to each speech discrimination test item, rather than simply marking it right or wrong, not only is a score available, but the examiner can then say something more specific about the communication problems the person has. If, for example, the client is making such errors as "fit" for "sit," the implications for the need to watch the speaker are obvious and can easily be illustrated to the client. If a "look and listen" presentation of the speech discrimination test is given and the person is still saying "fit" for "sit," the need for speechreading training becomes more evident. Or, if on the standard speech discrimination tests the client is substituting highly dissimilar consonants or vowels, the implication is that considerable distortion may be taking place and the need for aural rehabilitation services, as well as the nature of those services, is more readily seen. Such information is lost when the examiner seeks only a speech discrimination score and makes no attempt to relate to the types of errors responsible for the score. Even for the purpose of site of lesion testing, as well as for the purposes of the comparative evaluations of hearing aids, the examiner is likely throwing away potentially valuable information by not making note of the error responses.

Also of value in terms of rehabilitative implications is information obtained from administering speech discrimination tests (aided and/or unaided) at three intensity levels, i.e., 25 dB HL, 45 dB HL, and 30 dB SL (or whatever sensation level is needed to yield the most likely maximum score for the material used). The 25 dB HL is that fixed level which is approximately equal to the intensity level of what is called "faint level speech," such as in quiet conversation or intensity reduction due to the effect of distance. The 45 dB HL is that fixed level which is approximately equal to the intensity level of what is called "conversational speech." The third level refers to whatever intensity level above the person's threshold is likely to yield their maximum speech discrimination ability under optimum conditions. Again, both quantitative (speech discrimination score) and qualitative (specific error responses given) information can be of significant value, especially for rehabilitative purposes (and likewise for hearing aid comparisons). The same tests under various conditions of noise also can provide helpful direction to the need and nature of rehabilitation. Speech audiometric material, techniques, and interpretations are discussed in greater detail throughout this book. Therefore, no further elaboration is given here other than to emphasize again that when the examiner obtains only a speech discrimination score and fails to record the nature of the erroneous responses, much useful information—especially for rehabilitative purposes—is lost.

Assessment of Specific Communication Skills

Assessment of specific receptive communication skills can be made with various tests of speechreading skills, auditory skills, and/or combined mode (bisensory) skills. Since the focus of this chapter is related to materials and activities for improving specific communication skills, each of these areas will be treated separately with techniques for assessment and therapy discussed separately for each area.

SPEECHREADING SKILLS

Speechreading is a more inclusive term for lipreading. It may be defined as a receptive language skill involving the understanding of speech primarily through the use of visual cues. It is a skill that all adults already possess to at least some minimal extent. For the adult who acquires a hearing loss, speechreading skills become quite important as a means of supplementing (or even compensating for) the hearing loss. The extent to which this occurs, or can occur, varies markedly among individuals for a variety of reasons, which are discussed in detail by other authors (Jeffers & Barley, 1971; O'Neill & Oyer, 1961; Oyer & Frankmann, 1975).

Assessment of Speechreading Skills

Unfortunately, there is a lack of good, sensitive tools for the assessment of speechreading skills. The tests that are available do seem to be reliable in that individuals attain similar scores on repetitions of the test. Also, the tests which are available do appear to separate speechreaders into appropriate categories of "good," "fair," and "poor" speechreaders. However, anyone who has used these tests extensively in programs of aural rehabilitation no doubt has learned that they provide little sensitivity to real changes which occur as a consequence of therapy. A variety of other measures, subjective and objective, may confirm significant change in ease of communication with a given client but with no evident change in the score on the speechreading test per se. It is rare to observe marked change on these tests of speechreading when administered before and following a course of therapy. Typically such changes are seen only in instances of sudden severe hearing loss when one is able to assess speechreading skills shortly after the occurrence of the hearing loss and then again as time passes and/or therapy progresses. Even these marked changes appear to most likely occur only in fairly young adults. One should not conclude, however, that the available speechreading tests have no value. The clinician simply should interpret them cautiously and not be disillusioned by a lack of change in performance on the test. There are many other ways of assessing progress and change, keeping in mind that the primary goal is improvement in overall communication ability and not in speechreading alone. The aforementioned scales and questionnaires can be of considerable value in this regard, as can bisensory administrations of the speechreading tests. It is quite possible, and indeed likely, that a given client may well gain speechreading skill during the course of therapy and have it reflected only in overall communication ability but not in the score on the formal speechreading test given by visual mode only.

Information relevant to the development, purposes, and values of formal speechreading tests and the research pertaining thereto may be obtained by consulting Alpiner (1978), Jeffers and Barley (1971), O'Neill and Oyer (1961), and Oyer and Frankmann (1975). The main purpose of the present discussion is to describe and comment on the tests that are available and most commonly used and to describe other means of assessing speechreading skills. The particular tests used and the mode of presentation of those tests are a function of clinician preference and need.

The Utley Test of Lipreading is probably the most commonly used speechreading test. The test consists of three parts. Part I is a sentence test with two forms, which are roughly equated. Part II is a word test, and Part III is a story test. Part I, the sentence test, appears to be the most useful and most used of the three. The word test and the story test are of more limited value. Each form of the sentence test consists of 31 short phrases or sentences, which are basically common colloquial or idiomatic expressions. Because of the age of the test, some of the sentences are less colloquial today due mainly to sentence construction. The test may be scored on a verbatim basis or on a correct-message basis. The latter method of scoring is more practical and places greater emphasis on how well the person understands communication rather than on the more analytic word-for-word accuracy. The complete test is described in more detail by Jeffers and Barley (1971). The reader also would be advised to consult Alpiner (1978) for relevant discussion.

Also available for formal assessment of speechreading ability is the Barley Speechreading Test. Each of the two forms of this test consists of a group of sentences representing "everyday American speech." The test items were selected from the CID Everyday Sentences. Each form of the test consists of sentences of comparable length with a total of 125 words in each form. Scoring is done on a word-correct basis. This test is described in detail by Jeffers and Barley (1971).

Another tool for the formal assessment of speechreading ability is the Keaster Test of Lipreading, which is also detailed by Jeffers and Barley (1971). The revised form of this test is also referred to as the John Tracy Clinic Test. This test consists of two forms of 30 sentences each with a total of 188 words in each form. Scoring is done on a word-correct basis.

All of the above tests originally were devised as filmed tests of lipreading. It appears, however, that most clinicians make use of "live" presentations of these tests, a procedure that has obvious, but generally acceptable, limitations. Filmed and videotaped versions of such tests also have significant limitations as described by Alpiner (1978). This writer prefers the live mode of presentation. Care needs to be taken in such presentation to make note of the conditions and manner of the presentation as well as who presented the material. Based upon personal experiences with filmed and videotaped presentations of speechreading tests, it is this writer's view that live presentations are just as reliable and valid—if not more so—and that they provide more realistic information and avoid the many distractions and complaints of clients that are so characteristically associated with the recorded presentations. Clinically, the reliability of such presentations is surprisingly excellent, even with different presenters. Perhaps this observation is simply another reflection of the lack of sensitivity of these tests alluded to earlier. Nonetheless, since speechreading activities are typically presented in a live, face-to-face manner, the testing may as well occur in the same way. Again, however, the clinician needs to be aware of the kinds of controls that are necessary and the consequent limitations on interpreting the information.

A speechreading test for adults that appears to have good clinical utility and efficiency is a more recent one devised at the University of Denver Speech and Hearing Center. This test, The Denver Quick Test of Lipreading Ability (Alpiner, 1978), consists of 20 everyday expressions and is scored on a correct-message basis. Alpiner notes that this test does not appear to be any more sensitive to improvements in overall communication ability resulting from therapy than the previously described tests of lipreading. He further notes that he too has observed that such a phenomenon is not unusual with all of the formal tests of lipreading. Such observations do not preclude the utility of such tests, but do suggest caution in how they are used and interpreted. The use of these instruments for various research purposes becomes quite questionable.

Perhaps if clinicians would analyze changes in specific responses to test items, rather than look for changes in scores, much more helpful and meaningful information would be obtained. This writer has noted that in several instances when comparing pre- and posttherapy test results, the individual's speechreading score on the test did not change, but there was marked improvement in performance in terms of deriving meaning more closely related to what was actually said, or in terms of responding with items that were visually more similar to what was actually presented. Such changes, when combined with auditory information, could account for significant change in communication ability even though the speechreading score—based on visual-only presentation—did not change. This is an area of needed research. Just as in the case with auditory speech discrimination tests, clinicians are probably throwing away or ignoring very useful data by using only a score on speechreading tests. A test that comes closer to meeting this kind of need is the Lipreading Test for Phonemes (Binnie, Jackson, & Montgomery, 1976). The primary purpose of this test is to serve as a screening test to assess visual and auditory-visual confusions between consonants. Such a test can give indication of the extent to which the individual is able to differentiate homophenous categories of phonemes and thereby provide some direction as to the need for specific phoneme orientation and practice.

Another means of assessing speechreading skill and improvement is in the form of a Lipreading Profile as described by Binnie (1976). The rationale for his profile is that clinicians need some guidance regarding speechreading performance, which spans a wide variety of linguistically redundant cues. His profile includes the Lipreading Test for Phonemes described above and, in addition, includes six areas of visual intelligibility which typically receive attention during the rehabilitative process, i.e., PB Words, CID Sentences, Key Words, Sentence Deletion, Pseudo-Dialogue, and Automatic Speech. The reader should consult Binnie's description for further details.

Perhaps the best and most practical assessment of speechreading ability, at least for purposes of evaluating progress in therapy, is through careful sequencing of therapy material and collecting data on the performance of the individual with the material used for the speechreading training. Since the formal tests of speechreading typically do not reflect much change in performance, it becomes very important for the sake of accountability, if not for the sake of client and clinician morale and motivation, to have some means of demonstrating success on specific tasks and of assessing the effectiveness of the services provided. This approach can be used, though it typically need not be, for all material used in speechreading instruction and practice. Some material lends itself better to such analysis and data collection than does other material. At least some portion of the material used should be analyzed in such a way. For example, if one has a list of 100 common phrases or sentences for speechreading practice and mastery, an assessment of the person's performance on the entire list should be made prior to the introduction of the material and then again at the end of the carefully sequenced practice sessions. Procedures for incorporating such an approach into therapy are described in greater detail later. Such an analysis demonstrates the effect of practice and instruction and, if therapy is designed properly, results in demonstrable progress, which is most encouraging for both client and clinician. It also provides a more objective basis for describing changes in speechreading ability, with the assumption that there is a generalization and transfer effect of such accomplishment in terms of overall speechreading and communication ability.

Whether assessment of speechreading ability should be made by a combined sensory modality presentation or by vision alone is another important consideration in the evaluation process. The decision is best made on the basis of the clinician's purpose at the moment, but it is likely that both forms of assessment will provide the most useful information. Certainly the combined sensory modality is the ultimate goal. The merits of a bisensory approach, i.e., auditory-visual, in terms of both assessment and therapy, are discussed in a later section.

In summary, assessment of speechreading skill, and changes in that skill as a result of therapy, can be made in at least two main ways: by formal tests of speechreading, and by performance data collection on selected material. Each approach offers different information and each should be used in a given program of aural rehabilitation.

Materials and Activities for Enhancing Speechreading Skills

There is an abundance of commercially available materials for speechreading instruction and practice. The relevance and value of these materials vary, but they all can be used or adapted for given needs and can certainly stimulate ideas for clinician-designed materials and activities for a given client or group of clients. Such resources are included in the reference list for this chapter. The most useful resources for prepared materials of general applicability for speechreading training are, in this writer's experience, those of Broberg (1975), Haug and Haug (1977), Jeffers and Barley (1971), Nitchie (1950), and Ordman and Ralli (1976). A recent compilation of activities by Jeffers and Barley (1979) also appears to have good applicability. As implied earlier in this chapter, the most efficient and effective rehabilitation likely will result from adapting and tailoring the material to individual needs, not only in terms of the content of the material but also in terms of how the material is used and the extent to which the materials and activities relate to the various problem areas discussed in the section on case history information. Many of the commercially available materials were designed for general use and, more often than not, for lipreading classes or groups. Their use, without modification, is more relevant to those purposes. As one moves to more individualized rehabilitative efforts, the materials and the manner in which they are used need to be modified according to the manifested needs. It should be noted at this point that *any* of the materials developed for speechreading instruction and practice also can be used to great advantage for auditory/listening activities and/or bisensory therapy activities. Indeed, it is the preference of this writer not to dwell extensively on speechreading alone.

One of the first decisions the clinician typically faces in planning speechreading instruction and practice is the decision of whether, or to what extent, to dwell on the visual characteristics of individual phonemes. In this writer's view, extensive demonstration of and practice on isolated phonemes or words for purposes of speechreading is a questionable and typically unproductive use of valuable time. Speech is a dynamic, ongoing process. The visible characteristics of the individual phonemes vary considerably as a function of phonetic context, speaker, and speaking situation (conversational mode versus public speeches). Certainly an orientation to the visible aspects of speech is warranted, along with periodic reminders and relevant illustrations throughout the program of therapy. Most people are quite unaware of the visible characteristics of speech and, indeed, tend to be "letter" oriented as opposed to "sound" oriented with reference to speech. Therefore, general information on how the speech sounds ideally would appear on the lips, and how they are similar and dissimilar, can be of significant value. Undue emphasis and practice on this aspect, however, typically usurps time which can be better spent in more relevant and productive efforts. As is obvious, this writer advocates a more synthetic approach to aural rehabilitation. It should be stressed, however, that there is no published research that establishes superiority of any one approach over another. The final decision is made on the basis of personal experience, opinion, and preference. The client's opinions and preferences should not be ignored in making such decisions. This writer has found that clients can offer considerable valuable advice in deciding what approach is likely to work best for them. Some seem to need a more analytic approach, and the clinician should be open and flexible to such a need. Alpiner (1978) has investigated client feedback more formally and has summarized client preferences. His findings are quite consistent with this writer's experiences and should be used as a guide in making decisions about whether to use a traditional approach–whether analytic or synthetic—or what he calls a progressive approach. In providing an orientation to the visible characteristics of speech this writer prefers the basic classification and description of speech sounds of Nitchie (1950). His classification is quite easily understood by the general public. If one is going to use a more traditional approach and build speechreading activities around specific phonemes and key words, the Nitchie approach (Nitchie, 1950; Ordman & Ralli, 1976) is a very workable one. In this writer's view, time can usually be spent more wisely on more immediately relevant materials, but the final decision is influenced by the particular needs manifested and by such things as age of the client(s) and whether the clinician is using a group or individual format. Typically, the traditional approach tends to be preferred for elderly clients and for groups. This is not to say that it is the best approach for such situations; it is simply preferred. The extent to which one may need to provide concentrated orientation or practice on the visible characteristics of phonemes can be determined in a manner suggested by Binnie and colleagues (1976). Too much emphasis on the visible aspects of the various phonemes would seem to increase the risk of making the individuals too analytic in their attempts to understand speech. The extent to which such concern is valid is undetermined. One should remember that the visible characteristics of speech are a totally unnecessary and often absent requirement of speech, as is evidenced by any good ventriloquist.

There is a variety of prepared speechreading materials that this writer has found to be quite useful either as originally designed or with some modification. While the selection of which speech materials to be used is extremely important, the *ways* in which those materials are used and presented are equally important. Various materials that this writer has found to be particularly useful will be discussed, along with reference to ways in which such materials might best be used to maximize the relevance of the rehabilitative efforts.

Sequencing the Difficulty of Materials and Activities

Prior to the description and discussion of specific speech materials useful in speechreading training, it would be beneficial to consider the various ways in which any material can be used and presented. The most successful approach in terms of efficiency and effectiveness is going to be an approach in which the material used develops from easy to difficult. The principles and procedures discussed in this section are equally relevant to subsequent sections on auditory/listening training and bisensory training and should be reviewed with reference to those concerns.

Material can be sequenced from easy to difficult in terms of visibility, type of material (highly familiar versus unfamiliar; short versus lengthy, etc.), and in terms of the manner and conditions of presentation. With regard to visibility of material, the clinician can gradate the material selected by using a formula suggested by Sanders (1971) or a modification of his formula as personal experience might dictate. Sanders presents a way of calculating the percentage visibility of a word or sentence by assigning each phoneme the maximum visibility value given for its category. Clinicians wishing to employ this procedure should consult Sanders (1971) for the specific values and categories. This writer employs a modification that gives even less weight to the less visible vowels and consonants and slightly more weight to the more visible ones within each category. Such a modification allows a greater spread in the overall visibility scores for materials used, making it easier to sequence the materials more realistically. Clinicians can determine their own preference for modification of the visibility values. It should be noted that such assignment of values of visibility treats speech in a somewhat unrealistic way without consideration of coarticulatory factors, contextual cues, and other similarly important parameters. Such calculation of relative visibility does, however, give the clinician at least some general means of sequencing material from easy to difficult in terms of variations in visibility of the phonemes that comprise the material. Such sequencing better enables the clients to experience early success as they progress toward their goals, and it avoids some of the problems of random presentation of stimuli to be speechread.

Another way of sequencing any material used for improving communication skills is by beginning with highly familiar material and moving toward the use of less familiar material. Speech material may be familiar because of its content, e.g., colloquial forms and frequently used phrases, or because of the frequency of occurrence of the words which comprise the material, or because of the relevance of the vocabulary for the individual client. Clinicians can develop their own material based upon their own knowledge of frequently used phrases or by making use of such sources as Berger's compilation of the most common 100,000 words used in conversations (Berger, 1977c).

A third way of sequencing speech material used in speechreading training is the manner in which the material is presented for practice. No matter what material the clinician is using, whether of high visibility or low visibility, whether of high frequency of occurrence or low frequency of occurrence, the material can be presented in such a way as to progress from easy to difficult in a way that yields maximal success for the client. Indeed, within the limits of visibility and homopheneity of the material, if the client is making many errors it has to be viewed as the fault of the clinician for not breaking the task down into simpler and smaller steps. In other words, the material needs to be gradated in a way that allows the client success for each step of increasing difficulty. The easiest material to be understood is that which the client looks at on paper and then watches the clinician say. The clinician can move from the point where the client knows exactly what is going to be said and then, in successive stages, increase the range of choices—allowing mastery at each level—until the client has mastery of the set of material when the total material or component items are given in random order. Such a procedure, based on programmed learning principles, can be used with *any* material selected by the clinician and is applicable to auditory/listening training and bisensory training as well as to speechreading training. Such an approach provides a basis for both the clinician and the client to see progress and to determine that progress has definitely been made. As noted earlier in this chapter, any given material can be presented in its entirety first to get a baseline performance assessment. This can be followed by sequenced presentations as noted above, and then, at the end of the program, the entire material can be presented again for a final assessment. It is not necessary, or even desirable, to use all material in this manner. This approach, however, should be used with a significant portion of the material selected. As a result, the rehabilitative effort is more of a systematic, rather than a random, approach.

Once a given set of speech materials has been mastered in the manner described, other variations can be introduced to increase the difficulty. Such variations typically involve decreasing the redundancy of the material by simulating the daily problems of the individual (see section on case history information). Variations of rate, angle, distance, and lighting can be introduced. Visual and auditory distractions and/or a background of competing noises and/or messages can be introduced. Not only does such experience enable the hearing-impaired client to work toward mastery of selected, relevant material under these typical varying conditions, it also increases their tolerance, concentration, and confidence when they encounter such conditions in their daily lives. Their attitudes toward such situations begin to change as they are enabled to experience success and learn what their true limitations and abilities are. As this happens, the clients become more confident and relaxed, allowing them to focus their attention even better without the preoccupying and distracting fear of failure. The result is that they can become more effective communicators.

Another form of varying the difficulty of given material is through the use of different presenters. It is especially advantageous if the other presenters of material can include the spouse or other significant person(s) in the daily life of the hearing impaired client. Once the client has achieved a reasonable mastery of the material as presented by the clinician, he or she is ready to transfer that ability on the same material to other speakers. Such approaches also encourage considerable home practice on the selected material, which is also very important.

The difficulty of any given material can also be varied by the kind of responses required of the client. The typical response elicited is one of either writing down or repeating what the clinician said. Some form of accuracy check is needed. The clinician must avoid asking, "Did you get that?" Clients might report that they did not get the material when, indeed, they did or, more typically, they might report that they did understand when they did not. If a client answers "yes" to such a question it may be that he or she has no idea what was said and is bluffing, or it may be that a message was understood but it was the wrong message. To ask the client to write down or repeat the material is a good form of accuracy check and the clinician can decide how demanding to be in terms of message versus word-for-word accuracy. This form of check on accuracy, however, is not one that encourages a more realistic and appropriate conversational response on the part of the person with a hearing loss. A more realistic response to require of the client, and a more difficult one, is for the client to give a conversationally appropriate response, i.e., to contrive an answer to a question or, in response to a statement, to quickly reply with a statement that reflects an understanding of what was said by the clinician. If the clinician is concerned about more than just the accuracy of the general message, a highly specific and complete response could be required. For example, if the clinician asks, "How far do you live from town?," the client could answer simply, "Five miles," which would indicate that certainly the beginning of the question was understood and perhaps the second part. Had the client answered, "Five inches," it would be obvious that only the first part of the question was understood. To require an appropriate form of response, and yet check on accuracy of reception of the entire message, the client might be required to respond more specifically and completely, e.g., "I live five miles from town." This is an appropriate form of response in conversation and yet tells the clinician that the entire message was understood. Had the client answered the question by saying, "Sue lives five miles from Fountaintown," the clinician would have a better assessment of the accuracy of the reception of the entire question. The simple response, "Five miles," would have been an appropriate response and the clinician would never have been aware that the critical part of the question was misunderstood. This form of accuracy check should be used frequently, along with the typical repetition response, because it is more relevant to what the client should be doing every day. Many hearing-impaired persons become uneasy about correctly understanding people and tend to repeat what is said to them in order to avoid making an inappropriate response. Such repetitions are often annoying to the conversational partner. The more appropriate, but complete, form of response allows the conversational partner to know whether a misunderstanding has occurred, but without the imposition of repeats and responses to repeats. The requirement of the more appropriate forms of response in therapy also can help build confidence in the client, which greatly aids his or her daily communication.

Still another form of varying the difficulty of any given material is by introducing slight variations ranging from changing a word or two to completely paraphrasing the material. For example, if the particular sentence is "I saw him the other day," one could use a number of variations which would change the meaning, e.g., substituting "he" for "I," or "her" for "him," or "last week" for "the other day," and so on. Another variation of this is to have blanks that must be filled in. In this way the individual has some contextual cues on paper.

Finally, any material used, whether commercially available or designed by the clinician, can and should be used in situations which simulate, as nearly as possible, the daily experiences of the client, such as those referred to earlier in the section on case history information. One should not spend considerable time in therapy working on things the client is already able to do and which are not problem areas for the client. The effort should be directed toward those kinds of materials and situations which give the person the most difficulty on a day-to-day basis. The primary goal is to enable the hearing-impaired clients to function in their daily lives with a minimum of handicap. If that goal is to be realized, the materials and activities must be relevant. It should be stressed again that all of the foregoing comments and suggestions pertaining to the sequencing and presentation of speech material for practice, while not exhaustive, apply equally to auditory/listening training and bisensory training, and not just to speechreading training.

Useful Types of Materials and Activities in Speechreading Training

Given the foregoing discussion of how any speech material might be presented and sequenced,, a discussion of some of the more useful types of materials and activities is in order. Only those speech materials used somewhat frequently by this writer in providing aural rehabilitative services will be discussed. There are many other materials that may be of equal value and utility but which will not be discussed in this context. As implied earlier, if one is going to use a more traditional approach to speechreading instruction and practice wherein "lessons" are designed to focus on certain groups of phonemes, the Nitchie materials (Nitchie, 1950; Ordman & Ralli, 1976) are quite useful. Such materials are particularly useful with elderly clients and with individuals who have not had any previous exposure to speechreading instruction. Since this writer makes greater use of a more synthetic approach, i.e., one which spends more time on relevant general speech or highly tailored speech material, the supplementary materials included by Nitchie (1950) and in Ordman and Ralli (1976) are used more frequently. Nitchie (1950) presents a compilation of colloquial interrogative forms that can be quite useful in practice on speechreading skills as well as in other communication skills. Quick recognition of the correct interrogative is important to quick understanding of a question. Therefore, drill on various interrogatives, e.g., how, where, who, why, when, which, is judged to be a worthwhile expenditure of time. These interrogatives can be sequenced in a variety of ways, as described earlier, and can be presented in isolation or in the context of the full question. The remainder of the question can, of course, provide helpful contextual cues for the identification of the specific interrogative used. The response required of the client can vary according to the accuracy check procedure preferred by the clinician. An extension or variation of the use of questions, which has relevant value, is the development of a set of questions with various answers. The client is required to ask the question each time and the clinician(s) and/or members of a group have a set of various answers for the client to speechread. In this situation the client is prepared for the possible answers by knowing the topic of the question. For example, a question might be, "How long has it been raining?" Possible answers could include ones such as: (a) It has been raining since noon; (b) It has been raining for two hours; (c) since yesterday afternoon; (d) I think it has been raining since the day before yesterday; and so on. Several questions with various answers can be developed by the clinician. Again, the questions should be relevant either to the general daily living or the specific vocabulary/language needs of the given client(s). Such material can be used in a variety of ways, e.g., competing noise/message conditions, small group conversation simulations, and so on, as described earlier. Nitchie's book also has a compilation of common phrases, some of which need to be updated. Ordman and Ralli (1976) include in their lessons various groups of common phrases related to what people might typically say about certain topics or in certain situations, e.g., what people say about the weather. Considerable use can be made of this or similar material by combining all the groups of phrases in a separate compilation and requiring the clients to work toward mastery of the material using the various procedures of sequencing and presenting described earlier. It is also beneficial to arrange these or other such sentences according to their relative visibility. Such material is also excellent for home practice.

Another compilation of speech stimuli which this writer has used extensively is McDearmon's familiar phrases based on programmed learning principles (Jeffers & Barley, 1971). The list of 88 expressions are not necessarily highly familiar expressions per se, but they allegedly contain all the words comprising 50 percent of written English. This compilation is frequently used by this writer as one of the sets of material that clients are given to master. The client can take the material home and practice it with a friend, spouse, or other relative, and the clinician can spend a portion of each session on the material and can plot the progress toward mastery. Again, this material can be employed in the various ways and under the various conditions described earlier. If the clinician prefers, the client's performance with this material—or any other similar material—can be plotted in graph form to allow the client to see the progress from session to session. The clinician should establish a baseline score for all 88 phrases at the beginning of the therapy program and then plot the weekly progress. Such data can be extremely important in demonstrating change since, as noted earlier, the lipreading tests are generally not sensitive enough to reflect sufficient change to encourage and motivate clients. The McDearmon material also is quite useful in auditory/listening training and in bisensory training, and can be used in the same ways as described above.

A somewhat different but very useful activity which this writer has used for several years makes use of expanded sentences. One form of expanded sentence activity is based on research reported by Fisher and Kealey (1969). Their research involved sentences with blanks, such as "The ____ tree is ____ growing ____." They found that, in terms of speechreading, the most visible expansion was expansion by negation, e.g., "The tree is not growing." Listed in sequence from most visible to least visible expansions their results suggested the following order: (1) expansion by negation; (2) expansion of verb phrase; (3) expansion of noun phrase; (4) negation and noun phrase; (5) negation and verb phrase; (6) noun phrase and verb phrase; and (7) negation, noun phrase, and verb phrase. If one were to devise a set of expanded sentences which would be in order of visibility of expansion, it might be as follows: (1) The tree is growing; (2) The tree is not growing; (3) The tree is growing well; (4) The big tree is growing; (5) The big tree is not growing; (6) The tree is not growing well; and (7) The big tree is not growing well. Such research provides another form of sequencing the difficulty of material. This writer has devised several such expanded sentences for each basic sentence. A response sheet with the appropriate number of sentences with blanks is given the client. The client is asked to place a check mark where the expansion(s) occurred or to write in the specific word used to create the expansion. Clinicians can develop their own sets of sentences and response sheets and sequence them according to level of difficulty as they choose. Again, such material has utility beyond speechreading training alone. It can be used as an auditory/listening training activity or for combined mode presentations depending on the needs of the client(s). The various other conditions of presentation of material can also be employed with this material.

Another form of expanded sentence activity is that which simply continues to build on the original phrase or sentence. For example, one could start with "the tree" and expand it in ways such as follows: (1) the tree; (2) the maple tree; (3) the big maple tree; (4) the big maple tree is growing; (5) the big maple tree in the corner of the yard is growing; (6) the great big maple tree in the corner of the yard is growing; and so on. The writer once developed such a sentence the final form of which contained 56 words. Quite surprising was the fact that the clients not only followed the material, they were able to identify where the expansions occurred and generally were able to identify what the expansion was, even for the 56-word message. Needless to say, 56 words taxes the clinician's ability to present the material visibly and meaningfully. Such an activity is, however, an excellent way of increasing the client's ability to track lengthy material without giving up. It is somewhat easy, since the client is thoroughly familiar with the material after a few presentations and is alert for the expansion. Again, such material, clinician-designed, has utility beyond speechreading alone.

When using a synthetic approach, topic-centered speech material is probably the most frequent type of material used. Several commercially available books include such speech material. In addition to such material, clinicians can and should develop their own material according to the needs of the particular client(s). One can determine a vocabulary or set of topics that are unique to the client(s) being served. Such material can relate to job, school, home, leisure time activity, and so on. As a general rule, the younger the adult client, the more challenging and directly relevant the material must be. This is no doubt one of the reasons why so few younger adults avail themselves of aural rehabilitation services. The clinician must move beyond the "canned" material with such clientele and develop materials and activities uniquely designed for the particular individual seeking rehabilitation.

Elderly clients seem more inclined to want materials and activities that are of a more informative nature, and which are fun. Part of this is perhaps the important social needs which the aural rehabilitation groups can relate to. One can, however, meet this need and still work on some of the important materials described earlier. For example, a bingo game format can be used for the McDearmon phrases or for other similar material. The phrases are simply randomly placed on the bingo response sheet and a chip is placed over the phrase presented by the clinician. Other similarly enjoyable formats can be used for presenting relevant material. Materials and activities relevant to the needs of such clientele are described by Alpiner (1978), Broberg (1975), Fisher (1977; 1978), Hull (1977), Jeffers and Barley (1971), and Maurer and Rupp (1979).

One rarely finds speechreading material, or, for that matter, auditory/listening training material, which deals with the suprasegmental aspects of speech. Sanders (1971) does make some reference to these aspects, but mostly as they pertain to auditory skills. The suprasegmental aspects of speech, as described by Minifie, Hixon, and Williams (1973), are

> . . . changes in the intonational patterns of the voice (melody of the voice), changes in linguistic stress (relative emphasis given to syllable within an utterance), and changes in the durational characteristics of utterances (including pausal patterns, tempo and rate of syllable utterance). . . . (p. 281)

These features are called suprasegmental because they occur across several phonemes. While these features contribute to the vitality and variety in speech, they also contribute to the meaning of the message, sometimes conveying subtle shades of meaning. The suprasegmental features are typically thought of as auditory phenomena, but they also generally have a visible manifestation as well. Consequently, material that deals with these suprasegmental aspects of speech can be very useful in speechreading instruction and practice as well as for purposes of auditory/listening training and bisensory practice. For example, the simple word "oh" can convey quite a variety of meanings depending upon how it is said and the various facial expressions which accompany its utterance. Sentences can be developed to provide the client, with an opportunity to see and practice these suprasegmental features. In speechreading, the features that are most visible are the stress and durational characteristics, especially the latter. Vocal variety would not typically have any associated visible characteristics. The clinician can develop lists of sentences to practice suprasegmental features, although it is one of the less important activities. One of the difficulties with such material relates to a given clinician's ability to present the material correctly. A fair amount of practice and a little acting ability is sometimes necessary. An example of such a sentence is "What time did you arrive at the office today?" This same sentence can appear on a response sheet ten or fifteen times, with the client instructed to circle the word that was emphasized in order to convey a particular meaning. In the particular sentence given above any one word could be emphasized—except the word "what"—in order to change the meaning or intention of the question. Practice on such material, whether for speechreading or hearing or both, demonstrates to the client the variations in semantic intent of the message which can be conveyed auditorily or visually.

For additional approaches, methods, and materials for use in speechreading instruction and practice, the reader should consult Alpiner (1978) and Jeffers and Barley (1971). These two sources provide considerable practical suggestions along with helpful discussion of the various aspects of speechreading and the improvement of speechreading skills.

SPEECHEARING SKILLS

A troublesome aspect of the literature relating to aural rehabilitation has been the lack of parallel terms. Speechreading is a term that has become widely used to refer to the use of visual skills for understanding speech, as defined and described in previous sections. When one comes to the auditory or hearing portion of aural rehabilitation, however, a switch is made to the term "auditory training"—a training procedure rather than a skill. The terms *hearing* and *auditory skills* are really broader in scope than the auditory understanding of speech, just as *vision* and *visual skills* are broader in scope than the term *speechreading*. As a response to this cumbersome lack of parallelism in terminology, a term, which to the best of this writer's knowledge has not been coined, will be coined for the purposes of this chapter, i.e., *speechearing*, pronounced as a contraction of or blending of "speech" and "hearing". Speechearing is defined as a receptive language skill involving the understanding of speech primarily through auditory cues. *Speechearing training* would be narrower than *auditory training* but would be a significant part of or form of auditory training. Auditory training is defined by Sanders (1971) as "a systematic procedure designed to increase the amount of information that a person's hearing contributes to his total perception," and, so defined, includes auditory stimuli other than speech. Speechearing training would then be a systematic procedure designed to increase the amount of information that a person's hearing contributes to the understanding of speech.

Assessment of Speechearing Skills

Unlike the assessment of speechreading skills, there exists a wide range of instruments for assessing speechearing skills or abilities of an individual to use the sense of hearing for discriminating and/or understanding speech stimuli. Since such instruments are the primary topic of this book, this chapter will focus only on a few assessment procedures and tests that the writer most frequently employs as part of the aural rehabilitation process. It should be noted at this point that nearly all, if not all, of the speech audiometric instruments described throughout this book could be used, according to clinician preference, in a program of aural rehabilitation for purposes of assessment and/or therapy. A note of caution, however, is necessary for those who wish to use such instruments for therapy activities. Such use, without extensive adaptation, can void the validity of that instrument for the assessment of the individuals in question if they are thoroughly familiarized with the items on the test. As long as that limitation is recognized, the instruments can be employed in the therapy activities.

One of the forms of assessment that this writer finds helpful in a program of aural rehabilitation has been described earlier in the section discussing the audiologic test battery; the scores and erroneous responses on the standard speech discrimination tests administered at the three intensity levels. The reader may wish to review that section for its relevance here.

Another speechearing test that this writer frequently includes in aural rehabilitation activities is the KSU Speech Discrimination Test (Berger, 1977b). One of the reasons this test is used is that its multiple choice format and numerous forms adapt well to various rehabilitative activities designed to improve speechearing skills. The test consists of eight equated forms; each form contains 13 sentences. Within each form, the difficulty increases from the first to the last sentence, with a weighted scoring system. Each sentence contains a group of five phonetically similar key words from which the listener must select the presented word. These key words occur in various places within the sentences so that within each test form, no response position is used less than twice or more than three times. The format of this test lends itself well to the rehabilitative setting with the client circling the appropriate key word on the response sheet.

For the assessment of discrimination among consonants in an attempt to determine areas of need for specific speechearing training, this writer prefers the use of the Larsen Consonant Sound Discrimination Test (1950). This test, which is also discussed by Alpiner (1978) and Sanders (1971), was originally developed at the Deshon General Hospital for the Aural Rehabilitation Program of the Army and Navy. The response sheet for the test consists of 33 boxes or words. Each box compares words, usually five pairs, which include consonants of similar sounds. For example, Box 1 contrasts /*f*/ and /*ch*/ using the word pairs that follow: few/chew; fin/chin; filed/child; calf/catch; four/chore. The presenter pronounces one word of each pair and the listener circles the word perceived. The original Larsen Manual also includes additional supplementary auditory training materials, which makes a unique contribution to the profession today. There is a definite need for its reprinting and for a wider availability to clinicians who are attempting to assess and improve the speechearing skills of their clients.

Other useful assessment procedures similar to the Larsen Test, but which go a bit beyond it in terms of feature analysis information and its application to aural rehabilitation, are discussed by Binnie (1976). If one is assessing speechearing ability in order to gather information relevant to a need for aural rehabilitation, specific information about perceptual confusions and the types of distortions and errors the hearing-impaired person is experiencing and making becomes quite important. In addition to the tests and procedures described above and elsewhere throughout this book, the clinician can also make use of some of the auditory tasks developed as part of the increasing numbers of tests of auditory perception. Examination of those materials can enable clinicians to select items applicable to their needs and approaches.

As with speechreading assessment, a practical form of assessment of speechearing skills, especially for purposes of evaluating progress in therapy, is through the careful sequencing of the presentation of material and the collection of baseline performance data and progress data on the performance of the client for the particular material being used (see earlier discussion on sequencing of materials and activities).

In summary, assessment of speechearing skills, and changes in those skills as a result of therapy, can be made in at least two ways: by formal standardized tests of speechearing, and by performance data collection on selected material. Each approach offers different information. Both approaches have a valuable place in a program of aural rehabilitation. As in the case of speechreading tests, many of the speechearing tests do not reflect changes resulting from therapy and therefore the same cautions and recommendations apply here as discussed earlier.

Materials and Activities for Enhancing Speechearing Skills

This section deals with what is traditionally referred to as auditory training. However, as noted in the previous section, the narrower term *speechearing training* is used as a parallel to *speechreading training*. There are a variety of ways to enhance the ability of a hearing-impaired person to hear and understand speech. Only those methods and materials typically used by this writer will be detailed. For other approaches, the reader should consult Alpiner (1978), Haug and Haug (1977), Light (1978), Oyer (1966), Sanders (1971), and Smith and Karp (1978).

There are commercially available materials for speechearing training, but not nearly as many as are available for speechreading training. However, as noted earlier, *any* materials—whether designed for speechreading or speechearing—can be adapted and made useful for either of these aural rehabilitative purposes. Indeed, it is this writer's view that a significant portion of speechearing training in aural rehabilitation consists of what might be called listening training. Many of the hearing-impaired clients who seek help have unknowingly lost or abandoned the habit of listening. Due to difficulties in following conversations, and the associated discouragement, they no longer make a concerted effort to understand. This, of course, assumes they were good listeners prior to the hearing loss. Listening is an attitude or mental set that a person assumes in order to be maximally receptive to incoming information. So viewed, it applies equally to speechreading and speechearing. It is a conscious, deliberate attempt to maximize what is heard, or seen, and to understand what the speaker is trying to communicate. In this writer's view, much of speechearing training can best be directed toward improvement of listening skills as a primary goal. This is not to negate therapy activities directed toward improving the person's ability to use their hearing, distorted though it may be, for discriminating among specific speech sounds. Indeed, one of the decisions each clinician faces, as in the case of speechreading training, is the decision of whether, or to what extent, to dwell on the auditory characteristics and differences of individual phonemes. This writer is of the opinion that specific auditory training on discrimination of speech sounds is a potentially valid and productive activity, but extensive drill on such tasks is a questionable use of time. In the days of the Army and Navy aural rehabilitation programs, clients were available for considerable periods of time, as needed, on an individual basis. With today's constraints in terms of client availability, the time may better be spent in more immediately productive forms of rehabilitation. A certain amount of such drill and practice may well be warranted, but extensive expenditure of time on such discrimination tasks is difficult to justify unless it does not detract from other important aspects of the aural rehabilitation program. Reference was made in the previous section to procedures for determining specific phoneme discrimination problems and where confusions might exist. This determination is critical if one is to maximize the use of time by drilling only on those speech sounds which the individual is confusing. Likewise, consideration of such things as frequency of occurrence of the particular phonemes, as well as their visibility, can influence the decision whether to allocate time for such specific discrimination drills. If one is going to work on such skills, the materials developed by Kelly (1973) and Larsen (1950) are particularly useful, as are the various tests that emphasize certain frequency ranges of phonemes or discrimination among phonemes. A variety of such tests may be found in a compilation of speech audiometry materials by Berger (1977a). Such tests are also discussed elsewhere in other chapters of this book.

Since this writer advocates a more synthetic approach to working on specific communication skills in a program of aural rehabilitation, more effort is directed toward using the sense of hearing, and the ability to listen, to understand larger segments of speech under a variety of listening conditions and with various methods of presentation. These conditions and methods were described in detail in a previous section. Such activities are a critical part of the rehabilitative process. Relevance is a must. In the case of using hearing abilities and listening skills for understanding speech, the variety of acoustic conditions and competing noises the person encounters on a daily basis should be included in the rehabilitative effort. The need for such training in adjusting to a hearing aid is clear. Various speech materials can also be used extensively for telephone work. This writer has found that many clients assume they cannot understand speech over the telephone, only to find out after properly sequenced therapy activities that their ability to understand speech from the telephone is much greater than they thought possible. It should be noted here that there is good reason to believe that much of the improvement clients often experience is attributable to changes in attitude and confidence rather than improvement in specific auditory discrimination skills. This observation also pertains to other aspects of the aural rehabilitation program. If the proper sequencing of therapy activities leads to success and improvement and there is a marked change in performance, more than likely changes in both skills and attitude have occurred, with each contributing to the improvement of the other as therapy progresses. Clients typically seek rehabilitative services for the expressed purpose of improving specific visual and auditory skills—usually lipreading—and clinicians must relate to that request. With the proper design of therapy, however, changes in attitude and confidence will result and will contribute markedly to the improvement in overall communication ability.

In summary, speechearing training is a systematic effort to increase the amount of information that a person's hearing and listening skills contribute to the understanding of speech. A variety of relevant materials, commercially available and/or designed by the clinician, may be used. The critical factor in this training is sequencing of the materials and activities to make the experiences relevant and successful. It should be emphasized again that these same materials and activities are quite useful in a program of hearing aid orientation.

BISENSORY SPEECH PERCEPTION SKILLS

Bisensory (audio-visual) perception of speech refers to a receptive language skill involving the understanding of speech through the combined use of visual and auditory cues. The end goal of aural rehabilitation efforts directed toward specific communication skills is the improvement of the bisensory (audio-visual) perception of speech, not just speechreading or speechearing, but the combination of the two with their mutually supplementary nature. As the reader may have concluded from the overall orientation of this chapter, this writer advocates considerable bisensory presentation and practice, under varying conditions that simulate daily life. Some effort directed solely toward improvement of speechreading and/or speechearing is typically needed and justifiable, but the ultimate goal is the combination of the two sensory channels. Clinical experience, as well as research, clearly points to the supplementary nature of hearing and vision in the understanding of speech. It is critical for clients to understand, and see, that it is feasible to perform poorly on a speechreading task, and poorly on a speechearing task, but perform quite well on a bisensory task. The bisensory performance is more than the sum of the separate senses. A given client is likely to be more reliant on one sense than the other, as a function of the degree and nature of the hearing loss, or as a function of the visual acuity and clarity. In some instances, the two senses may contribute somewhat equally. In other instances, the speechreading skills may be secondary and serve to aid the speechearing abilities, or vice versa. Or, the relative contribution of each sensory channel may vary from one situation to another, such as in conditions of noise or conditions of darkness or other interference with vision. Clients need to be aware of these points and need to have carefully sequenced therapy activities directed to these combined skills.

Assessment of Bisensory Skills

The simplest way to assess bisensory speech perception skills is by simply employing a "look and listen" mode of presentation with any of the speechreading or speechearing tests and then comparing the results with the unisensory presentation. It must be remembered, however, that such usage is not necessarily included as part of the design of a given test and results may vary accordingly. If, as discussed earlier in this chapter, audiologists would simply record the responses given on speech discrimination tests rather than marking an item right or wrong, considerable valuable information could be collected regarding the potential contribution of speechreading in a given case. Of course, if the audiologist would go one step further and also administer the test as a "look and listen" task, the importance of bisensory perception or the need for rehabilitation, would be more immediately evident. This approach can be extremely valuable in hearing aid selection procedures and in making decisions regarding the relative contributions of a hearing aid to a person's total perception of speech, especially in instances where the individual in question has little or no measurable speech discrimination or speechearing ability. The comparison of visual-only performance with audio-visual performance may show marked improvement under the bisensory condition. Even though the individual may have little or no usable residual hearing when assessed auditorily, that hearing, with a hearing aid, may provide a critical and badly needed supplement to the speechreading skills and result in a significant improvement in overall perception. There is a definite facilitory interaction of the two senses. The various efforts at bisensory evaluation approaches and techniques are discussed by Alpiner (1978). For further information on bisensory research, the reader should consult Binnie (1973; 1976), Hutton (1960), Oyer and Frankmann (1975), and Sanders (1971).

Materials and Activities for Enhancing Bisensory Speech Perception Skills

It should be noted that while the research on bisensory perception of speech is clear and consistent in the demonstration of the superiority of the bisensory versus unisensory (whether auditory or visual) mode of presentation, that superiority relates strictly to the reception/perception of speech information. The superiority of the bisensory approach for purposes of learning certain tasks, as opposed to simply receiving/perceiving information, is a different consideration, and one on which the research is less clear. It appears that intersensory inhibition concerns are more likely to pertain to the learning process than to the simple reception/perception of speech. These two phenomena should be kept separate and the research interpreted accordingly. In the rehabilitation of hearing-impaired adults, the concern is with the improvement of the total reception of speech and the role of the combined senses in contributing to that end goal.

Therapy activities and materials for enhancing bisensory reception/perception of speech need not really be any different than those described in detail under the preceding sections on speechreading and speechearing. Again, the critical aspects are the sequencing and the relevance of the materials and activities. As is commonly recognized, hard-of-hearing adults report the greatest difficulty in small group conversations and in conditions of competing noise and/or competing messages. As the signal-to-noise ratio decreases (with noise being defined more broadly in terms of visual and/or auditory interference) the importance of the supplementing sensory channel increases. Erber (1977) has demonstrated the importance of bisensory presentation in instances of reduced optical clarity, suggesting optical blurring as a potential technique in bisensory and speechearing training activities. Likewise, Montgomery (1977) developed a technique for improving a client's ability to process the visual and auditory aspects of speech simultaneously, whereby, through the use of a two-room arrangement, he artificially separated consonants from vowels in running speech to reduce the amount of consonant information presented auditorily and to force the client to develop skills for lipreading consonants in the presence of vowel sounds. His research demonstrated significant improvement in performance with training. It is toward such ends that therapy should be directed, using any of the sources of materials described earlier and/or using speech material which the clinician tailors to the specific daily needs of the client(s) who seek service. The new material developed by Jeffers and Barley (1979) is designed for bisensory presentation and training and should prove useful. Likewise, Smith and Karp (1978) should be consulted for additional ideas.

It should be noted here that in those instances where no hearing or no vision is available as a supplement, there is ample research to support the facilitory nature of the tactile sense (Oyer & Frankmann, 1975). Cutaneous stimulation, such as with a bone conduction vibrator or other higher fidelity tactile stimulator, can be a significant supplement to the remaining sense of hearing or vision.

In summary, since the end goal of rehabilitative services directed toward communication skills is to maximize the ability to use the incoming auditory and visual information for purposes of achieving the best possible total reception/perception of speech for a given individual, the combination of sensory information and its mutual facilitation should receive significant attention in the rehabilitative effort. The clinician should compare the performances of a given client on speechreading tasks, speechearing tasks, and bisensory tasks, and seek to improve each, but with the primary goal being improvement of the combined audio-visual reception/perception of speech, especially as it relates to the daily needs of the individual client.

REFERENCES

Alpiner, J. G., Ed. *Handbook of adult rehabilitative audiology.* Baltimore: Williams and Wilkins, 1978.

Berger, K. W. *Speech audiometry materials.* Kent, Ohio: Herald Publishing House, 1977a.

Berger, K. W. *The K. S. U. speech discrimination test.* Kent, Ohio: Herald Publishing House, 1977b.

Berger, K. W. *The most common 100,000 words used in conversations.* Kent, Ohio: Herald Publishing House, 1977c.

Binnie, C. A. Bi-sensory articulation functions for normal hearing and sensorineural hearing loss patients. *Journal of the Academy of Rehabilitative Audiology,* 1973, *6,* 43–53.

Binnie, C. A. Relevant aural rehabilitation. In J. Northern (Ed.), *Hearing disorders.* Boston: Little, Brown and Company, 1976, pp. 213–227.

Binnie, C. A., Jackson, P. L., & Montgomery, A. A. Visual intelligibility of consonants: a lipreading screening test with implications for aural rehabilitation. *Journal of Speech and Hearing Disorders,* 1976, *41,* 530–539.

Broberg, R. F. *Over-fifty nifties: lipreading practice material for senior citizens.* Washington, D. C.: The A. G. Bell Association for the Deaf, 1975.

Erber, N. P. Auditory-visual perception of speech. *Journal of Speech and Hearing Disorders,* 1975, *40,* 481–492.

Erber, N. P. *Auditory-visual perception of speech with reduced optical clarity.* Paper given before the American Speech and Hearing Association, Chicago, Illinois, 1977.

Fisher, C. G., & Kealey, M. S. *The visibility of three methods of expanding simple English sentences.* Paper given before the American Speech and Hearing Association, Chicago, Illinois, 1969.

Fisher, M. *Lipreading for a more active life.* Washington, D. C.: A. G. Bell Association for the Deaf, 1977.

Fisher, M. *Lively lipreading lessons.* Washington, D. C.: A. G. Bell Association for the Deaf, 1978.

Garstecki, D. C. A behavioral approach toward adult hearing aid orientation. *Journal of the Academy of Rehabilitative Audiology,* 1974, *7,* 9–17.

Giolas, T. G., Owens, E., Lamb, S., & Schubert, E. D. Hearing Performance Inventory. *Journal of Speech and Hearing Disorders,* 1979, *44,* 169–195.

Haug, O., & Haug, S. *Help for the hard of hearing.* Springfield, Illinois: C. C. Thomas, 1977.

Hull, R. H. *Hearing impairment among aging persons.* Lincoln, Nebraska: Cliff Notes, Inc, 1977.

Hutton, C. A diagnostic approach to combined techniques in aural rehabilitation. *Journal of Speech and Hearing Disorders,* 1960, *25,* 267–272.

Jeffers, J., & Barley, M. *Speechreading (lipreading).* Springfield, Illinois: C. C. Thomas, 1971.

Jeffers, J., & Barley, M. *Look, now hear this: combined auditory training and speechreading instruction.* Springfield, Illinois: C. C. Thomas, 1979.

Kelly, J. D. *Clinician's handbook for auditory training.* Washington, D. C.: A. G. Bell Association for the Deaf, 1973.

Larsen, L. L. *Consonant sound discrimination.* Bloomington, Indiana: Indiana University Press, 1950.

Light, J. B. *The Joy of listening: an auditory training program.* Washington, D. C: A. G. Bell Association for the Deaf, 1978.

Maurer, J. F., & Rupp, R. R. *Hearing and aging: tactics for intervention.* New York: Grune & Stratton, 1979.

Minifie, F. D., Hixon, T. J., & Williams, F. *Normal aspects of speech, hearing and language.* Englewood Cliffs, New Jersey: Prentice-Hall, 1973.

Montgomery, A. A. *Assessment of a new auditory-visual integration training technique.* Paper given before the American Speech and Hearing Association, Chicago, Illinois, 1977.

Nitchie, E. H. *New lessons in lipreading.* Philadelphia: Lippincott, 1950.

O'Neill, J. J., & Oyer, H. J. *Visual communication for the hard of hearing.* Englewood Cliffs, New Jersey: Prentice-Hall, 1961.

Ordman, K. A. & Ralli, M. P. *What people say: the Nitchie School basic course in lipreading.* Washington, D. C.: A. G. Bell Association for the Deaf, 1976.

Oyer, H. J. *Auditory communication for the hard of hearing.* Englewood Cliffs, New Jersey: Prentice Hall, 1966.

Oyer, H. J., & Frankmann, J. P. *The aural rehabilitation process: a conceptual framework analysis.* New York: Holt, Rinehart, and Winston, 1975.

Ross, M. *Principles of aural rehabilitation.* Indianapolis: Bobbs-Merrill, 1972.

Sanders, D. *Aural rehabilitation.* Englewood Cliffs, New Jersey: Prentice-Hall, 1971.

Sanders, D. A. Hearing aid orientation and counseling. In M. C. Pollack (Ed.), *Amplification for the hearing-impaired,* (1st ed.). New York: Grune & Stratton, 1975, pp. 323–372.

Smith, C. R., & Karp, A. *A workbook in auditory training for adults.* Springfield, Illinois: C. C. Thomas, 1978.

Robert L. McCroskey, Ph.D.
Roger N. Kasten, Ph.D.

14

Assessment of Central Auditory Processing

History has never been kind to yesterday's knowledge, and it is foolish to expect that tomorrow's history will be any kinder to today's knowledge. To advance the science and the art of assessing human auditory function, a written record must be available to summarize what has transpired, to state what is current, and to stimulate questions in the minds of readers. It is the task of students and professionals to be informed and to reach for the future while practicing and questioning the best of what is.

Information is the basis of creativity, but it can also restrict thought if the consumer does not bring a critical mind to the issue. Consider, for example, the expressed fact in earlier audiology texts that the pinnae serve little or no function (Newby, 1958; O'Neill & Oyer, 1966; Newby, 1972). This so-called fact has become such a part of the accepted store of knowledge, that it seems to have eliminated any need for further attention to the pinnae by later authors (Gerber, 1977; Northern & Downs, 1978; Martin, 1978; Ross & Giolas, 1978). Evidence of the role of the pinnae in auditory localization, however, has been available for more than 15 years (Batteau, 1964).

Historically, audiologists have given so much attention to *identifying* auditory disorders that attention to the manner in which the auditory system processes spoken events has suffered. For a moment or two, it seems appropriate to state the obvious. The processing of speech proceeds from the reception of speech. Speech is an outward manifestation of a language and, therefore, the understanding of auditory processing of speech is inextricably bound to the language. Speech is the acoustic reality of language. It is tangible and measurable in terms of frequency *composition,* intensity *variations,* and temporal *patterns.* However, a moment's reflection on the most common procedure for determining whether an auditory system is within normal limits will reveal that only the dimensions of frequency and intensity are in regular use. The audiometer has become the standard for auditory screening by health professionals in several disciplines. The recent addition of tympanometry, acoustic reflex, and ABR testing as companion procedures are valuable, but attention remains focused on frequency and intensity. One might ask why there are so many children with apparently normal auditory sensitivity—at least for frequency and intensity—who exhibit a variety of problems associated with the comprehension of a verbal message. A puzzling situation is not to be shrugged off as just one of those exceptions that proves the rule, nor is it to be dismissed from mind by assuming that some artifact in the situation or the equipment caused the aberrant behavior. Unusual behaviors in otherwise cooperative clients offer opportunities for discovery of new information about audition. The base of professional knowledge is not so secure that scientific inquiry may be postponed through clichés or through assigning new labels to old problems and feeling satisfied. The present chapter will, along with other protocols, introduce two new procedures for assessing an almost forgotten dimension—time—in the evaluation of central auditory competence.

This discussion is organized according to three age groups: (a) preschool; (b) elementary school; and (c) adult. Each will contain a review of common procedures that relate to central auditory processing. In addition, new data on auditory behavior across the three categories will be presented.

PRESCHOOL YEARS

Infants (To Three Years)

There has been a tendency to view behavioral characteristics as maturational byproducts rather than viewing development as a dynamic neuroexperiential confluence that grows because each contributes to the other. As one thinks of infant audition and of ways to assess its states, its progress, and its potential, one must recognize that every auditory experience has the possibility of changing the way in which that auditory system will respond to the next stimulation.

PRENATAL

Sound affects fetal heart rate at 28 weeks gestational age. The potential of prenatal audition is barely entering the consciousness of most audiologists. Nonetheless, if auditory experience contributes to the ability of an organism to use succeeding auditory experiences, then audiologists, linguists, and developmentalists must focus attention on those earliest moments of responsiveness to sound. The premature baby, by gestational age rather than weight, offers opportunities for looking at auditory processing at a time when the infant has yet to reach an auditory age (AA) of zero. An AA of zero is arbitrarily defined as the moment of full-term birth.

Physiological reactions to the presence of sound are in common use by the few individuals who have studied fetal responsiveness to acoustic stimulation. Perhaps the best known work is that of Johannson, Wedenberg, and Westin (1964), in which they report that the fetus should be responsive to sound, as evidenced by altered heart rate, by 28 weeks gestation. It must be noted that other data suggest that such responses may not be detected consistently until approximately 32 weeks of age (Tanaka & Arayama, 1969). Even experimental extinction and spontaneous recovery have been measured in fetuses over 28 weeks gestation (Spelt, 1938). For those who feel that the assessment of auditory function in neonates and infants is not a profitable use of time, or that there may be little utility in the efforts, further reading is suggested in the area of behavioral embryology.

It is assumed that fetal responses are a reflection of brainstem participation and, while this involves the central auditory system, the extent of cortical participation in such responses is unknown. It is reasonable to assume that there is reception of such information at the level of the cortex and that there is distribution of such auditorily based signals from Heschl's area to other cortical centers so that eventually associations with visual, acoustic, and motoric events will take place.

NEONATAL—ONE MONTH

The issue of whether language emerges from genetic direction or evolves through auditory experiences remains an unclear issue. The truth may be that each is correct and neither can function without the other. It may be that humans, like some insects, may be composed of homologous units containing key genes that execute decisions resulting in cloning of cells that are committed to a line of development (Garcia-Bellido et al., 1979), but being committed to a line of development does not guarantee that the purpose for which the system has been dedicated will be fulfilled unless those cells receive appropriate stimulation and experiential nourishment.

Responsiveness to sound is characteristic of this age group. Among the most common stimuli for assessing auditory sensitivity by behavioral means are narrow band noise (Vicon Apriton, Telesensory Crib-o-Gram), warbled pure tones (Rudmose Warblet, Zenith Neometer), steady state pure tones (H. C. Scott Phonic Ear), steady-state triangular waves (DiaHab Miniometer), and noise makers (Down's Kit). It has been traditional to report that signal intensities of at least 90 dB are needed in order to elicit responses from newborn infants. This assumption is based on the known noise levels of the nurseries and on data that suggests that noise *in utero* is in excess of 70 dB, and therefore it is unlikely that an infant will sort out a lesser signal from the background noise–particularly if it is at or below the level of the acoustic environment before birth. Levels of 90 dB and 100 dB SPL have been designed into all of the instruments cited (except the Miniometer, which has a maximum intensity of 70 dB SPL, because the emphasis in hearing screening has been on the detection of children with severe or profound hearing losses. High-frequency stimuli at high intensities will certainly pass all but the most severely involved children, but the milder losses are certainly more prevalent and contribute to a variety of linguistic and learning problems that confound developmental and educational progress.

It is no longer appropriate to develop tests that will ensure a passing performance by all but the most severely damaged. The early work of European scholars and educators of the deaf (Ewing & Ewing, 1944; Wedenberg, 1956; Tervoort, 1964; van Uden, 1967; van Uden, 1968) helped create an awareness of the need for early instruction of children with *severe* hearing problems. This gave impetus to the screening techniques that are aimed at detecting deafness rather than levels of auditory competence. Auditory competence is acquired through experience with sound and both the peripheral end organ and the transmission systems must perform well in order for normal auditory processing to emerge.

There is an obligation to look at more than mere presence or absence of responses to high intensity signals—and those only among babies born at risk. There are risks among the babies who are not in intensive care units and it is these more subtle differences that must be detected, since these may be more amenable to correction or compensation if appropriate intervention is available. More effort needs to be directed at the minimal intensities to which newborns will respond and to all measurable temporal components associated with the stimuli and the responses. It has already been demonstrated that stimuli of 500 and 3000 Hz presented at intensities of 50 and 70 dB SPL are adequate to elicit responses from neonates (McCroskey & Yarbrough, 1967).

Audiologists must guard against the kind of intellectual inbreeding that comes from reading only journals that are specialty-specific. Creativity often is engendered by multidisciplinary views of a given problem; thus, a fact viewed from one perspective may appear absolute, but when viewed from another perspective may be labeled as an artifact.

The full creative force of speech-language-hearing specialists will be thwarted as long as health care providers believe that severe auditory deficits are the only ones that need to be detected, that effective educational programs for families are not available, and that there is validity to the concept of a prelingual period in the life of an infant. Auditory perception is the receiving, processing, and classifying of such sensory information for coding into familiar symbols (Rupp, 1978), and this process begins with earliest sensory input. Published annotated bibliographies of representative test procedures (McCroskey & Bell, 1965; McCroskey & Cory, 1969; and McCroskey & Deines, 1974) indicate that neonates and infants are not only responsive to auditory stimulation, but are capable of making considerable numbers of discriminations among speech stimuli.

The topic of infant competence is beginning to receive more attention, as exemplified by the work of Horowitz (1979), who has used a large black and white checkerboard to hold the visual attention of young infants while presenting acoustic stimuli. In contrast to existing assumptions about the fleeting attention span of all infants, her data indicate most infants can retain attention for several minutes.

The question before audiologists and otologists is one of distinguishing responses that are reflexive from those that represent more centrally mediated responses. The most common concept of the central auditory system includes everything from the cochlear nuclei to and including the cortex. Topp (1977) includes all of the eighth cranial nerve in the central system. A satisfactory model is not yet available for separating end-organ deficiencies (which result in reduced stimulation of the neural system) from the reflexive and the timing functions provided by the brainstem, or from the cognitive and controlling functions of cortical structures. This deficit is illustrated to some extent by the work of Miltenberger et al. (1978) and Snow et al. (1977). Central processing should involve more than a simple, organismic response to a signal and, perhaps, more than simple discrimination of events. The central responses of real interest must give evidence that the organism has received, discriminated, and attached significance to the event.

Auditory age is a viable concept and its relationship with chronologi-

cal age has significance for the development of intervention strategies. In the disciplines other than audiology, one is accustomed to such comparisons as physiological age with chronological age; thus, a person of 60 years may be said to have the blood pressure of a 20-year-old person. Among psychologists, it is even more common to compare mental age with chronological age (CA) and infer something about the ability of a person to function in various settings. It is proposed that Auditory Age (AA) is a viable concept, whether one is considering infants (McCroskey, 1967b) or elderly persons (McCroskey, 1979), and that the relationship of AA to CA has significance for the development of intervention strategies at all ages.

Localization is a response that can be observed and measured in the 0–1-month-old infant. Murphy (1961) described stages of development of auditory localization. He reports that the turning of the eyes toward the sound source is observable by one month of age. Indeed, this response is observable within the first 24 hours of life for some infants. Murphy also observed that localization to the right occurs first in 60 percent of the English babies he tested. This affinity for directionality to the right appears to emerge by twelve hours of age (Turkewitz, 1977). Northern and Downs (1978) also report a maturational scale for sound localization, which suggests that American infants may not be as advanced auditorily as English babies, but the differences may be more attributable to stimuli and technique than to nationality. It is noteworthy that Murphy's data contain a caution with respect to the more commonly used startle responses. He suggests that auditory reflexes may reflect basil neural pathways and that even a severely impaired infant may startle early in life but fail to give any response a month or two later. Localization is taken to imply binaural hearing, but where the infant actually becomes selective in making responses, i.e., reacts differently to the voice of a parent than to other nonrewarding acoustic events of equal or greater intensity, it is evident that the signal has traversed the central auditory pathway and cortical participation has occurred.

Startle responses and other reflexive responses to sound of moderate intensity have been demonstrated. Murphy (1962) has described the performance of one premature infant, in which it was possible to obtain reactions to pure tones at intensities of 50–60 dB during the first hour of life and on each of five successive days. Whether one is dealing with routine screening in a hospital nursery or addressing only the *at risk* babies, such responses indicate that the auditory pathway involving the ear, the organ of Corti, the basilar membrane, and the neural connections in the brainstem are complete and responsive to stimulation. Repeated presentations of a stimulus that initially elicits a startle response may permit inferences regarding cortical participation. For example, if there is selective inhibition of the startle to a given stimulus, this is evidence that the infant may have determined the nonsignificance of that event and no longer responds even though the intensity may be in excess of other, less familiar acoustic events that yield the startle response. In all likelihood, it is this observation that has lead other researchers to test procedures involving respiration, high-amplitude sucking (HAS), and heart rate (HR).

The startle response is observable as an overall body response—sometimes confused with the Moro Reflex—that is a frequent product of a high-intensity (75 dB SPL or greater) signal that is usually characterized by a short rise time. Recently, there has been some criticism of describing the massive startle response of infants as a Moro Reflex (Gerber, 1977). According to Dorland's *Medical Dictionary,* the Moro Reflex is characterized by the arms being suddenly thrown outward in an embracing attitude as a result of placing an infant on a table, then forcibly striking the table on either side of the infant's head. The vibratory component would stimulate activity of the muscles of the neck and lead to the response, whether the acoustic stimulus were present or not. In practice, audiologists do not impose the direct vibratory stimulation of the infant, and in that sense the criterion for the Moro Reflex is not met; rather, care is taken to avoid touching the infant, the crib, or the person holding the infant. Only the acoustic event intrudes after a period of quiet, but is often sufficient to evoke the same behavioral reactions that characterize the Moro Reflex.

A common response to an unexpected sound is a vigorous eye blink, which is referred to as the auropalpebral reflex (APR). This reflex may be accompanied by an overall body response or startle reaction. Perhaps the most definitive report on APR is that of Fröding (1960), in which he reports on 2,000 children who were examined during the first 30 minutes of life. Only those eventually proven to be severely damaged failed to show the APR in response to acoustic stimulation (white noise at 126–133 dB SPL). The APR is expected to appear when an unanticipated acoustic event with a short rise time, and a duration not greater than 5 msec is presented at approximately 60 dB above the true threshold of the predominate frequency being presented. Inferences can be drawn when the APR is observed; for example, if the APR is observed at a signal intensity of 80 dB SPL, and threshold plus 60 dB is required for the APR, then the threshold for that stimulus would probably not be greater than 20 dB SPL. The observance of an APR on initial presentation of the stimulus provides information about that portion of the central auditory system that begins with the olivary nuclei and extends to that portion of the spinal system in which the reflex arc is completed. Repeated presentations of the stimulus should yield diminishing strengths of response and lead to the inference that learning (perhaps in conjunction with habituation or adaptation), possibly at the cortical level, has taken place and that higher centers in the central processing system have begun to exercise control.

A high-amplitude sucking (HAS) paradigm has been used to study auditory discrimination capabilities in infants. Butterfield and Cairns (1974) have described the HAS procedure as one in which an infant is allowed to suck on a pacifier that is wired to yield a graphic display of the strength of the sucking. After base-line data are obtained, a speech stimulus is programmed to be presented immediately following each high-amplitude suck. Initially, this leads to an increase in HAS, but thereafter there is a response decrement. When the response strength falls below a predetermined level, some aspect of the speech stimulus is altered and if the stimulus change is discriminated by the infant, then there is a shift in the strength of sucking. An earlier experiment by Eimas and his colleagues (1971) used the HAS paradigm to determine whether infants, between one and four months of age, could distinguish between the synthetically produced monosyllables *pa* and *ba*. They concluded that infants perceive speech stimuli in a categorical and linguistically relevant manner.

Respiration audiometry holds promise for assessing more than simple sensitivity to sound. Bradford (1975) employed respiration audiometry and was able to obtain thresholds of zero dB for 24 out of 25 infants under one month of age. His stimuli were pure tones of 1,000 and 3,000 Hz. Retests at four months of age revealed the same thresholds for 23 of the infants. It would seem that the technique could be used to assess voice recognition, sensitivity to intonational patterns, and for discrimination among speech sounds. Bradford's data were collected while infants were in a relaxed sleep following feeding. It has been the experience of the present authors, also, that the quiet period immediately following feeding is an ideal time for assessing auditory function in newborns and infants. A very deep sleep presents as many problems as an awake and active baby can present, although the awake state does not preclude the use of respiration audiometry (Suzuki et al., 1964).

Heart rate has been shown to alter in response to sound in neonates. A technique closely related to other physiologic responses to sound is one involving analysis of heart rate (Clifton, Graham, & Hattan, 1968). Standard electrocardiographic procedures can be used to monitor heart rate (HR) during control periods and periods of stimulation. In 1962, Bartoshuk studied the decrement in HR under various conditions and concluded that variations in cardiac acceleration are directly related to stimulus intensity and that the response decrement may represent selective habituation, which may be a form of discrimination learning. Later, Bartoshuk (1964) looked at newborns between 24 and 100 hours of age as they responded to four intensities of a 1000 Hz tone in five complete cycles of ascending and descending series. He found an approximately linear relation between cardiac responses plotted on a log scale and stimulus intensity in decibels. It seems unlikely that the simple reflex arc at the subcortical level, which has been implicated as the possible mechanism for startle responses to sound, could also account for the less direct and less obvious cardiac response to acoustic stimulation. The possibility of cortical participation seems more likely and this procedure could be a better indicator of the integrity of the auditory processing system, including more than the end organ and the brainstem systems.

Auditory brainstem responses (ABR) appear to be a viable means of assessing the transmission system from the cochlea to the cortex. Most graphic displays are two-dimensional and show the amplitude of response at the nuclei of the ascending auditory pathway during the first 10 msec following the onset of a series of click-stimuli (Lev & Sohmer, 1972). Procedures involving evoked brainstem potentials have been viewed as reflecting the maturation of the auditory system; for example, of the six or seven waves that are regularly observed in normal adults, the newborn infant typically exhibits only waves I, III, and V (Salamy & McKean, 1976). Further, in all discernable waves, the central response latency to the stimulus is delayed relative to a mature auditory system. With maturation, the wave form begins to take on adult characteristics and exhibits shorter latency at one year of age. Such procedures appear to give useful information regarding the integrity of the brainstem system, but the administration of the test requires sedation of the infant and this introduces some risk. The results of this test procedure are usually displayed in a two-dimensional plot, but Williston (1978) has introduced a three-dimensional display that has the potential for improving the diagnostic capability of ABR tests, because it provides more information on the temporal–spatial relationships for these wave forms.

Intentional use of audition occurs within the first month of life. Infant proclivity for sound is illustrated in the work of Butterfield (1968), who used an instrumented pacifier nipple to allow one-day-old infants to control the onset and offset of various types of music by their sucking activity. It was concluded that infants are not passive in their hearing function and that their auditory systems are not only functioning in a way that permits inferences regarding the end organ and brainstem participation, but in a way that implies cortical participation—if the emergence of preferential selection of music may be accepted as reflecting cortical function.

Auditory experience leads to auditory responsiveness. Auditory experience from the earliest moments (including the time the fetus spends in a sound-treated womb) will have its influence on the psychoneurologic development of the auditory system. Neurologically, it has been demonstrated that the diameter of the auditory neurons in animals can be diminished as a function of auditory deprivation and that the process is not completely reversible with later auditory stimulation (Stein & Schuckman, 1973; Webster & Webster, 1977).

Auditory experience leads to auditory responsiveness. McCroskey and Herman (1971) developed a tape recorded auditory experience program comprised of noise makers that were in common use for auditory screening (bell, buzzer, and whistle) and music. Each of 32 awake and alert infants was placed in a spring-mounted tray upon which was attached a photocell that was responsive to a light source. Infant movements varied the distance between the light source and the photocell, which created a corresponding variation in voltage that was fed to a strip-chart recorder in order to give a graphic display of movement. The auditory experience program was played for ten minutes on each of the first three days of life. It was found that some infants could be described as low-responders at the outset, while others were clearly high-responding individuals. For those in the former group, neither the increase in the number of responses nor the increase in the magnitude of those responses achieved statistical significance. On the other hand, the high-responding neonates increased significantly the *number* of their responses, but the magnitude of movements remained essentially the same. It would have been appropriate to use speech as a stimulus, also, particularly in view of the work of Condon and Sander (1974), in which they made careful analysis of motion pictures taken of infants while listening to speech. Their data indicate that the total organization of infant behavior is synchronized with speech patterns. Even nonverbal communication, involving facial and manual gestures, are imitated by infants between 12 and 21 days of age (Meltzoff & Moore, 1977). This matching process generally is thought to appear after eight months of age, but that position is no longer tenable.

There can be no doubt that acoustic input from the earliest moments not only contributes to the capacity of the auditory transmission system but leads to the proliferation of neuronal interconnections at the cortical level where the time-frequency-intensity patterns of the infant's native language are stored. Anything that disrupts or distorts the early auditory experience introduces a language delay if not a language disability.

It would be presumptuous to describe a protocol for the assessing of an auditory system for speech–language development at this time. There are insufficient data on the *normal* auditory responses to complex auditory events to warrant specific conclusions. This whole area invites the researcher and the clinician to ask questions. A review of this section shows that auditory discrimination between CV syllables is possible at one month of age (Eimas et al., 1971), that vocal contours are discriminable (Morse, 1974), that organization of infant behavior appears synchronized with speech patterns of adults (Condon & Sander, 1974), that auditory stimulation affects positively the responsiveness of neonates (McCroskey & Herman, 1971), that neonates actively select preferred acoustic stimuli (Friedlander, 1970), and that discrimination of speech sounds improve with age (Eilers et al., 1977).

Because of the emerging evidence of a relationship between early intermittant conductive hearing losses and the development of the auditory system, and the linguistic and educational implications of such impairments, it is appropriate to include reference to a relatively recent addition to test procedures in the United States, i.e., immittance testing (both tympanometry and acoustic reflex test). The significance of being able to monitor middle ear problems during these early and important days is not appreciated entirely, but the emerging data suggest that the effect could be profound (Webster & Webster, 1977). Proposed guidelines for immittance testing have been published recently (ASHA, 1979). Some of the problems associated with obtaining tympanagrams and acoustic reflexes during the early days or weeks of life are related to the assumption that vernix caseosum blood may fill the ear canal initially, as well as the fact that the external auditory canal is flexible and can give misleading results. Other problems relate to the body position of the infant during reflex testing (Faires & McCroskey, 1978). According to Jaffe (1977), the newborn tympanic membrane can be examined immediately after delivery and, while there may be debris in the canal initially, it quickly dehydrates and inspection is possible.

It would appear from preliminary data that the capacity for temporal discrimination proceeds in a systematic manner as the auditory age of the infant increases. It is appropriate that temporal analysis proceed as an isolated phyllodium at the present time in order to provide the background needed for later study of the interacting effects of time with frequency and intensity—as occurs in spoken events. Both real-time and perceptual-time in continuous speech must be studied in the future. Perceptual-time analysis by the auditory system is an integral part of speech (in which the real-time of syntactic units varies greatly while relative time within an utterance follows the established real-time rules). Where the auditory age of a developing child falls behind the chronologic age, one can expect delayed speech at best and at worst severe learning problems or mental retardation.

NEONATAL—TWO TO FOUR MONTHS

It has been demonstrated that by one month of age infants can perform intentional acts in order to cause auditory input. This is well ahead of the earliest age at which Bates et al. (1975) and Yoder (1979) say that a child begins to engage in intentional behavior, i.e., the controlling of the environment. Indeed, these data challenge Piaget's concept of the preintentional period in infancy. It is probably unnecessary to state that all the auditory behaviors reflecting central participation that were cited for one month of age can be demonstrated in these older infants. The ability of infants to differentiate their environment appears to be well established (Lewis & Freedle, 1973). Indeed, infants can discriminate mismatched objects and their sounds by the fourth month (Lyons-Ruth, 1977).

INFANT: FOUR TO SIX MONTHS

No response equals no information. The fourth month may present some problems with respect to auditory responsiveness. These writers have had several experiences with four-month-old infants who were unresponsive to the common infant auditory screening devices and, indeed, were unresponsive to sounds presented at maximum intensities in standard soundfield testing situations. Experienced audiologists are familiar with the phrase that a child appears to be "too deaf to be deaf." The rule under which the present writers operate is: *no response equals no information.* In the presence of no information, no conclusions are to be drawn. It is not rare to find a completely unresponsive four-month-old infant who, when retested in two to four weeks, will give completely normal responses. No longitudinal study of such infants has been conducted to determine whether the initial unresponsiveness is a predictor of a more subtle problem that will surface later.

At five months of age, vocal contours are discriminable (Morse, 1974), and imitation of intonational patterns of a child's native language is beginning to emerge (Nakazima, 1962; Weir, 1966). Arising out of tonal contrasts is a demonstrated ability to detect vowel differences (Trehub, 1973). Whether natural or synthetic speech is employed, cortical participation is implicated clearly.

INFANT: SIX TO TWELVE MONTHS

Speed and accuracy of localization may be predictive of ear–brain integrity. At six months of age, infants will localize a variety of acoustic stimuli whether they are comprised of pure tones, speech, or complex noises. In general, infants will localize quickly to a low-intensity signal presented at the left or right of the head, but they are not yet proficient in localizing in any plane other than the horizontal one. Speech–sound discriminations are beginning to be quite accurate (Eilers et al., 1977). Between six months and twelve months of age, localizaiton is a very effective technique for determining auditory sensitivity, but it is more important to be aware that the speed and accuracy of localization gives valuable information on the maturation and efficiency with which the auditory system (from the pinnae through the cortex) functions. Between the age of six months, at which time the infant simply localizes to the left or right without particular attention to the azimuth of the signal, and twelve months, the infant will localize directly to the sound source regardless of the azimuth from which the stimulus originates. Experience shows that the composition of the stimulus is not critical, although the younger infant will respond more accurately to a triangular wave form than to a pure tone, and will respond better to speech signals (minimally voiced syllables, whispered syllables, or whispered sibilant sounds) than to pure tones.

Speed and accuracy of localization may be predictive of ear–brain efficiency/integrity. In the section on test procedures for school-aged children, reference will again be made to localization skills. At this early age, the localization is static, i.e., the sound source is stationary and the infant needs only to locate it visually. Test procedures to be described later involve dynamic auditory localization (auditory tracking) with the subject following an invisible sound source.

Beginning at seven months of age, it is also possible to use play audiometry as well as techniques involving conditioned orienting responses (COR). Thompson and Thompson (1972) found that a 3000 Hz pure tone produced fewer responses than could be obtained with speech, filtered speech, white noise, or filtered noise. They also found that play audiometry (using speech or speech-type spectra) yielded more responses than did COR, regardless of the stimulus used.

Wilson and Diefendorf (1979) utilized computer generated speech tokens, as well as separately generated formant segments of the same speech–sound tokens, with infants approximately eight months old. In this approach, the infant is trained to respond to a given diotically presented speech sound, but not to respond to other speech sounds or to isolated formants of speech sounds. Subsequently, when the two formant components of the conditioned speech sound are presented dichotically, and the infant responds appropriately, central auditory fusion has been demonstrated.

Adequate hearing from birth through seven months of age is a critical prerequisite to normal language function. It has been demonstrated that infants begin to take on the vocal characteristics of their native languages by five months of age. It is possible to identify, in many instances, the native language of the infant by the vocalization patterns that emerge around seven months of age (Nakazima, 1962; Tervoort, 1964). In fact, infants can imitate intonational patterns produced by parents by the eighth month (Nakazima, 1962).

By nine months of age, regardless of the language from which the infants come, there is clear response to persons calling them by name.

The infants can imitate intonational patterns but they do not imitate words, syllables, or phonemes, as a rule (Nakazima, 1970). Usually by eight months of age and certainly by nine months of age, infants are able to distinguish the intent of a message by the intonational contour of the utterance (Kaplin, 1969). It is very likely that the intonational patterns of speech are the source of the imitated body movements noted by Condon and Sander (1974). While this may seem remote in relation to the utterance of syntactically accurate sentences, the intonational patterns are viewed as the raw materials out of which language and speech will emerge.

CHILD: 12 TO 36 MONTHS

Most of the test procedures that yielded valid responses for neonates can be applied to this age group. The selection of the specific test procedures depends upon the condition and status of the infant; for example, there are techniques that depend upon an infant's being confined to a crib (Simmons, 1977) or attached to an apparatus (Gidoll, 1952; Bradford, 1975; Davis, 1976), but in some instances mobility and willingness to sit still for the duration of a test become important factors in the overall protocol.

Test procedures involving localization can be conducted rather easily with the infant seated comfortably on a parent's lap while stimuli are presented from the various directions and angles specified by Murphy (1961). A modified Ewing procedure (Ewing & Ewing, 1944) is employed using the triangular waves of the Miniometer as stimuli instead of tissue paper or rattles. Additionally, the use of whispered phonemes or syllables as well as voiced phonemes or syllables, as recommended by the Ewings, are frequent supplements to the tonal presentation of the Miniometer. These speech-like stimuli are uttered at minimum possible intensities from positions slightly behind and to the right and left of the infant's head. With practice, it is possible for signal intensities to be as low as 35 dB SPL. The voiced stimuli will sample hearing at the fundamental frequency of the speaker, and the unvoiced sibilants will sample the frequency range around 3000 Hz. Speech-like stimuli are sometimes the only stimuli to which a child may respond voluntarily.

A hand raised, an earphone touched, a marble dropped, or a picture identified may be the most objective indication that central processing has occurred. Play audiometry begins to emerge as a useful technique for identifying auditory sensitivity, but more importantly, most infants can identify some body parts and common objects. These words can form the basis for a speech reception threshold. Indeed, a picture identification technique can be introduced using both single words and short sentences composed of carrier phrases (show me the ____; point to the ____;

where's the ____; etc.) plus single words that are in the known vocabulary of the child. Sound field testing, using simple spoken commands, is easily accomplished (Sweitzer, 1977) beginning around 18 months. With some infants, earphones can be used and ear-specific performance measured. Sweitzer (1977) feels that the speech detection threshold should be about 6 dB better than the speech reception threshold.

Eilers et al. (1977) attempted to study developmental changes in speech discrimination in infants up to 18 months of age. Their procedure is called Visually Reinforced Infant Speech Discrimination (VRISD) and involves a lighted, animated toy animal as the reinforcer. The stimuli were CV pairs that were naturally spoken as the infant was seated on the parent's lap. A distraction technique similar to that of the Ewings was employed while the stimulus pairs and the reinforcements were administrated. They report that 90 percent of the infants can be tested with this procedure. They project that a tangible reinforcer could be used with infants from eight months of age through 36–48 months of age. Again, it is demonstrated that discrimination of speech events can be quantified, even in children under three years of age. Occasionally, it is forgotten that tangible reinforcement operant-conditioned audiometry (TROCA) is a tested and established procedure for working with retarded or otherwise difficult-to-test individuals (Fulton, 1971; Lloyd & Cox, 1975).

Variations on the peep show (Dix & Hallpike, 1947) have been employed for several years with success. In many respects, the work of Dix and Hallpike with infants beginning at two years of age was the forerunner of many of the current visual reinforcement approaches. The COR technique, for those who have the equipment and facilities, is established as an acceptable procedure (Suzuki et al., 1972). This procedure can be used with speech stimuli, narrow band noise, and pure tones.

Auditory temporal behaviors have emerged as significant indicators of central auditory dysfunction. The work of Beasley et al. (1976), and Berlin (1976) have demonstrated that the adult auditory system can be stressed by compressing the speech signal and overloading the processing system. Individuals whose temporal capacities do not fall within normal limits break down more rapidly under these accelerated speech conditions. Extensive effort has been directed toward the time relationship of different simultaneous speech events, and stimuli that are different but altered in relative intensity. It has been found that there are tolerance limits for both, and that abnormal auditory systems perform differently than do normal systems.

Earlier work in the area of delayed auditory feedback indicated that normal listeners become attuned to the arrival times of their own speech at their two ears. Asymmetries of the head contribute to asymmetrical arrival times of the voice signal from the vocal tract to the two ears. The relative speed of transmission of bone-conducted internal speech in relation to air-conducted external side-tone means that the auditory system in many cases must adapt to four arrival times of the same signal and cope with the apparent confusion.

McCroskey (1957) demonstrated that the intelligibility of a speech signal was improved by adding the bone-conducted component to the mouth-emitted signal while maintaining the appropriate temporal asymmetry between the two and elevating the bone-conducted signal above the air-conducted counterpart. In the normal course of events, a speaker is able to listen to these multiple signals and, by some means, sort them out and attend to the critical frequency–intensity–time composite. Since intensity has been demonstrated to alter transmission time (Mokotoff et al., 1977) and neuronal involvement shifts with frequencies being transmitted, the importance of the time dimension takes on added significance. In the case of continuous speech, there is a continuous shift of the frequency spectrum, along with the intensity changes that are part of the inherent characteristic of the various phonemes. The auditory system must not only learn to interpret the relative durations of the voiced and unvoiced phonemes, but it must be able to detect frequency transitions that are of no more than 50 msec duration and be able to discriminate interphonemic pause relationships or voice-onset times of the magnitude of 20 msec (Eimas, 1971). Unfortunately, the dimension of time remains virtually unexplored and therefore is virtually ignored.

An area can be ignored only where there is sufficient information to demonstrate that it is not relevant; areas of minimal information must be explored completely. Mokotoff et al. (1977) used auditory evoked brainstem responses (ABR) with an infant at 25.5 weeks gestational age with complications. The infant was seen periodically thereafter up to 14 months of age. The initial results indicated no responses at less than 50 dB HL, and they remained relatively consistent, with the most recent hearing level at 40 dB. Thus, periphreral hearing impairment, whether conductive or cochlear in nature, may be detected in the responsiveness of the brainstem. The impact of early conductive hearing losses has been summarized by Katz (1978), and the value of a technique assessing the transmission portion of the central auditory system has clear importance for the development of medical, audiological, and educational strategies.

In the section dealing with children between three years of age and six years of age, there is reference to a new auditory fusion test that has been used recently at Wichita State University. Specific data are available on the auditory fusion of children from three years of age upward (see Fig. 14-1), and it appears possible to project the probable temporal integrity of children below the age of three. Based upon the slope of the curve, it is hypothesized that the minimal silent interval between two acoustic

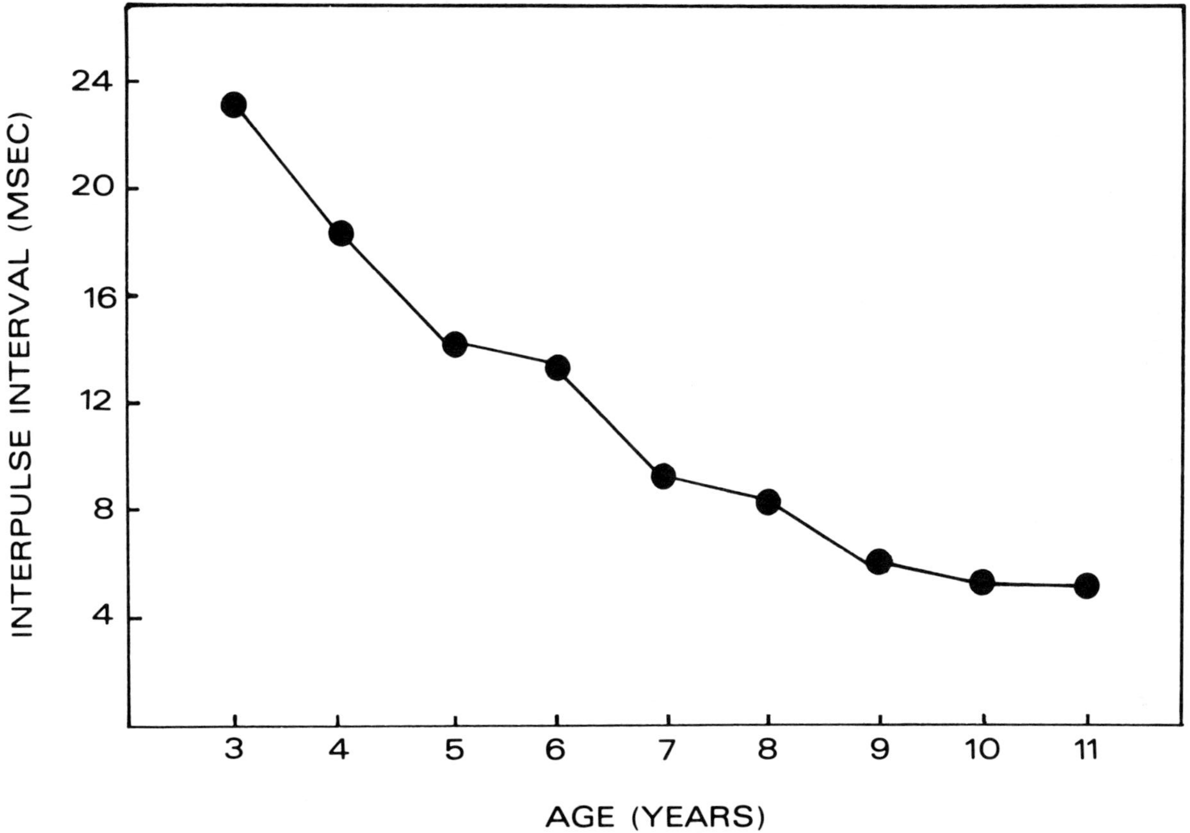

Fig. 14-1. A summary of mean auditory fusion points (data pooled for five frequencies, three intensities, and ascending–descending orders) for children from three to twelve years of age (N=135).

events that is detectable by a one-month-old infant, where the signal intensity is at least 40 dB but not greater than 60 dB SL, will be 40 msec. This is greater than the interval suggested by the Eimas et al. (1971) data.

The auditory timing capacity of an infant controls the speaking rate of parents. One of the most obvious facts of the auditory timing function of infants and very young children is that they process unfamiliar spoken messages more slowly than older children and adults. In addition, their affinity for the significance of intonational patterns, as noted by Weir, (1966), Morse, (1974), and Nakazima (1962), is amply illustrated by the vocal animation of adults as they try to communicate with young children. This is an area of minimal information and therefore demands full exploration. Such exploration is in progress at this time with older listeners (Divenyi & Hirsh, 1978). In an attempt to ascertain the relationship between speaker rate and complexity of message, and the age or grade level of listeners, Cuda (1976) analyzed random samples of speech from teachers at the first, third, and sixth grade levels. It was found that rate of utterance increased across these grade levels and that mean length of utterance increased significantly between the first and third grades, while the complexity of the utterance continued to increase across the three grade levels sampled. It is assumed that listeners shaped the manner of speech by the teacher. This is a common phenomenon and is illustrated when one attempts to talk to a person whose native language is different and the speaker tries to overcome the language barrier with volume, slow speech, and increased melody.

CHILD: THREE TO SIX YEARS

In addition to all techniques identified in previous sections, this age group has matured sufficiently to make it easier to use speech stimuli in a variety of forms (expanded/compressed, S/N ratios, dichotic, filtered, etc.) and with a variety of responses (picture selection, object manipulation, repetition, hemispheric representation, etc.).

The efficiency with which the central auditory system processes the dimension of time is critical in the acquisition of normal verbal skills. Throughout the chapter there has been reference to the neglected area of time in almost all procedures for assessing auditory function. This section is no exception. Clinical observation shows that the rate of speech among very young children is significantly slower than that of adults, and that the speech rate accelerates as one moves from preshcool through primary grades to intermediate or secondary school levels. Because the orientation has been one of looking at physical maturation as establishing the limits of motoric performance, there has been little or no attention given to the possible influence of auditory processing as the determiner of motoric performance in the area of speech production. Again, clinical observation as well as parental observation led to the conclusion that speech production may be slow for the young child. If slower speech production were the product only of a relatively immature motor system, then there should be no effect on auditory comprehension—since reception, transmission, and understanding require no motor response. Under such a circumstance, it would be expected that children would understand speech delivered at adult rates, provided the vocabulary was within their experiences. Common sense suggested that this was not the case and the auditory system itself was not behaving as rapidly in the time domain as it would later in life. These notions, together with the knowledge that pause time within words as well as pause times at word or phrase junctures were critical to the acquisition of an ability to form verbal composites, led to the hypothesis that, along with the necessity for learning frequency and intensity patterns, there was a need to detect very brief pauses and assimilate them as a part of the linguistic process.

A test was developed in which two brief pulses of sound were separated by a varying silent interval. The child's task was simply to say whether *one* or *two* tones had been detected. McCroskey and Davis (1976) reported the results of an investigation using 135 children between the ages of three and twelve years. Their data indicate a strong maturational effect on auditory temporal processing (see Fig. 14-1) with plateauing of this skill beginning at nine years of age. This is of considerable interest because this is also the age that is cited by Chomsky (1969) as the time of mastery of language skills. This same age was identified by McCroskey and Cory (1968) in an earlier investigation of 92 children between the ages of three and 15 years, in which it was found that for each three-year increment in age, the threshold for detecting durational differences between tones was halved and age nine, again, was the first age at which any child was able to establish the durational equality of two tones. The auditory task used by McCroskey and Cory was more difficult than the later one employed by McCroskey and Davis (1976); it was forced-choice procedure in which the listener had to state whether the short or the long tone came first. The equipment was programmed to make the discrimination more difficult with each successive correct ordering of the stimuli and to make the task easier after two consecutive erroneous judgments. A recording attenuator was used to perform control functions and to plot a Bekesy-like audiogram for time (temperogram). The important element is that age nine emerges in all three independent investigations as the time at which the auditory system is able to perform with adult-like efficiency in the time domain.

SCHOOL-AGE CHILDREN

Auditory processing disabilities may result from peripheral or central disorders. As consideration is extended to children over the age of five years, a sizable number of evaluation vehicles have been described in the literature relating to auditory processing. Prior to a strict consideration of these test vehicles, however, some consideration should be given to the possible generator(s) of auditory processing problems.

Excellent descriptions of the anatomical structure and function of the central auditory nervous system have been provided by Snow et al. (1977), and by Willeford and Billger (1978). In neither of these reports do the authors hypothesize regarding the specific lesion or disorder that results in a specific auditory processing problem, but rather they present a generalized coverage of the total central auditory nervous system and leave the specificity to the reader. An additional report of central auditory performance and function has been presented by Duane (1977). Once again, readers are presented with the available information and are at liberty to draw their own conclusions regarding the loci of auditory processing deficits.

It is, of course, fascinating to speculate on the physiologic bases for auditory processing problems. Many long and interesting discussions have been held comparing the performance and probable site of lesion in children having auditory perceptual problems and with children having "aphasic" manifestations. It has been suggested that aphasic children possess a central nervous system *lesion,* while learning disabled or auditory perceptually disabled children possess a central nervous system *dysfunction.* These differentiations, while easy to verbalize, are frequently very difficult to conceptualize. While it is often true that the child with auditory preceptual problems and the child with aphasia appear to be on far ends of a long continuum, it appears tenuous at best to attempt to establish physiologic similarities between the two conditions.

One cannot help but speculate that some percentage or degree of auditory perceptual deficit may result, not from a preexisting central auditory nervous system disorder, but rather from a peripheral disorder. Recently, Katz (1978) discussed the deleterious effect of conductive hearing loss in children. He pointed out in a series of conclusions that conductive hearing losses tend to act primarily like earplugs and, thus, ". . . deprive the auditory system of normal activity." He also points out that this deprivation may involve the retrocochlear system and the brain. The greater or longer the deprivation the more extreme may be the retrocochlear signs. He further states that, ". . . disruption in auditory perception and language (presumably cerebral functions) are associated with fluctuating hearing loss, especially unilateral problems and with early age of onset."

Partial support for Katz's conclusions can be found in the work of Omer (1972). She evaluated 153 children with learning problems who scored normal or better on the Weschler Intelligence Scale for Children and who were below grade level placement in at least one academic subject. Each child was evaluated with conventional audiometric testing and also with the Peabody Picture Vocabulary Test (PPVT) to provide a measurement of receptive vocabulary. Her findings revealed that 41 percent of the children were below their chronological ages in vocabulary development. Of those children with speech discrimination scores in the 90–100 percent range, 64 percent scored at or above their chronological age on the PPVT, while those with speech discrimination in the 85–89 percent range revealed only 42 percent at or above their chronological ages. Further, she was able to suggest, on the basis of the PPVT and speech discrimination scores, that speech reception thresholds in the 10–14 dB range may well have a handicapping effect on the auditory verbal performance of the child. While the pure-tone test is not a test of central auditory processing, it may alert the audiologist to such a possibility.

Further support for Katz's position comes from the work from Hardin and Kasten (1976). They evaluated the auditory functioning of a group of learning disabled (LD) and regular classroom children by means of tympanometry. They found a significantly greater incidence of previous middle ear disorders among LD children than among the regular classroom children. Thus, it may be concluded that a significantly greater number of the LD children experienced periods of transitory conductive hearing loss than did their counterparts in the regular classroom. Hardin and Kasten further pointed out that those LD children whose better binaural pure-tone averages were worse than 10 dB HL scored significantly poorer on the auditory–vocal association and grammatical closure subtests of the Illinois Test of Psycholinguistic Abilities than did their LD counterparts whose better binaural pure-tone averages were better than 10 dB HL. The presence of an apparently diminished auditory performance following a history of mild threshold elevations has been pointed out forcefully by Northern and Downs (1978). Thus, it would appear that serious consideration must be given to the impact of mild hearing losses or previous transitory mild hearing losses when evaluating the overall auditory performance of a child with an auditory perceptual disorder.

Evaluation Techniques

It is somewhat difficult to select an appropriate starting point for a discussion of evaluative vehicles when so little is known about the disorder being evaluated. Indeed, an evaluation of the subtests of the more popularly used test vehicles reveals a diversity of terms referring to the specific disorder being evaluated. This may be due in part to the fact that extensive research does not exist to document specific disorder syndromes under the umbrella heading of auditory processing disorders. It may also be due in part to "the nature of the beast." By this it is meant that children give the appearance of manifesting specific problems on the basis of the academic placements they receive, the types of teaching environments in which they are located, and the remediation procedures attempted with them. At this point in the state of the art, it appears difficult to determine whether each specifically identified disability is a true deficit or is a reflection of the environment in which the child has been placed.

One of the most commonly used test vehicles, perhaps because of its longevity in the field, is the Illinois Test of Psycholinguistic Abilities (Kirk et al., 1968). This test, with the six auditory subtests designed to measure reception, association, auditory sequential memory, grammatic closure, auditory closure, and sound blending, has been used extensively by speech and language pathologists, psychologists, and audiologists. There can be little doubt that the results of the ITPA have been extremely useful in identifying children whose auditory performance deviated somewhat from normal. Unfortunately, several authors (Burns & Watson, 1973; Willeford, 1976; Kasten and Griffin, 1979) have questioned the accuracy of the ITPA in identifying potential auditory processing disorders. In addition, Drichta (1976) has pointed out that the auditory subtests do not appear to sample independent processing abilities. That is, the individual subtests appear to be sampling an overlapping auditory continuum. This may be due in part to the fact that the ITPA is an auditory test delivered via live voice. Thus, the overall accuracy of the test results can be influenced by the skill or lack of skill of the test administrator. A number of practitioners, including the authors, have observed test–retest ITPA scores showing dramatic changes in performance in both directions. If it is reasonable to question the validity of the retest scores on the basis of the tester competence, it becomes equally reasonable to question the validity of the initial test performance. These comments are not made to negate the value of the ITPA as a diagnostic tool, but rather to urge caution in the interpretation and gospel adherance to test scores.

The Goldman-Fristoe-Woodcock Auditory Skills Test Battery (Goldman et al., 1970; Woodcock, 1976) and the composite Auditory Perceptual Test (Butler, et al., 1973) provide auditory test sequences that are presented via magnetic tape. This type of presentation clearly eliminates major elements inherent in live-voice presentations; however, neither test provides rigorous definition for test administration. Both tests are to be administered at a comfortable listening level in a controlled auditory environment. Obviously, both of these definitions are open to individual interpretation and the reliability or accuracy of any given set of results is somewhat dependent on the ability of the administrator or on the environment in which the test is administered. Given the great diversity of individuals who might well be administering this pair of recorded test materials, one must indeed question the reliability of presentation levels or environmental test noise levels that could be encountered. One further comment must be made regarding the reliability of the Goldman-Fristoe-Woodcock test (GFW). Schubert et al. (1973) compared the performance on Katz's Staggered Spondaic Word Test (Brunt, 1972) with the noise subtest of the GFW. The Staggered Spondiac Word Test has been found to be a highly reliable vehicle for identifying both pathological and normal auditory functioning. Of significance to this discussion is the report that subjects who scored within the normal range on the SSW Test distributed themselves within the range from the first to the 99th percentile on the GFW. Schubert et al. point out that they found very poor test–retest reliability on the noise subtests (NS) of the GFW. In fact, they state, "The GFW cannot with our population be considered a reliable nor a valid measure of central auditory function." The implications of these findings are cause for concern.

It is altogether possible that the SSW and NS–GFW are sampling different aspects of auditory performance. This would explain the lack of agreement between these two evaluation vehicles, but it would not explain the broad range of scores that contributed to the lack of test–retest reliability on the NS–GFW. These statements are not made to diminish the potential value of results from the GFW battery but, again, rather to highlight the necessity for a cautious interpretation of results.

It has been observed that some users of the GFW confront children with a continuous presentation of the full battery, without apparent concern for possible physical and psychological overloading of this system. While data do not presently exist to confirm our impressions, it is likely that subject fatigue influences scores in the latter half of the test battery. Unfortunately, this same criticism must be voiced regarding the Composite Auditory Perception Test. Barring explicit instructions to the contrary, it appears that all too often these lengthy test batteries are administered at the convenience of the tester rather than according to the stamina of the child. While individual speech-type tests are not considered to be particularly fatiguing, a prolonged series of demanding speech presentations can easily become an overwhelming and bewildering experience for the young perceptually impaired child.

An example of the type of results that can be obtained with the GFW is given in Table 14-1. These results were obtained from a seven-year, seven-month-old girl whose mother and teacher both complained that she did not appear to understand or attend to speech as well as expected, particularly in a noisy situation.

Table 14-1
Type of Results With the Goldman-Fristoe-Woodcock Test

Subtest	Percentile	Age Equivalency
Selective attention	2	5–3
Diagnostic discrimination	92	14–2
Recognition memory	64	8–6
Memory for content	7	5–11
Memory for sequence	10	5–7
Sound mimicry	—	below 3–8
Sound recognition	26	6–8
Sound analysis	46	7–5
Sound blending	22	6–4
Sound–symbol association	45	7–1
Reading of symbols	19	6–7
Spelling of sounds	10	7–0

It can be seen readily that this complete test battery attempts—through the use of words, dissected words, partial words, nonsense syllables, and word symbols—to sample performance across a substantial number of specific areas within the perceptual process. There is little doubt that the various subtests of the GFW, as well as the Composite Auditory Perception Test, sample different aspects of auditory performance, but there is legitimate room for question as to whether the samples within each categorical label are exclusive to, or representative of, that specific label.

Two of the more exciting approaches to the measurement of auditory processing disorders involve the Flowers-Costello Tests of Auditory Abilities (Flowers et al., 1973) and the Willeford Test Battery (Willeford, 1976; Willeford & Billger, 1978). These two tests present two distinct advantages over previously mentioned test batteries. To begin with, both tests are recorded on magnetic tape and are administered under earphones with strict instructions regarding presentation intensity and environment. In addition, and in some respects more importantly, the specific subtests are named according to the content of the subtest rather than the specific disability allegedly being evaluated. As a result, users of either the Flowers-Costello or the Willeford test are not able to apply stereotype labels to children on the basis of the test results, unless the test administrator provides a firm justification for the labels being applied.

It has become almost commonplace to examine reports written to summarize the results of previously discussed test batteries and find statements such as, "The results of the ITPA reveal that the child has a deficit in auditory association," or "With the Composite Auditory Perception Test, the child had particular difficulty with auditory synthesis," or "The child displayed particular difficulty with memory for sequence with the Goldman-Fristoe-Woodcock test." It is easy for these definitive statements to flow from the pen of the naive, but supposedly expert, test administrator. This task is made even easier since the three test constructions have provided convenient labels that can be applied to the children. This is not so much a wholehearted criticism of the three tests involved as it is a criticism of manner in which the test results are used. Given a convenient subtest name, the administrator can now point an impressively professional finger at the child and provide an equally impressive and professional-sounding label to the child and the child's problem. Whether this label accurately describes the child or not is a moot question; the reasoning seems to be that if a child scores poorly on a specific subtest, it is fair to apply the label from that subtest to the child.

With the Flowers-Costello and the Willeford Test Battery, on the other hand, the test administrator is forced to describe the precipitating behaviors, the specific test performance, the inferred capabilities or disabilities, and then state conclusions as to the nature of the problem and suggest recommendations for remediation. It would appear that tests of these types will demand a far more accurate description of the test stimuli, the child's response patterns to these stimuli, and the significance of the response patterns. Both of these tests have in common the fact that they have borrowed judiciously from previous speech-type evaluation vehicles used with individuals possessing central auditory nervous system *pathologies*. Also, both tests rely heavily upon varying types of two-eared performance, including speech performance in the presence of competition.

The Flowers-Costello test consists of two subtests: one presenting low-pass filtered speech and one presenting full-spectrum speech in the presence of a competing message. Both tests utilize incomplete sentences and require the subject to point to a picture that will complete the meaning of the sentence.

The Willeford Test Battery consisted originally of four subtests with the recent addition of two further subtests, each designed to evaluate specific aspects of auditory function. One of the subtests requires the identification of dichotically presented competing sentences. A primary sentence is presented to one ear at 35 dB sensation level (SL) while a competition sentence is presented to the other ear at a 50 dB SL. The task is to identify the content and at least paraphrase the meaning of the primary sentence. Willeford strongly suggests that this test samples temporal lobe function as originally described by Ohta et al. (1967). Norms developed by Willeford for this subtest reveal a definite age effect in the five to nine year range, with ear dominence apparently stabilizing following the ninth year. This effect is closely correlated with the earlier discussion on temporal discrimination found in a previous section (Child three to six years) and with data by Tallal (1978).

The second subtest consists of consonant–nucleus–consonant words, which are presented monotically and are low-pass filtered with a 500 Hz cut-off. This subtest, according to the suggestion of Bocca and Calearo (1963), should be sensitive to functioning of the lower centers of the temporal lobes. Once again Willeford's norms revealed a distinct age effect, but this subtest is not sensitive to "earedness" as was the earlier subtests.

The third subtest in the Willeford battery involves a binaural fusion task patterned after the classical approach of Matzker (1959). This subtest is designed in such a way that the recipient simultaneously receives a two-syllable word that is low-pass filtered (500–700 Hz) in one ear and high-pass filtered (1900–2100 Hz) in the other ear. The low-pass filtered portion is typically presented at an intensity 30 dB greater than the 500 Hz pure-tone threshold, and the high-pass filtered signal is typically presented 30 dB above the 2000 Hz pure-tone threshold. Willeford arbitrarily has assigned the score for a given two-eared presentation to the ear receiving the low-frequency signal. This subtest is constructed in such a way that the normal-hearing listener would have significant difficulty responding correctly to either ear independently, but is able to perform quite adequately when the two segments are presented simultaneously in separate ears. Once again, Willeford points out that there is a maturational effect in the binaural fusion task in the range from five to nine years, but performance tends to stabilize and variability diminishes beyond the nine-year level.

The fourth subtest in the Willeford battery involves the presentation of sentence material that alternates rapidly from ear to ear. The speech signal switches between ears every 300 msec, and the materials are presented in each ear at 30 dB SL. This is the one subtest that does not display a maturational effect, in that normal five-year-olds are able to perform as well as adults. With this particular subtest, Willeford arbitrarily assigns the performance score to the ear in which the sentence item is initiated. He does point out, however, that the alternating speech subtest is the least sensitive of the four original subtests.

Recently, Willeford has added two additional subtests to the battery. These include one subtest that utilizes time compressed speech and one subtest consisting of synthetic sentence identification with an ipsilateral competing message as described by Jerger and Jerger (1975). At the time of this writing, comprehensive data from the use of these two subtests are not yet available.

The Willeford Test Battery is intriguing as a measure of auditory processing ability, since the subtests have been designed to sample integrity and performance at varying levels within the central auditory nervous system. Thus, a deficit in performance of the binaural fusion subtest might suggest a brainstem disorder. A deficit in performance on the competing sentence subtest could suggest a high-level temporal lobe disorder, while a performance deficit with the synthetic sentence identification subtest might suggest either a brainstem or a temporal lobe disorder, depending upon the pattern of the results. Clearly, Willeford is able to present a meaningful argument for the necessity of using a carefully constructed series of speech tests designed to sample performance at varying levels within the central auditory nervous system. An additional benefit of the Willeford battery is that these results do not lend themselves to the application of specific labels to individuals with deficit scoring patterns. Rather, performance must be described and then discussed in relation to a child's observed auditory performance problems. In this way, the examiner is forced to describe a *child* with a problem rather than to describe a problem within a child.

No discussion of tests of auditory performance would be complete without a detailed description of the Staggered Spondaic Word Test (SSW) as presented by Katz (1962, 1968, 1970, 1973, 1979). This excellent test has probably been used more extensively and with a broader based population than any other single test of central auditory nervous system performance. It utilizes conventional spondaic words that are presented in such a manner that the first syllable of one word is presented to one ear in quiet. Simultaneously, with the presentation of the second syllable of that spondaic word, the first syllable of another spondaic word is presented to the opposite ear. The second syllable of the second spondaic word is then presented in quiet. Thus, for each presentation, a score can be obtained for the right ear with no competition, the right ear with competition, the left ear with competition, and the left ear with no competition. This test has been described in detail in several textbooks (Brunt, 1972; Katz, 1977; White, 1977; Brunt, 1978), and is available commercially (Katz, 1973).

Space does not permit a detailed discussion of the utility of the SSW Test. Needless to say, it has proven to be highly sensitive to the subtle disorders characterized by auditory processing problems. Katz reports that the test has been used with children down to age five, but there is a distinct maturational effect with a right ear dominance and increased variability below the age of eleven. Nonetheless, the SSW Test must be considered as a valuable addition to the armamentarium of tests available for the evaluation of selected auditory processing disorders. The user should become familiar with the test through an examination of the textbooks previously cited and through a search of the comprehensive bibliographies contained in these textbooks. The Staggered Spondaic Word Test can then be put to use with the knowledge that it is brief, well controlled, and highly reliable.

No attempt will be made to discuss or describe the many less well-known tests or subtests that have been utilized in attempting to discover and describe auditory processing disorders. The majority of these lesser known tests have utilized a variety of speech stimuli that are very similar to those stimuli previously described. Rather, it seems appropriate at this point in time to consider some alternative methods of evaluating the performance of individuals with suspected auditory processing disorders.

DYNAMIC AUDITORY LOCALIZATION

Accurate auditory tracking of a moving signal is a reflection of an efficient binaural integration of sound. Batteau (1961) has suggested that the pinnae contribute to a differential arrival time for different bands of frequencies within a complex signal, and it is this division that contributes to the localization of sound in space. Previous investigations (McCroskey & Davis, 1976; McCroskey & Kidder, 1980) have demonstrated that LD children have auditory fusion points that are different according to stimulus frequencies, in contrast to the uniform fusion points of normal children. Based on the previous studies, it was hypothesized that the LD child would be less efficient in the tracking of a moving acoustic stimulus. This hypothesis was confirmed (Devens, Hoyer, & McCroskey, 1976, 1978) and it is suggested that Dynamic Auditory Localization (tracking) is a potentially useful addition to procedures for assessing central auditory processing.

SPEECH IN COMPETITION

General background noise affects LD children adversely; meaningful background noise is an auditory disaster. It is an accepted and established fact that the ability to respond correctly to speech presentations diminishes as the intensity of a competing message increases. It matters little whether the individual has normal hearing, a mild auditory disorder, or a recognized and diagnosed pathology; speech performance will deteriorate as the intensity of the competition is increased. Competing signals consisting of white noise, speech spectrum noise, cold running speech, highly similar speech, cafeteria noise, or cocktail party noise have all shown similar effects. Different competitions require different message-to-competition ratios in order to influence speech reception to a similar degree, but the general pattern of the effect maintains across types of competition. It has been suggested frequently (Myklebust, 1954; Katz & Illmer, 1972; Kasten & Griffin, 1976) that chilren with learning disabilities or auditory processing disorders have more difficulty attending to or discriminating speech in the presence of competition than do normal children. In fact, Clements (1969) described the child with learning disabilities as ". . . drawn to irrelevant stimuli in his environment . . . ." Myklebust (1954), in discussing children who were later to be described as having learning disabilities, refers to the problems these children have with both auditory and visual competition. He relates competition to distractibility and describes distractibility as ". . . the incapacity to maintain sustained attention to one activity with fleeting attention to irrelevant and minor details."

Tarnopol (1969) considered auditory figure-ground to be an important consideration for children with learning disabilities. He strongly suggested the standardization of an auditory figure-ground test that could be used in diagnosing and describing children with learning disabilities. He proposed a speech-in-noise test as a method of measuring auditory figure-ground intactness. Katz and Illmer (1972) point out that approximately 60 percent of the children referred to them for learning problems demonstrated poor performance in speech-in-noise tasks. They discussed the hyperactive child who seems to be able to hear adequately, but who generally is unable to cooperate or follow instructions. They suggested that these children may well be the types of children who are classified as having behavioral problems but who primarily have difficulties discriminating speech-in-noise. Katz and Illmer then go on to discuss the fact that, in controlled observations, they were able to chart systematically an increase in hyperactivity as background noise levels increased in intensity. They refer to this whole pattern as auditory foreground–background confusion.

These same types of observations are relatively common in the literature of special education. Many have observed the performance of children with learning disabilities and have reported these particular types of auditory difficulties, but very little appears to have been done to quantify the absence or presence of a specific masking, confusion, or distraction effect.

With this in mind, Kasten and Griffin (1976) designed a preliminary investigation to evaluate the influence of auditory distractibility upon children in learning disability classrooms and children in regular public school classrooms. Forty children placed in self-contained learning disability (LD) classrooms were compared with a like number of children from regular classrooms. All children had hearing sensitivity within normal limits. The speech discrimination task involved listening to and repeating PBK monosyllabic words. Each child listened to one list in quiet, one list in the presence of multiply recorded classroom babble, and one list in the presence of a staggered choral reading of *The Cat in the Hat* (Seuss, 1957). The primary PBK words were presented at 65 dB SPL while the competition was presented at a level of 6 dB less intense. This particular primary-to-secondary ratio was selected as being representative of typical classroom levels according to the findings of McCroskey and Devens (1975). The two background competitions were selected to represent noise environments typically encountered in the educational setting. Specifically, one environment consisted of an ongoing noise babble while the other environment consisted of a very meaningful and highly intelliglble speech signal.

Interestingly, small but statistically significant differences were found between the two groups of the presentation in quiet with the LD children scoring slightly poorer. Even more interesting was the fact that the classroom babble reduced performance by at least 30 percent for all students and no significant differences were seen between the LD and the regular classroom children. This held true for separate analyses of grades one through three (Level I), three through six (Level II), and for the analysis of the total group. With the choral reading of *The Cat in the Hat,* however, the LD children performed significantly poorer whether the analysis was done at Level I, Level II, or with the total group. It is significant to note that, with signal-to-noise (S/N) held constant, the nonmeaningful, rather generalized classroom babble affected both groups of children similarly, while the highly meaningful content of the choral reading background had a significantly greater effect upon the LD children than upon the regular classroom chilren. It would appear that a distracting competition offers a far more difficult task for LD children than does a generalized type of nonmeaningful noise, such as that used in audiometric evaluations or employed in some of the commercially available tests of auditory perception.

Having observed that a meaningful or distracting type of competition at a S/N ratio of +6 dB had a more deleterious effect for LD children than for regular classroom children, Carlin and Kasten (1977) attempted to determine the approximate S/N ratio at which LD children began to demonstrate their deficiency. They evaluated 54 children from self-contained LD classes and 54 matched regular classroom children utilizing the Word Intelligibility by Picture Identification Test (Ross & Learman, 1971), with this primary signal presented at 65 dB SPL. The competition was again a choral reading or *the Cat in the Hat* and the competition was presented at S/N ratios at +6, +12, and +18 dB. At +18 dB, the most favorable S/N ratio, the LD children performed slightly poorer than the regular classroom children across grade levels. The regular classroom children yielded performance levels that were essentially identical for the +18 and +12 S/N ratios, while the LD children demonstrated an increasing deficit in performance at the +12 dB level. At the +6 dB setting, the most difficult S/N ratio, the regular classroom children began to show a deficit in performance, while the LD children demonstrated a disparity even greater than at the two previous S/N ratios. It should be noted that the performance levels of LD children were significantly poorer than those of the regular classroom children at each S/N ratio, but the magnitude of the discrepancy increased as the S/N ratio became more detrimental. One interesting tendency was noted. As the children increased in age, the discrepancy in performance between the two groups tended to diminish, but remained significantly different at each age level.

One further evaluation of auditory distractibility was carried out by Mueller and Kasten (1978). They evaluated the performance of a large group of third-grade children involved in a remedial reading program with a matched group of regular classroom children possessing no reading difficulties. Their protocol involved a more complex sentence type auditory task that called for the children to attend, discriminate, process, retain, and respond. The stimulus materials contained three levels of auditory complexity and consisted of items such as, "Point to the cup," or "Point to the cup before you point to the star," or "After you point to the cup, point to the star." Primary sentences were presented at 65 dB SPL and the auditory distraction (*The Cat in the Hat*) was presented at at S/N ratio of +6 dB. The reading-disabled children performed significantly poorer than the nonreading-disabled children in quiet, and in the presence of the speech distraction the difference between the two groups was more obvious. The deficit suffered by the reading disabled children also increased in magnitude as the level of auditory complexity increased.

One clear indication appears to emerge from the results of these three investigations. A speech discrimination task or a speech processing task in the presence of a meaningful speech distraction holds genuine promise as a quick screening device for the presence of auditory processing problems. Further, it would appear that a meaningful speech distraction provides a more sensitive probe for subtle processing disorders than would a more conventional nonmeaningful competing noise.

TIME-ALTERED SPEECH

For a number of years, investigators have expressed interest in the use of time-compressed speech for the purpose of assessing central auditory function (Calearo & Lazzaroni, 1957; Bocca & Calearo, 1963; Kurdzeil & Noffsinger, 1973; Beasley et al., 1976; Konkle et al., 1977), or as a means of evaluating children with speech and language or reading problems (Orchik & Oeschlager, 1974; Ormson & Williams, 1975).

Each auditory system has an optimal listening rate; defective auditory systems have critical listening rates. The data presented on the effects of time-compressed (accelerated) speech are but samples of current thinking. For a more complete review, the reader is referred to the three-volume anthology and bibliography of Duker (1974). The amount of literature on time-expanded (slowed) speech is quite minimal. Yet, the obvious progression for clinically oriented researchers would be to move from the detrimental effects of compressed speech to the potential beneficial effects of expanded speech. It seems reasonable that, if an auditory system has some basic defect and is unable to process speech satisfactorily when communication is at a normal or faster-than-normal rate, it might be possible to *facilitate* communication if the same information were presented at some slower-than-normal rate. It was under this assumption that McCroskey instigated a series of investigations that have spanned two decades.

The effect of expanded speech upon auditory comprehension by LD children has been tested, and the data indicate that while compressed speech leads to decreased comprehension, moderately expanded speech leads to improved comprehension of simple sentences (McCroskey & Thompson, 1973). The data also indicate that there is a potential rollover effect if the rate of speech is expanded too much. The inference drawn by McCroskey and Thompson is that there may be a critical listening rate for the LD child and that if the input rate either exceeds or fails to reach that optimum, comprehension suffers. Expansion and compression, leading to rate-altered speech, can be accomplished with electromechanical systems (Fairbanks et al., 1954) or microprocessors (Cramer & Talambiras, 1971). Both methods have been employed to: (a) accomplish rate alteration; (b) retain normal pitch of voice; and (c) maintain relative time values within utterances.

Optimal listening rate will vary according to the level of linguistic difficulty in the message. It should be noted that current research plans call for the development of an interactive computer-controlled program in which children can respond continuously to verbal material; the ongoing analyses of their response accuracy will dictate the degree of expansion or compression that is required to arrive at optimal performance by listeners. The outcome will be a Bekesy-like audiogram, except that the dimensions will be response accuracy versus rate-of-speech rather than an intensity-by-frequency display.

Normal children were assumed to be able to cope with a wide range of speaking rates, particularly if the stimuli were simple, active, affirmative, declarative sentences; however, it was important to verify their responses to the test procedures used by McCroskey and Thompson (1973). A group of 40 first graders in regular classrooms were presented with the same stimulus materials. The initial results indicated that speech expansion resulted in improved auditory processing of simple sentences, and this was *not* the expected outcome, since it had been hypothesized that normal children would handle a variety of speech rates with equal facility.

The researchers were convinced that normal children should be able to accommodate the variety of rates that must be a part of every child's experience and still sort out the linguistic and articulatory codes that lead to verbal competence. It was decided to review the data on file for each of the children. It was found that nine of the children had been flagged for special assistance during the next school year because of potential reading problems. The data for these nine children were deleted; the analyses then yielded a result indicating that rate did not influence auditory comprehension (the children achieved at least 97 percent accuracy on the compressed speech and were 100 percent correct on expanded speech). The data on this small sample suggested that if larger numbers were tested, the difference might achieve significance—in favor of slowed speech—even among children who were considered to be completely normal.

Nelson (1976) tested 360 elementary school children with the same basic procedure employed, with the added factors of sentence difficulty and age levels included. Her results show that auditory comprehension improves with age from age six through age nine, and the degree of comprehension (as measured by a picture-selection task) is related to the speed at which the sentences are delivered as well as to the complexity of the sentences. As these data were reviewed, it became apparent that there was a potential difference between those who used Standard English (SE) and those who used Black English (BE). Eighty children in each category, equally divided across the age range from six through nine comprised a matched sample drawn from the original 360 subjects. These data showed that BE-speaking chidren have greater difficulty comprehending SE than do SE-speaking children, and that a significant effect of rate of speech was found for the BE-speaking group only. In other words, Standard English spoken at a rate slower than normal (175 wpm was chosen as the normal rate for virtually all these studies) facilitated comprehension of SE, but did not bring it to a point of equality (Nelson & McCroskey, 1978). The data from the study of 360 chidren were not reanalyzed with the BE data deleted in order to determine whether the rate effect would no longer obtain.

The assessing of central auditory processing by means of rate-altered speech has included other populations demonstrating verbal deficiencies. Previous experience with the six-year-old children who had been flagged as having potential reading problems suggested the need for specific investigation of older children diagnosed as reading disordered. Subsequently, 120 children equally divided according to classifications of normal or reading disordered, were tested under the same conditions that had been employed previously. The results indicate that children with reading disorders performed significantly less well than their counterparts for all

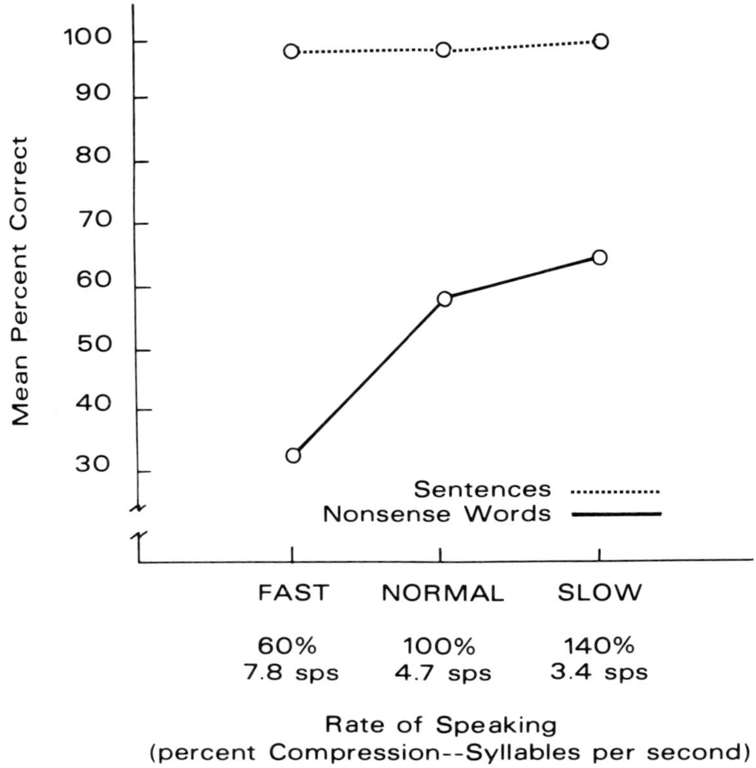

Fig. 14-2. A comparison of the effects of speaking rate upon the auditory comprehension of sentences and nonsense words by first-grade listeners.

levels of linguistic difficulty, and that speaking rate significantly affected sentence comprehension for the reading disordered children only (McCroskey & Thompson-Nelson, 1973).

The full impact of rate of speaking upon auditory reception of verbal information is illustrated by comparing performance with simple sentences versus nonsense words under conditions of varying rates of speaking (McCroskey & Hagler, 1975). Whether one is speaking of initial learning of a language or the acquisition of the second language or dialect, Fig. 14-2 illustrates the impact of speaking rate upon recognition of unfamiliar verbal material, in contrast to the effect of rate upon familiar verbal material. The implication for developmentalists and for speech-language pathologists who work with language impaired and articulatory deficient children is clear. If optimum listening rates can be identified, then instruction can take place under most favorable conditions for a given listener.

The original stimulus and response materials (McCroskey & Thompson, 1973) were used in an informal pilot investigation of 23 trainable mentally retarded children who were between seven and 14 years of age. In contrast to the LD children who showed improved auditory comprehension as rate of speaking was reduced somewhat (but experienced a decrement in comprehension with further expansion of the signal), the TMR listener showed highest comprehension at the slowest speaking rate. Since 175 wpm was the original speaking rate and the maximum expansion was 180 percent, it was decided that a follow-up investigation using a slower initial speaking rate (150 wpm) and a greater degree of expansion (225 percent) would be employed in order to attempt to find the optimal listening rate for sentences for TMR listeners.

Rate of speaking has a profound effect upon auditory verbal processing and comprehension; this brings into question the interpretation of results from all tests that are orally administered or contain orally presented tasks. Schroder and McCroskey (1975) looked at the effects of speech expansion upon auditory comprehension of 40 TMR listeners. Half of the subjects were drawn from a sheltered workshop program and half from a special classroom in a regular elementary school. The stimulus materials were four equated sets of seven sentences each, plus practice sentences; all sentences were recorded at four rate-altered conditions (150, 112, 75, and 56 wpm). All sentences were heard at all four rates by all children. For each sentence heard, the children touched one of four line drawings situated in equally sized quadrants on 8½ by 11 inch paper. Each picture was situated over a microswitch to permit measuring response latency as well as response accuracy. The results indicate both statistically and educationally significant advantages to using a speaking rate that is markedly slower than even a slow normal rate. The data show that auditory comprehension improves by approximately 25 percent when the word-per-minute rate is reduced to at least 75 wpm and, further, the response latency is shortened by approximately .75 seconds. There are two elements that are significant and deserve additional research: (a) the ability to receive and understand the meaning of a spoken sentence improves dramatically under conditions of extensive speech expansion; and (b) previously held notions about the limited auditory memory span of mentally retarded subjects may be an artifact of rate of central auditory processing rather than a pure reflection of memory span. The latter statement is based on the fact that all MR subjects had shorter response latencies when the same sentences were simply made longer in duration (slowed down), with content held constant. This was true whether the timing for the latency was measured from the beginning of the utterance or from the end of the utterance to the response. The implications of these data, as well as those collected on LD and reading-disordered subjects are profound. Indeed, the results of this auditory processing test bring into serious question the validity of virtually all instruments that rely upon orally given instructions or orally administered subtests for the testing of intelligence.

The slow processing of spoken verbal material by TMR listeners is hypothesized to represent very poor auditory temporal integration; the poor educational performance exhibited by retarded children may reflect the temporal overloading of the transmission and processing systems as much as, if not more than, the assumed limitations of intellect. This auditory processing test obviously does not separate the influence of time from the influence of language and the two are somewhat confounded. It was out of this background that the new nonlinguistic test of temporal efficiency (auditory fusion) was developed (McCroskey & Davis, 1976). The general area of auditory fusion has been studied in terms of auditory flutter, where the rate of tone interruption is accelerated until the tone is heard as a steady-state sound (Chapman et al., 1955), and in terms of a unified or composite perception of independent verbal stimuli dichotically delivered to the two ears (Berlin & Lowe, 1972).

Audiologic data regarding auditory processing generally have not been made available for use in special education literature. It should be born in mind that the evaluation and remediation of auditory processing disorders are not the exclusive domain of the audiologist. Children described as learning disabled or as having an auditory processing disorder typically are not found in the audiology clinic but rather in classrooms where they attempt to master and understand academic subjects. With this thought in mind, it seems reasonable to expect that the literature from the field of general education or special education would have relatively detailed descriptions regarding the manifestations of auditory processing problems and the remediation of these problems. A sampling of some of the more recent and well-respected textbooks concerning the education of learning disabled or exceptional children reveals, however, that this is not always true.

Myers and Hammill (1969) present a relatively brief and general discussion of auditory processing disorders. Dunn (1973) provides a surface description of the manifestations of auditory processing problems. Bryan and Bryan (1975) offer a very short but insightful section dealing with assumptions concerning auditory processing, but offer little useful information in terms of measuring or remediating these problems. Haring and Bateman (1977) discuss the relationship (or lack of relationship) between auditory perceptual problems and reading disabilities, and also provide a very brief description of one selected auditory perception program. Hammill and Bartell (1978) briefly describe two commercially available tests for auditory processing and present two pages of activities for the teacher to assess informally the integrity of the auditory processing system. Mann et al. (1978) provide a very basic and very limited discussion of auditory processing disorders as they relate primarily to language problems. Salvia and Ysseldyke (1978) summarize pertinent published data from selected test manuals, but present few suggestions or interpretations regarding the material discussed. Meyen (1978) makes mention of auditory processing disorders, but tends not to go beyond this initial introduction. Adamson and Adamson (1979) refer to auditory processing disorders, but tend to stay away from any meaningful discussion of this problem area.

The above comments are not made in criticism of these writers in the area of special education. Special educators are confronted with a myriad of educational, perceptual, motoric, and psychological problems, and they tend (as do most other writers) to concentrate upon their areas of expertise. We would hope that the writers in the field of special education would turn to the audiologists for primary information relative to the identification and remediation of auditory processing disorders. Unfortunately, audiologists have provided special educators with only limited guidance and direction.

It is apparent that the ramifications of the subtle influences of auditory processing disorders are just beginning to be identified. It is necessary that discoveries and accomplishments be shared with colleagues in allied professional fields. With an active exchange of information, the gap between professionals in communicative disorders and special education can be reduced. It is an unfortunate fact that the professional literature in special education contains almost no contributions from the field of audiology and the professional literature in audiology is essentially devoid of contributions from writers in special education. These two fields of professional endeavor must learn how to benefit from the achievements and mistakes of each other in order to develop and utilize meaningful evaluation and remediation tools for children with auditory processing problems.

ADULTS

Extensive research has been carried out relating to the identification or diagnosis of central auditory nervous system *pathologies* and this material is covered in other portions of this book. The study of auditory *processing* disorders within the adult population is a specialty area characterized by a relative lack of professional literature. There appears to have been a general lack of interest in the identification or description of the more subtle disorders. This is not meant to imply that there is no interest in the adult with auditory processing disorders, but rather that the identification of children during the formative and educational years appears to be viewed as more critical. This is also not meant to imply that adults do not have auditory processing disorders, but rather that adults are in a better position to develop and use appropriate coping behaviors.

Interest in central auditory pathologies has been concentrated primarily with the adult population because central auditory pathologies may be life-threatening and because a greater number of such pathologies are found among the adult population than among the child population. Interest in central auditory *processing* disorders has not been as concentrated with the adult population, because processing disorders are usually not life-threatening, as it has with children because they appear to be more vulnerable (educationally and socially) and have rigid auditory demands placed upon them in the educational setting.

One point should be clearly understood. There is no body of literature to indicate that central auditory processing disorders can be outgrown. Stated differently, it is reasonable to assume that a school-age child with a central auditory processing disorder will become an adult with a central auditory processing disorder. If this situation actually exists, it is legitimate to ask why so little time and effort has been expended upon the adult population. To begin with, it must be remembered that much of today's adult population attended school in an era that preceeded the recognition of, or even the acknowledgement of, auditory processing disorders. Thus, today's adults with auditory processing disorders may have been looked upon as children who were inattentive, slow to respond, daydreamers, distractable, or even mildly retarded. Indeed, since their present adult auditory functioning is not different than it has been throughout their entire lives, they tend to see no reason for a diagnostic work-up or for rehabilitative management.

Adults have far greater freedom of choice when it comes to individual life style than do children. They are free to choose a life style that will allow them to circumvent their auditory processing problems while children are forced to return to the same auditory educational environment day after day. Adults are free to develop occupational pursuits that place no demands upon the auditory system, while children are required to receive, discriminate, process, store, and utilize new auditory information on almost an hourly basis. In short, adults can develop coping behaviors and can place themselves in favorable auditory environments so that the existence of an auditory processing problem does not become a major drawback in their accepted life style. These particular options are rarely open to the school-age child.

Obviously, there is a desperate need for comprehensive research relating to the auditory processing ability of allegedly normal, near-normal or possibly disordered adults. It will be necessary to follow carefully a known population of children with auditory processing disorders in order to plot the manifestations of these disorders as a function of advancing years. This type of approach will ultimately allow definitive statements regarding the existance and significance of these disorders as a result of adult maturation.

Finally, it should be kept in mind that the identification and description of an auditory processing disorder in an adult does not present any new or unique problems. All evaluative tools previously described are available and useable with the adult population. Assuming a reasonable competence with speech and language, both speech and nonspeech stimuli should be able to be utilized without difficulty. Indeed, identification of auditory behaviors that deviate from the norm should be easier in the adult population since an age effect will probably not need to be considered in test interpretation (where CA and AA are below 70 years).

Much of the effort directed toward evaluating auditory processing and auditory perception has been through the use of test instruments or devices that are designed to give objective indications of the efficiency of an auditory system. An interesting inventory of hearing performance has been developed recently by Giolas et al. (1979). Basically, the individual assesses his own auditory performance by making judgments of his ability to understand speech in such settings as: face-to-face meetings, group settings, through standard communications systems, against noisy backgrounds, etc. It was not surprising that the correlation between self-ratings and ratings by spouses were far from unity (they ranged from 0–0.67), but it does raise a question as to which set of judges was more accurate. The important element is the development of a self-rating system, which samples perceived performance in a variety of settings; there are both diagnostic and rehabilitative implications for the use of such an inventory.

Labels have been attached to the problems associated with aging listening systems, e.g., presbycusis, phonemic regression, etc., but these labels do not offer clues as to the underlying factors that interfere with the transmission (routing) and perception (comprehension) of the spoken events. The concept of Auditory Age, based upon performance on the Wichita Auditory Fusion Test, suggests that the temporal integrity of the auditory system begins to decline in the fifth decade of life. This trend toward temporal deterioration increases in the sixth and seventh decades of life (see Fig. 14-3), as does individual variability as illustrated by the standard deviations in Fig. 14-3. Indeed, increasing variability is characteristic as one moves toward the extremes of age. This supports the concept of an Auditory Age (AA) based upon auditory fusion; for example, not all elderly persons exhibit the speech discrimination problems that one frequently associates with advancing age. These individuals would exhibit auditory fusion characteristics that are more like those of persons in the fifth or sixth decade of life; thus, having an AA of 40 or 50. The

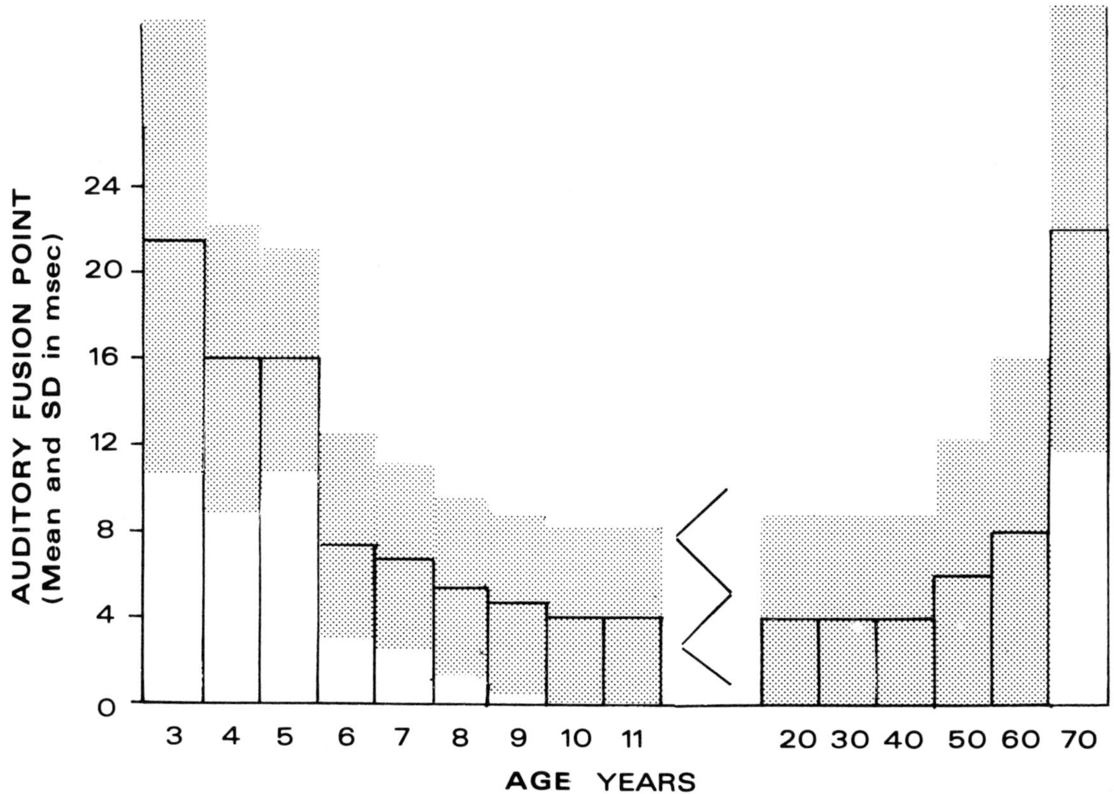

Fig. 14-3. A summary of mean auditory fusion points (for 1000 Hz stimulus tones and 60 dB SL) and standard deviations (shaded areas) for persons between two and eighty years of age (N=700).

value of making such determinations about temporal integrity may not lie in a preventive area but rather in the quality of counseling that can be done to help the individual understand his own limitations and to assist the family in compensating for those limitations.

The possibility of a prophylactic procedure may emerge when it is possible to detect the onset of deterioration. It is not possible at this time to define the specific roles of the vertical circuit of interneurons that are arranged in a particular spatial configuration and that transform cranial nerve data into a state of knowing or comprehending. It is known that experience leads to the proliferation of circuits of nerve cells, but it is also recognized that the rich array of incoming nerve fibers carrying sensory information into the spiny stellate cells in the cortex are lost with advancing age, and that the blood supply to the brain is altered with advancing age (Lassen et al., 1978).

Auditory fusion data have been collected on persons from the third year of life through the seventh decade of life (McCroskey and Davis, 1976; McCroskey and Schmitt, 1979). Figure 14-4 combines data from three investigations in order to illustrate an interesting relationship among normal, young learning disabled, and adult listeners with a mean age of 73 years. Auditory fusion data have been collected on normal, reading-disordered (McCroskey & Kidder, 1980) and trainable mentally retarded (Schroder & McCroskey, 1975), and in none of these sample populations has it been found that auditory fusion values vary according to the frequency of the stimulus tone employed. The only exceptions have been among the learning disabled and the elderly. With these two populations, it has been found that temporal processing is different for different frequencies. Considering the complex interrelationships of time, frequency, and intensity in an ongoing speech event, it would seem likely that a system handling different frequencies within a complex event in an inconsistent manner could lead to confusion. Indeed, the possibility of auditory reversals, not unlike reversals in reading, might be expected to occur.

Compressed speech has been used to stress the auditory system in order to detect processing difficulties. This is an acceptable practice, but for those who are interested in rehabilitative measures with aged persons, there is a need for information regarding the optimal rate at which the system can function. It is recommended that audiologists not only look for the rate which causes problems, but also look for those rates that can be handled comfortably by the listener. Expanded speech has already been shown to facilitate auditory comprehension by persons with reading disorders, mental retardation, and learning disabilities. The data are somewhat equivocal for elderly individuals (McCroskey & Schmitt, 1978), but the data seem clear that there are optimal age-related speaking

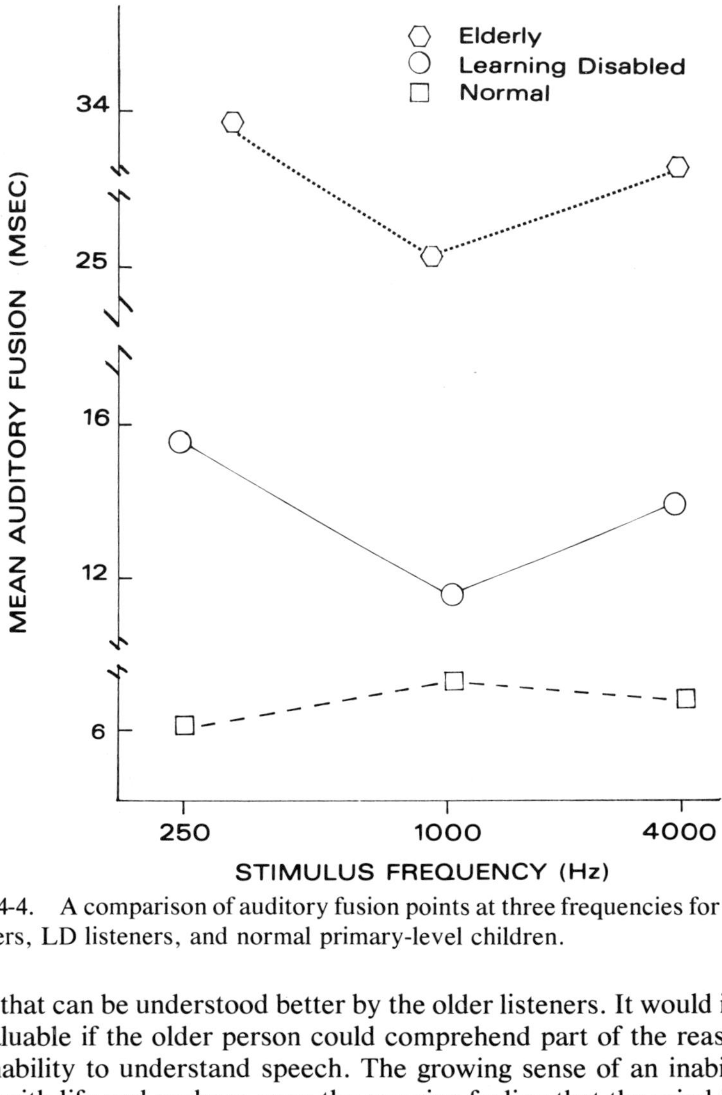

Fig. 14-4. A comparison of auditory fusion points at three frequencies for elderly listeners, LD listeners, and normal primary-level children.

rates that can be understood better by the older listeners. It would indeed be valuable if the older person could comprehend part of the reason for his inability to understand speech. The growing sense of an inability to cope with life and perhaps even the growing feeling that the mind is slipping can be altered if there is understanding of the alterations in temporal functions that have occurred. The elderly person is again in command of the environment by informing listeners that things must proceed more slowly if he is to understand fully. In addition, the counseling that can be done with families would be invaluable to the continued self-respect of the aging person in family and social settings.

The ability of the aging individual to deal with speech discrimination also received some attention. Gaeth, in 1948, described a phenomenon that he termed "phonemic regression." He discussed and described those aging individuals whose discrimination abilities were markedly poorer than would be anticipated on the bases of pure-tone audiograms. Since that time, phonemic regression has been considered to be at least a part of the auditory syndrome affecting many aging individuals.

Kasten and Thomas (1978), however, examined a group of hearing-impaired individuals over the age of 70 who would be described, by conventional test procedures, as displaying phonemic regression. They also presented to these aging individuals conventional monosyllabic word discrimination tests accompanied by a structured positive or negative reinforcement schedule relative to their performance. They found that reinforcement, reflecting either good or poor performance, functioned to improve discrimination scores by approximately 30 percent. Seventeen of the 18 subjects demonstrated a significant improvement of performance under both reinforcement schedules, and test–retest evaluation revealed essentially identical performance levels. Kasten and Thomas suggested that phonemic regression, as typically defined, appears to be an auditory manifestation of a nonauditory deficit. They postulated that increased motivation, increased attention, presence of reinforcement, increased interest, or a combination of these factors were responsible for the improvement observed over the conventional test scores. In short, phonemic regression appears to be, at least in part, a function of the test environment rather than actual performance ability.

Jerger and Hayes (1977) pointed out a decreasing ability on the part of older individuals to respond correctly to synthetic sentences at 0 dB message-to-competition ratio as opposed to conventional monosyllabic words, with the deficit increasing with increasing age. Of particular interest is the fact that their aging subjects tended to respond more like individuals with central auditory pathologies than any other group of subjects. It might be hypothesized from the data of Jerger and Hayes that the aging individuals, with the synthetic sentence task, tended to function as though they possessed a form of auditory processing disorder.

Indeed, Kasten (1979), Hull (1979), and McCroskey (1979) have suggested, on the bases of the available literature, that many aging individuals tend to function auditorily in a manner that is strikingly similar to that of the learning-disabled child. Additional research will be needed to verify their observations. It should be apparent, however, when we review the performance of aging individuals on the auditory fusion task and on selected speech processing tasks, that the performance of aging persons does demonstrate some real similarities with the performance of the young learning-disabled individuals (see Fig. 14-4).

For a number of years, these authors have been totally disenchanted with the word "presbycusis" as a disorder description. The use of the word presbycusis implies that all aging individuals are affected with the same auditory disorder. It is highly probably that aging individuals experience the same multiplicity of auditory problems experienced by the total younger population. The task of the audiologist is to devise a speech protocol, possibly similar to that of Jerger and Hayes, that will allow a distinguishing differentiation among the various disabilities.

SUMMARY

The authors have attempted to provide an overview of auditory processing from the seventh month of gestation through the seventh decade in chronological age. At the ends of the scale, it has been demonstrated that listening systems develop or decay rapidly and possibly in accordance with the kinds of acoustic stimulation they receive. Communicative interactions between neonates and adults emerge early. It has been emphasized that the trend toward detection of disorders, rather than assessment of processing behaviors, is in need of change. Finally, the presumed inadequacies of the aging ear may be looked at in a different way and lead to more effective counseling and rehabilitation.

REFERENCES

Adamson, W., & Adamson, K. *A handbook for specific learning disabilities,* New York: Gardner Press, 1979.

ASHA Subcommittee on Impedance Measurement. Guidelines for acoustic immittance screening of middle-ear function. *ASHA,* 1979, *21,* 283–288.

Bartoshuk, A. K. Human neonatal cardiac acceleration of sound: habituation and dishabituation. *Perceptual and Motor Skills,* 1962, *15,* 15–27.

Bartoshuk, A. K. Human neonatal cardiac responses to sound: a power function. *Psychonomic Science,* 1964, *1,* 151–152.

Bates, E., Camaioni, L., & Volterra, V. The acquisition of performatives prior to speech. *Merrill-Palmer Quarterly,* 1975, *21,* 205–226.

Batteau, D. W. The role of the pinna in human localization. Final report, contract N123—(60540) 35401A, United States Naval Ordnance Test Station, China Lake, California, 1964.

Beasley, D. S., Maki, J. E., & Orchik, D. J. Children's perception of time-compressed speech on two measures of speech discrimination. *Journal of Speech and Hearing Disorders,* 1976, *41,* 216–225.

Berlin, C. I. New developments in evaluating central auditory mechanisms. *Annals of Rhinology and Laryngology,* 1976, *85,* 833–841.

Berlin, C. I., & Lowe, S. S. Temporal and dichotic factors in central auditory testing. In J. Katz (Ed.), *Handbook of clinical audiology.* Baltimore: Williams and Wilkins Company, 1972, pp. 280–312.

Bocca, E., & Calearo, C. Central hearing processes. In J. Jerger (Ed.), *Modern developments in audiology*. New York: Academic Press, 1963, pp. 337–370.

Bradford, L. J. Respiration audiometry. In L. J. Bradford (Ed.), *Physiological measures of the audio-vestibular system*. New York: Academic Press, 1975, pp. 249–317.

Brunt, M. The staggered spondaic word (SSW) test. In J. Katz (Ed.), *Handbook of clinical audiology*. Baltimore: Williams and Wilkins, 1972, pp. 334–356.

Brunt, M. The staggered spondaic word test. In J. Katz (Ed.), *Handbook of clinical audiology*. Baltimore: Williams and Wilkins, 1978, pp. 262–275.

Bryan, T., & Bryan, J. *Understanding learning disabilities*. Sherman Oaks, California: Alfred Publishing Company, 1975.

Burns, G., & Watson, B. Factor analysis of the revised ITPA with underachieving children. *Journal of Learning Disabilities*, 1973, *6*, 371–376.

Butler, K., Hedrick, D., & Manning, C. *Composite Auditory Perceptual Test*. Hayward, California: Alameda County School Department, 1973.

Butterfield, G. An extended version of modification of sucking with auditory feedback. Working Paper #43, Bureau of Child Research Laboratory, Children's Rehabilitation Unit, University of Kansas Medical Center, 1968.

Butterfield, E. C., & Cairns, G. F. Discussion summary—infant reception research. In R. Schiefelbusch, & L. Lloyd (Eds.), *Language perspectives–acquisition, retardation, and intervention*. Baltimore: University Park Press, 1974, pp. 75–102.

Calearo, C., & Lazzaroni, A. Speech intelligibility in relation to the speed of the message. *Larngoscope*, 1957, *67*, 410–419.

Carlin, M., & Kasten, R. *Listening skills of children in regular and learning disability classrooms*. Paper presented before the American Speech and Hearing Association, Chicago, Illinois, 1977.

Chapman, L. F., Symmes, D., & Halstead, W. C. Auditory flutter fusion in patient with cortical abalations. *Journal of Comparative Physiology and Psychology*, 1955, *48*, 421–425.

Chomsky, C. *The acquisition of syntax in children from 5 to 10*. Cambridge, Massachusetts: The M.I.T. Press, 1969.

Clements, S. A new look at learning disabilities. In L. Tarnopol (Ed.), *Learning disabilities: introduction to education and medical management*. Springfield; Charles C. Thomas, 1969, pp. 31–40.

Clifton, R. K., Graham, F. K., & Hatton, H. M. Newborn heart rate response and response habituation as a function of stimulus duration. *Journal of Experimental Child Psychology*, 1968, *6*, 265–278.

Condon, W. S., & Sander, L. W. Getting the rhythm of human speech. *Science News*, 1974, *105*, 21.

Cramer, H. L. & Talambiras, R. P. The braided-speech method of time-compressing speech. In E. Foulke (Ed.), *Proceedings of second Louisville conference on rate and/or frequency controlled speech*. Louisville, Kentucky: University of Louisville, 1971, pp. 206–218.

Cuda, R. A. *Analysis of speaking rate, syntactic complexity and speaking style of public school teachers*. Unpublished thesis, Wichita State University, Wichita, Kansas, 1976.

Davis, H. Principles of electric response audiometry. *Annals of Otology, Rhinology, and Laryngology*, Supplement 28, 1976, *85*, 1–96.

Devens, J. S., Hoyer, E. A., & McCroskey, R. L. Technical note: an apparatus for exploring auditory localization. *Journal of the American Audiological Society*, 1976, *2*, 68–70.

Devens, J. S., Hoyer, E. A. & McCroskey, R. L. Dynamic auditory localization by normal and learning disability children. *Journal of the American Audiological Society*, 1978, *3*, 172–178.

Divenyi, P. L., & Hirsh, I. J. Some figural properties of auditory patterns. *Journal of the Acoustical Society of America,* 1978, *64,* 1369–1385.

Dix, M. R. & Hallpike, C. S. The peepshow technique for pure tone audiometry in young children. *British Medical Journal,* 1947, *2,* 719–723.

Downs, M. P., & Sterritt, G. M. Identification audiometry for neonates: a preliminary report. *Journal of Auditory Research,* 1964, *4,* 69–80.

Drichta, C. E. *The relationship of psycholinguistic ability and the rates of preferred listening, speaking, and comprehension to age and sex.* Unpublished doctoral dissertation, Wichita State University, Wichita, Kansas, 1976.

Duane, D. A neurologic perspective of central auditory dysfunction. In R. Keith (Ed.), *Central auditory dysfunction,* New York: Grune & Stratton, 1977, pp.1–42.

Duker, S. *Time-compressed speech: an anthology and bibliography in three volumes.* Metuchen, New Jersey: The Scarecrow Press, 1974.

Dunn, L. *Exceptional children in the schools.* New York: Holt, Rinehart and Winston, 1973.

Eilers, R. E., Wilson, W. R., & Moore, J. J. Developmental changes in speech discrimination in infants. *Journal of Speech and Hearing Research,* 1977, *20,* 766–780.

Eimas, P., Siqueland, E., Jusczyk, P., & Vigorit, J. Speech perception in infants. *Science,* 1971, *171,* 303–306.

Ewing, I. R., & Ewing, A. W. G. The ascertainment of deafness in infancy and early childhood. *Journal of Laryngology and Otology,* 1944, *59,* 309–333.

Fairbanks, H., Everitt, W. L., & Jaeger, R. P. Method for time or frequency compression-expansion of speech. *Transactions of the Institute of Radio Engineers, Professional Group on Audio,* 1954, *AU-2,* 7–12.

Faires, S. L., & McCroskey, R. L. Effect of body position upon acoustic reflex in human newborns. *Journal of Allied Health and Behavioral Science,* 1978, *1,* 50–70.

Flowers, A., Costello, M. & Small, V. *Flowers-Costello test of central auditory abilities.* Dearborn, Michigan: Perceptual Learning Systems, 1973.

Friedlander, B. Z. Receptive language development in infancy. *Merrill-Palmer Quarterly of Behavior and Development,* 1970, *16,* 7–51.

Fröding, C. A. Acoustic investigation of newborn infants. *Acta Otolaryngologica,* 1960, *52,* 31–40.

Fulton, R. T. A program of developmental research in audiologic procedures. *Journal of the Kansas Speech and Hearing Association,* 1971, *11,* 25–30.

Gaeth, J. *A study of phonemic regression in relation to hearing loss.* Unpublished doctoral dissertation, Northwestern University, Chicago, Illinois, 1948.

Garcia-Bellido, A., Lawrence, P. A., & Morata, G. Compartments in animal development. *Scientific American,* 1979, *241,* 102–110.

Gerber, S. *Audiometry in infancy.* New York: Grune and Stratton, 1977.

Gidoll, S. H. Qualitative determination of hearing to audiometric frequencies in the electroencephalogram: preliminary report. *Archives of Otolaryngology,* 1952, *55,* 597–601.

Giolas, T. G., Owens, E., Lamb, S. H., & Schubert, E. D. Hearing performance inventory. *Journal of Speech and Hearing Disorders,* 1969, *44,* 169–195.

Goldman, R., Fristoe, M., & Woodcock, R. *Test of auditory discrimination.* Circle Pines, Minnesota: American Guidance Service, 1970.

Hammill, D., & Bartel, N. *Teaching children with learning and behavior problems* 2nd ed. Boston: Allyn and Bacon, 1978.

Hardin, M., & Kasten, R. *Auditory capabilities of children in learning disabled classrooms.* Paper presented before the Kansas Council for Exceptional Children, Wichita, Kansas, 1976.

Haring, N., & Bateman, B. *Teaching the learning disabled child.* Englewood Cliffs, New Jersey: Prentice-Hall, 1977.

Horowitz, F. D. *Mothers and infants and the development of communicative competence.* Paper given before the Convention of the Kansas Speech and Hearing Association, Overland Park, Kansas, 1979.

Hoverston, G. H., & Moncur, J. P. Stimuli and intensity factors in testing infants. *Journal of Speech and Hearing Research,* 1969, *12,* 687–702.

Hull, R. *Aging and auditory disorders.* Paper presented before the Aspen Symposium on Communication problems of the aging, Aspen, Colorado, 1979.

Jaffee, B. F. History and physical examination for evaluating hearing loss in children. In B. B. Jaffee (Ed.), *Hearing loss in children.* Baltimore: University Park Press, 1977, pp. 152–181.

Jerger, J., & Hayes, D. Diagnostic speech audiometry. *Archives of Otolaryngology,* 1977, *103,* 216–222.

Jerger, J., & Jerger, S. Clinical validity of central auditory tests. *Scandinavian Journal of Audiology,* 1975, *4,* 147–163.

Johansson, B., Wedenberg, E., & Westin, B. Measurement of tone response by human foetus. *Acta Otolaryngologica (Stockholm),* 1964, *57,* 188–192.

Kaplan, E. L. The role of intonation in the aquisition of language. Doctoral dissertation, Cornell University, Ithaca, New York, 1969.

Kasten, R. *The current status of hearing aids and the elderly.* Paper presented before the Aspen symposium on communication problems of the aging, Aspen, Colorado, 1979.

Kasten, R., & Griffin, B. *Auditory processing of meaningful speech in the presence of competing message in normal children and children exhibiting learning disabilities.* Paper presented before the Convenion of the American Speech and Hearing Association, Atlanta, 1979.

Kasten, R., & Thomas, P. *A study of auditory discrimination abilities among aging individuals.* Unpublished paper, 1978.

Katz, J. The use of staggered spondaic words for assessing the integrity of the central auditory nervous system. *Journal of Auditory Research,* 1962, *2,* 327–337.

Katz, J. The SSW test—an interim report. *Journal of Speech and Hearing Disorders,* 1968, *33,* 132–146.

Katz, J. Differential diagnosis of auditory impairments. In R. Fulton & L. Lloyd (Eds.), *Audiometry for the retarded.* Baltimore: Williams and Wilkins, 1970, pp. 97–124.

Katz, J., & Illmer, R. Auditory perception in children with learning disabilities. In J. Katz, (Ed.), *Handbook of clinical audiology.* Baltimore: Williams and Wilkins, 1972, pp. 540–563.

Katz, J. *The SSW test manual.* Brentwood, Missouri: Auditec of St. Louis, 1973.

Katz, J. The staggered spondiac word test. In R. Keith (Ed.), *Central auditory dysfunction.* New York: Grune and Stratton, 1977, pp. 103–128.

Katz, J. The effects of conductive hearing loss on auditory function. *ASHA,* 1978, *20,* 879–886.

Katz, J. *Age related changes in central auditory function.* Paper presented before the Aspen Symposium on Communication Problems of the Aging, Aspen, Colorado, 1979.

Kirk, S., McCarthy, J., & Kirk, W. *Illinois test of psycholinguistic abilities.* Champaign, Illinois: University of Illinois Press, 1968.

Konkle, D. F., Beasley, D. S., & Bess, F. H. Intelligibility of time-altered speech in relation to chronological age. *Journal of Speech and Hearing Research,* 1977, *20,* 106–115.

Kurdzeil, S., & Noffsinger, D. *Performance of cortical lesion patients on forty percent and sixty percent time-compressed speech materials.* Paper presented before the American Speech and Hearing Association, Detroit, Michigan, 1973.

Lassen, N. A., Ingvar, D. H. & Skinhøj, E. Brain function and blood flow. *Scientific American,* 1978, *239,* 62–71.

Lev, A., & Sohmer, H. Sources of averaged neural responses recorded in animal and human subjects during cochlear audiometry. *Archiv für Klinishe und Experimentelle Ohren-Nasenund Kehlkopfheilkunde,* 1972, *201,* 79–90.

Lewis M., & Freedle, R. Mother–infant dyad: the cradle of meaning. In P. Pliner, L. Krames, & T. Alloway (Eds.), *Communication and affect: language and thought.* New York: Academic Press, 1973, pp. 127–155.

Lloyd, L. L., & Cox, B. P. Behavioral audiometry with children. In M. Glasscock (Ed.), Sensorineural hearing loss in children. *Otolaryngologic Clinics of North America,* 1975, *8,* 89–107.

Lyons-Ruth, K. Bimodal perception in infancy: response to auditory-visual incongruity. *Child Development,* 1977, *48,* 820–827.

Mann, L., Goodman, L., & Wiederholt, J. *Teaching the learning-disabled adolescent.* Boston: Houghton-Mifflin Company, 1978.

Martin, F. N. *Pediatric audiology,* Englewood Cliffs, New Jersey: Prentice-Hall, Inc., 1978.

Matzker, J. Two new methods for the assessment of central auditory functions in case of brain disease. *Annals of Otology, Rhinology, and Laryngology,* 1959, *68,* 1185–1187.

McCroskey, R. L. *Effects of bone conducted side tone upon speech intelligibility.* Paper given before American Speech and Hearing Association, Cincinnati, Ohio, 1957.

McCroskey, R. L. Preschool training. In I. S. Fusfeld (Ed.), *A Handbook in readings in education of the deaf and post school implications.* Springfield, Illinois: C. C. Thomas, 1967a, pp. 56–61.

McCroskey, R. L. Early education of infants with severe auditory impairments. *Proceedings of International Conference on Aural Education of the Deaf:* Vol. 2, Washington, D. C.: The Volta Bureau, 1967b, pp. 1891–1905.

McCroskey, R. L. Some characteristics of Temporal Auditory Behavior Among Elderly Persons. In M. Henoch (Ed.), *Aural rehabilitation for the elderly.* New York: Grune and Stratton, 1979, pp. 149–168.

McCroskey, R. L., & Bell, M. M. An annotated bibliography of publications on testing hearing of infants. *Volta Review,* 1965, *67,* 548–592.

McCroskey, R. L., & Cory, M. W. *Duration discrimination by normal children from three to sixteen years of age.* Paper given before American Speech and Hearing Association, Denver, Colorado, 1968.

McCroskey, R. L., & Cory, M. W. An Annoted Bibliography of Publications on Testing the Hearing of Infants: II. *Volta Review,* 1969, *71,* 27–33.

McCroskey, R. L., & Davis, S. M. Auditory Fusion: Developmental trends. Scientific Exhibit, American Speech and Hearing Association, Houston, Texas, 1976.

McCroskey, R. L., & Deines, R. R. An annotated bibliography of testing the hearing of infants. *Volta Review,* 1974, *76,* 436–444.

McCroskey, R. L., & Devens, J. S. Acoustical Characteristics of public school classrooms constructed between 1890 and 1960. In J. Mowrey (Ed.), *Proceedings of the technical program. NOISEXPO.* Bay Village, Ohio: Acoustical Publications, 1975, pp. 101–104.

McCroskey, R. L., & Hagler, P. *Auditory comprehension of rate-altered nonsense words.* Paper given before American Speech and Hearing Association, Las Vegas, Nevada, 1974.

McCroskey, R. L., & Herman, N. Some effects of certain auditory experiences upon responsiveness of human neonates. *Journal of the Kansas Speech and Hearing Association,* 1971, *11,* 68–76.

McCroskey, R. L., & Kidder, H. C. Auditory fusion among learning disabled, reading disabled, and normal children. *Journal of Learning Disabilities,* 1980, 13, 69–76.

McCroskey, R. L., & Nelson, N. W. The Wichita studies on comprehension of rate-controlled speech. In E. Foulke (Ed.), *Proceedings of the third Louisville conference on rate controlled speech.* New York: American Foundation for the Blind, Inc., 1975, pp. 60–81.

McCroskey, R. L., & Schmitt, J. F. A pilot study of auditory temporal processing among elderly adults. Final report: Wichita State University grant, 3399–22. Wichita, Kansas, 1978.

McCroskey, R. L., & Thompson, N. W. Comprehension of rate controlled speech by children with specific learning disabilities, *Journal of Learning Disabilities,* 1973, *6,* 29–35.

McCroskey, R. L., & Thompson-Nelson, N. W. *Comprehension of rate-controlled sentences of varying linguistic complexity by children with reading disorders.* Paper given before the American Speech and Hearing Association, Detroit, Michigan, 1973.

McCroskey, R. L., & Yarbrough, S. B. *An auditory screening procedure for human neonates.* Paper given before the American Speech and Hearing Association, Chicago, Illinois, 1967.

Meltzoff, A., & Moore, M. D. Initiation of facial and manual gestures by human neonates. *Science,* 1977, *198,* 75–78.

Meyen, E. *Exceptional children and youth, an introduction.* Denver: Love Publishing Company, 1978.

Miltenberger, G. E. Central auditory testing with peripheral hearing loss. *Archives of Otolaryngology,* 1978, *104,* 11–15.

Mokotoff, B., Schulman-Galambos, C., & Galambos, R. Brainstem auditory evoked responses in children. *Archives of Otolaryngology,* 1977, *103,* 38–43.

Morse, P. A. Infant speech perception: a preliminary model and review of the literature. In R. Schiefelbusch, & L. Lloyd (Eds.), *Language perspectives–acquisition, retardation, and intervention.* Baltimore: University Park Press, 1974, pp. 19–53.

Mueller, K., Kasten, R. *Auditory processing skills of reading disabled children.* Paper given before the American Speech and Hearing Association, San Francisco, California, 1978.

Murphy, K. P. Development of hearing in babies. *Hearing News,* 1961, *29,* 9–11.

Murphy, K. P. Ascertainment of deafness in children. *Panorama,* 1962, *3,* 4.

Myers, P., & Hammill, D. *Methods for learning disorders.* New York: John Wiley & Sons, 1969.

Myklebust, H. *Auditory disorders in children.* New York: Grune and Stratton, 1954.

Nakazima, S. A comparative study of the speech development of Japanese and American English in childhood. *Studies in Phonology,* 1962, *3,* 27–39.

Nelson, N. W. Comprehension of spoken language by normal children as a function of speaking rate, sentence difficulty, and listener age and sex. *Child Development,* 1976, *47,* 299–303.

Nelson, N. W., & McCroskey, R. L. Comprehension of Standard English at varied speaking rates by children whose major dialect is Black English. *Journal of Communication Disorders,* 1978, *11,* 37–50.

Newby, H. A. *Audiology.* New York: Appleton-Century-Crofts, 1958.

Newby, H. A. *Audiology* (2nd Ed.). New York: Appleton-Century-Crofts, 1972.

Northern, J. L., & Downs, M. P. *Hearing in children.* Baltimore: Williams and Wilkins Co, 1978.

Ohta, F., Hayashi, R., & Morimoto, M. Differential diagnosis of retrocochlear deafness: binaural fusion test and binaural separation test. *Journal of International Audiology,* 1967, *6,* 58–62.

Omer, J. The incidence of hearing impairment in students identified as learning-disabled. *Language, Speech, and Hearing Services in Schools,* 1972, *3,* 34–40.

O'Neill, J., & Oyer, H. *Applied audiometry.* New York: Dodd, Mead and Co., 1966.

Orchic, D., & Oeschlager, M. *Time-compressed speech discrimination in children: its relationship to articulation ability.* Paper given before the American Speech and Hearing Association, Las Vegas, Nevada, 1974.

Ormson, K., & Williams, D. *Central auditory function as assessed by time-compressed speech with elementary school age children having articulation and reading problems.* Paper given before the American Speech and Hearing Association, Washington, D.C., 1975.

Ross, M., & Giolas, T. *Auditory management of hearing-impaired children.* Baltimore: University Park Press, 1978.

Ross, M., & Lerman, J. A picture identification test for hearing-impaired children. *Journal of Speech and Hearing Research,* 1970, *13,* 44–53.

Ross, M., & Lerman, J. *Word intelligibility by picture identification.* Pittsburgh: Stanwix House, 1971.

Rupp, R. Evaluation of auditory perception in children. *Audiology: An audio journal for continuing education,* 1978, *3,* 7.

Salamy, A., & McKean, C. M. Postnatal development of human brainstem potentials during the first year of life. *Electroencephalography and Clinical Neurophysiology,* 1976, *40,* 148–426.

Salvia, J., & Ysseldyke, J. *Assessment in special and remedial eduction.* Dallas: Houghton-Mifflin, 1978.

Schroder, T., & McCroskey, R. L. *Comprehension of time-expanded speech by mentally retarded children.* Paper given before the American Speech and Hearing Association, Chicago, Illinois, 1975.

Schubert, G., Meyer, R., & Schmidt, J. Evaluation of the noise subtest of the Goldman-Fristoe-Woodcock test of auditory discrimination. *Journal of Auditory Research,* 1973, *13,* 42–44.

Simmons, F. B. Automated screening test for newborns: the crib-o-gram. In B. F. Jaffe (Ed.), *Hearing loss in children.* Baltimore: University Park Press, 1977, pp. 89–98.

Snow, J., Rintelmann, W., Miller, J., & Konkle, D. Central auditory imperception. *Laryngoscope,* 1977, *87,* 1450–1471.

Spelt, D. K. Conditioned responses in the human fetus in utero. *Psychological Bulletin,* 1938, *35,* 712–713.

Spralding, J. E., & Reid, M. J. An operant audiometric procedure for difficult-to-test patients. *Journal of Speech and Hearing Disorders,* 1968, *33,* 236–247.

Stein, B. E. & Schuckman, H. Effects of sensory restriction upon the responses to cortical stimulation in rats. *Journal of Comparative Physiology and Psychology,* 1973, *82*, 182–187.

Seuss, Dr. (pseud) *The Cat In The Hat.* New York: Beginner Books, 1957.

Suzuki, T., Ogiby, Y., & Takei, T. Basic properties of conditioned orientating reflex audiometry. *Minerva Otolaringologica,* 1972, *22*, 181–186.

Suzuki, T., Kamijo, Y., & Kuichi, W. Auditory test of newbord infants. *Annals of Otolaryngology,* 1964, *73*, 914–923.

Sweitzer, R. S. Audiologic evaluation of the infant and young child. In B. F. Jaffe (Ed.), *Hearing loss in children.* Baltimore: University Park Press, 1977, pp. 101–131.

Tallal, P. An experimental investigation of the role of auditory temporal processing in normal and disordered language development. In A. Caramazza & E. B. Zurif (Eds.), *Language acquisition and language breakdown.* Baltimore: Johns Hopkins University Press, 1978, p. 50.

Tanaka, Y., & Arayama, T. Fetal responses to acoustic stimuli. *Practica Oto-rhino-laryngologica,* 1969, *31*, 269–273.

Tarnopol, L. *Learning disabilities: introduction to education and medical management.* Springfield: Charles C. Thomas, 1969.

Tervoort, B. Personal communication, 1964.

Thompson, M., & Thompson, G. Response of infants and young children as a function of auditory stimuli and test methods. *Journal of Speech and Hearing Research,* 1972, *15*, 699–707.

Thompson, G., Wilson, W. R., & Moore, J. M. Application of visual reinforcement audiometry (VRA) to low-functioning children. *Journal of Speech and Hearing Disorders,* 1979, *44,* 80–90.

Topp, S. Abnormal central auditory processing. In B. F. Jaffe (Ed.), *Hearing loss in children.* Baltimore: University Park Press, 1977, pp. 490–501.

Trehub, S. E. Infant's sensitivety to vowel and tonal contract. *Developmental Psychology,* 1973, *9*, 91–96.

Turkewitz, G. The development of lateral differentiation in the human infant. In S. Dimond & D. Blizard (Eds.), *Evolution and lateralization of the brain.* New York: New York Academy of Science, 1977.

van Uden, A. *A world of language for deaf children, part 1.* St. Michielsgestel, The Netherlands: Institute for the Deaf, 1968.

Webster, D. B., & Webster, M. Neonatal sound deprivation affects brain stem auditory nuclei. *Archives of Otolaryngology,* 1977, *103*, 392–396.

Wedenberg, E. Auditory tests in newbord infants. *Acta Otolaryngologica,* 1956, *46*, 446–461.

Weir, R. H. Some questions on the child's learning of phonology. In F. Smith & G. Miller (Eds.), *The genesis of language.* Cambridge, Massachusetts: M.I.T. Press, 1966, pp. 153–168.

White, E. Children's performance on the SSW test and Willeford battery: interim clinical data. In R. Keith (Ed.), *Central auditory dysfunction.* New York: Grune and Stratton, 1977, pp. 319–340.

Willeford, J. Central auditory function in children with learning disabilities. *Audiology and Hearing Education*, 1976, *2*, 12–20.

Willeford, J., & Billger, J. Auditory perception in children with learning disabilities. In J. Katz (Ed.), *Handbook of clinical audiology.* Baltimore: Williams and Wilkins, 1978, pp. 410–425.

Willston, J. *A new look at evoked potentials.* Paper given before the American Auditory Society, San Francisco, California, 1978.

Wilson, W. R., & Diefendorf, A. Personal communication, 1979.

Woodcock, R. *Goldman-Fristoe-Woodcock auditory skills test battery–technical manual.* Circle Pines, Minnesota: American Guidance Service, 1976.

Yoder, D. *Communication behavior in severely and profoundly handicapped children: assessment and intervention.* Paper given before the Kansas Speech and Hearing Association, Overland Park, Kansas, 1979.

Debara L. Tucci, M. S.
Roger A. Ruth, Ph. D.
Zahrl G. Schoeny, Ph. D.

15

Calibration for Speech Audiometry

The importance of calibration as a means of specifying the physical properties of the stimulus and of evaluating the stability of test instrumentation used in auditory assessment is well established. Quantification of the speech stimulus with its transient properties and spectral complexity requires a rigorous approach to calibration. Implementation of a comprehensive calibration procedure for use in speech audiometry requires that the clinician: (1) understand the need for specification of the speech signal, and related instrumentation in the test environment; (2) adhere to the current standards; and (3) develop uniform and functional clinical calibration procedures to insure the accuracy of speech test results and transfer of clinical information between facilities.

The focus of this chapter will be practical in nature in order to provide a calibration program that will both fulfill the requirements of the current and proposed standards and offer supplemental procedures for conditions not dealt with in these standards.

INSTRUMENTATION

The typical test apparatus which may be used for speech audiometry is illustrated in Fig. 15-1. As shown here, the input stimulus is modified by an amplifier, attenuator, and switching network. In the case of the live

We wish to thank David Lilly, William Melnick, and Ernest Nilo for their helpful comments on an earlier draft of this chapter.

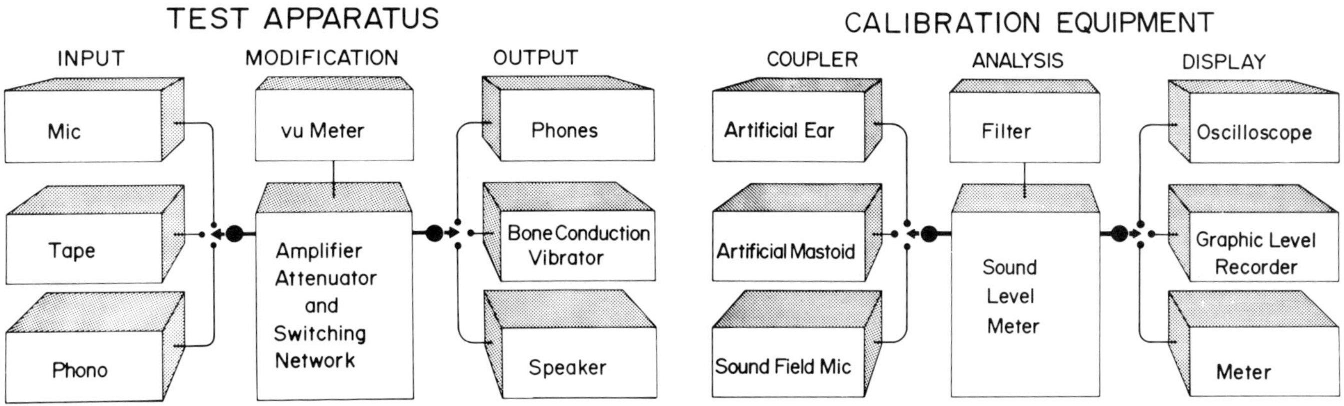

Fig. 15-1. Block diagram of instrumentation used in speech audiometry, including appropriate calibration equipment. Use of the bone vibrator for presentation of the speech signal and of the artificial mastoid for such calibration is an optional component of this system. In addition, it is recognized that the storage oscilloscope and graphic level recorder are not readily available in most clinical facilities, and may be considered optional items for minimal calibration requirements. These instruments, however, are necessary for an exhaustive calibration of the speech signal.

voice (microphone) presentation, the standard volume indicator (VU meter) serves to monitor the talker's vocal output during the test procedure. Transducer characteristics are evaluated through the measurement of signal properties at each of the output sources conventionally used for speech testing, including earphone, loudspeaker, and, in some cases, bone vibrator.

Instrumentation used for physical calibration of this equipment is shown in the second portion of the figure. The sound level meter is an essential component of the system used for signal assessment. In order to make measurements from the earphone or loudspeaker, the sound level meter is coupled to the signal output source by means of the artificial ear or soundfield microphone, respectively. For bone vibrator calibration, an artificial mastoid is coupled to the transducer and the output is measured in voltage or decibel change. This may be accomplished with either a sound level meter or voltmeter. The artificial ear and artificial mastoid are devices that simulate the critical characteristics of the human ear or the human headbone for signals presented via the corresponding transducers. An adequately standardized coupler for soundfield measurements is not available. However, the KEMAR anthropometric manikin (Burkhard & Sachs, 1975), with the Zwislocki coupler (Zwislocki, 1971) may be used for this purpose. The oscilloscope and graphic level recorder, although not necessary for routine calibration, will allow visualization of the speech signal, and thus permit a more thorough evaluation of acoustical output.

The typical sound level meter is composed of a microphone, amplifier, optional weighting network and external filter connection, RMS rectifier, and display meter. Weighting networks provide standardized frequency responses for use in acoustical measurements. The "A" weighting was designed to approximate the response of the normal-hearing human at relatively low sound pressure levels, and is the most widely used of the weighting networks. External filter sets provide the capability of analyzing spectral composition, which is especially important for evaluation of speech signals. Furthermore, use of the external filter is necessary for measurement of ambient noise levels in the test environment.

Microphones used for soundfield measurements are designed and factory calibrated for either free-field, pressure, or random-incidence response. The type of microphone used will dictate the manner in which it is properly placed in the soundfield relative to the sound source. For example, for measurement of sound pressure levels the free-field-type microphone should be pointing directly at the sound source, while the pressure type microphone should be oriented perpendicular to sound flow. When making measurements in the soundfield, the sound level meter is held

Table 15-1
Partial Listing of Most Commonly Encountered Sources of Instrumentation Error Associated With Speech Audiometry and Most Significant Resultant Signal Alterations

	Potential Sources of Error	Potential Problems
Tape	Bias	Distortion, poor S/N ratio change in frequency response
	Head alignment	Loss of signal, distortion
	Capstan	Wow, flutter, noise
	Tape speed	Overall shift in frequency
	Magnitized heads	Distorition, poor S/N ratio change in frequency response
Phono	Needlewear	Altered spectrum, distortion, excessive record wear
	Tracking force	Change in fidelity of reproduction, record wear, faulty tracking
	Turntable speed	Frequency displacement
Mic	Aging and damage to internal components	Reduction of signal, change in frequency response, distortion
Control circuity	Attenuator nonlinearity	Inaccurate intensity output
	Noisy attenuator and/or switching network	Spurious transients and unwanted noise
	Aberrant amplification	Distortion, poor S/N ratio change in frequency response
Phones	Aging and damage to internal components	Reduction of signal, change in frequency response, distortion
	Deterioration of cushion	Change in acoustical coupling
Bone vibrator	Damaged electro-mechanical element	Reduction of signal, change in frequency response, distortion
Speaker	Damage to internal components	Loss of signal, change in frequency response, distortion
	Crossover network	Loss of signal, change in frequency response, distortion
Connecting cords	Faulty wiring	Impropoer polarity, reduction of signal, hum
	Break in continuity from use	Intermittency or loss of signal, static

away from the body, and always with the microphone between the tester and the sound source.

Many of the abnormal stimulus conditions revealed by thorough calibration may be due to either improper use or connection of equipment, or damage due to equipment wear. These problems may be avoided by attending to potential sources of error as part of the general calibration procedure. Some of these possible error sources, and their resulting signal alterations are listed in Table 15-1.

CALIBRATION PROCEDURES

Procedures outlined in this section are based on the proposed document of the American National Standards Institute, "Specification for Audiometers" (working draft, May 1978), unless otherwise noted. Although these are not official, but proposed standards, they are discussed here because they address the issues involved in speech calibration more thoroughly than the present standards, and are likely to be accepted as the new standard in the near future. Furthermore, the procedures outlined here also meet the requirements of the current ANSI S3.6-1969 standard.

Ambient Noise Measurements

The ambient noise levels in the test environment must be assessed according to the American National Standards Institute "Criteria for Permissable Ambient Noise during Audiometric Testing" (ANSI S3.1-1977). Table 15-2 provides the maximum acceptable noise levels as measured with an octave band filter for both the ear covered (earphone testing) and

Table 15-2
Maximum Permissable Ambient Noise Levels in dB SPL (*re* 20 μPa) as Per the ANSI S3.1-1977 Standard for Speech Audiometry With Soundfield, Bone Vibrator (Unoccluded Ear), and Earphone Presentation

Test Tone Frequency (Hz)	250	500	750	1000	1500	2000	3000	4000
Octave band levels: ears uncovered	18.5	14.5	12.5	14.0	10.5	8.5	8.5	9.0
Octave band levels: ears covered (earphones)	23.0	21.5	22.5	29.5	29.0	34.5	39.0	42.0

ear uncovered (soundfield and bone conduction testing, with unoccluded ear) conditions. Although it is important to measure noise levels at all frequencies used for pure-tone testing, noise in the frequency bands above 4000 Hz need not be considered for speech testing. In the event that octave band analysis is not available, it is possible to evaluate noise levels using the "A" weighting on the sound level meter, as discussed by Killion and Studebaker (1978).

Earphone Calibration

INTENSITY

Intensity calibration is accomplished by use of a 1000 Hz pure tone routed through the proper input channel (either microphone, phonograph, or tape player). The 1000 Hz calibration tone on the tape or disc recording is used for this purpose. A suggested procedure for calibrating the microphone circuit is as follows. The calibration signal is presented to the microphone through a standard earphone positioned approximately four to six inches from the audiometer microphone. This signal may be generated either by the second channel of a two channel audiometer or by a portable audiometer. The calibration tone is delivered to the audiometer microphone at a level of approximately 74 dB SPL as measured by a sound level meter.

When calibrating any of the three input sources, the VU meter is adjusted to zero. The sound pressure level developed within the artificial ear must be 12.5dB (± 3dB) above the standard reference value for a 1000 Hz pure tone. For example, with the audiometer attenuator adjusted to 70 dB HL, the output of a TDH-49 earphone should be 90 dB SPL (7.5 dB reference threshold), whereas the output of a TDH-39 earphone should be 89.5 dB (7.0 dB reference threshold). This same procedure should be completed for each input source used and for each earphone.

ATTENUATOR INTERVALS AND LINEARITY

The attenuator dial used for speech testing must have intervals of 2.5 dB or less. When compared to the designated difference between two successive dial readings, the measured sound pressure level difference should compare to within 1 dB or three-tenths of the dial interval, whichever is smaller. While electrical linearity measurements may be made throughout the range of attenuation, acoustical measurements of linearity typically may be obtained only to 40 or 50 dB HL, depending upon instrumentation used and the ambient environment.

While the standard specifically requires the capacity for a 2.5-dB dial interval, many audiometers in current usage attenuate only in 5-dB steps. In the event that 5-dB steps are used, the same criterion for calibration tolerances should be applied.

FREQUENCY RESPONSE

A specific requirement of the speech audiometer or speech circuit of a diagnostic audiometer is that it yield a relatively flat frequency response throughout the "speech range" of 250–4000 Hz. In the case of a recorded speech input (either tape recorder or phonograph), a standard recording of tones is used for the calibration procedure. With an attenuator setting of 100 dB HL or the maximum level of the audiometer, whichever is less, the output is measured at the earphone for the frequency range covered on the test tape or disc recording. The sound pressure levels at the earphone must not differ from that at 1000 Hz by more than ± 5 dB within the range from 200–4000 Hz.

In order to evaluate frequency response with a live-voice microphone, pure tones of 74 dB SPL are developed proximal to the audiometer microphone, at an orientation and distance recommended by the manufacturer for that specific microphone (approximately four to six inches). At each of the test frequencies, including 250, 500, 750, 1000, 2000, 3000, and 4000 Hz, the sound pressure level measured through the earphone must not differ from that at 1000 Hz by more than ± 5 dB.

OVERALL DISTORTION

Nonlinear distortion is the process by which the waveform of the signal output is altered relative to the signal input, and is manifest by the presence of energy at frequencies other than those of the original stimulus. Although intermodulation, transient, and harmonic distortion measurements should all be used to fully describe the presence of nonlinearities in the instrumentation (Beranek, 1949), only harmonic distortion measurements have been standardized for purposes of audiometric calibration.

The procedure for assessment of harmonic distortion in the speech audiometer is as follows. The input stimulus is a pure tone having no harmonic exceeding 1 percent of the amplitude of the fundamental frequency. With the signal input through the proper source, the VU meter is adjusted to zero and the output level of the sound level meter is noted. The level of the stimulus is then increased 9 dB as shown on the sound level meter. The VU meter in this case will be maximally deflected, thus insuring assessment of distortion at levels that may be associated with peak intensity of the speech signal. At the maximum output of the audiometer (not to exceed 120 dB SPL), harmonics of the following frequen-

Table 15-3
Approximate Values for Conversion of Decibel Difference Between Fundamental Frequency and Second Harmonic to Percent Distortion

Difference Between Fundamental and Second Harmonic (dB)	% Distortion	Difference Between Fundamental and Second Harmonic (dB)	% Distortion
40	1	29	3.6
39	1.1	28	4
38	1.3	27	4.5
37	1.4	26	5
36	1.6	25	5.6
35	1.8	24	6.3
34	2	23	7
33	2.2	22	8
32	2.5	21	9
31	2.8	20	10
30	3.2		

cies are measured: 250, 500, 1000, 2000, and 4000 Hz. No harmonic may exceed 3 percent of the amplitude of the fundamental. Table 15-3 provides approximate percentage harmonic distortion based on measured decibel difference.

EQUIPMENT GENERATED NOISE

Excessive equipment generated noise is easily identified with subjective listening checks. Because minimal levels of internally generated noise could interfere with threshold testing, however, it is important to follow the physical measurement procedure. Output level of the audiometer is measured with no signal input at an attenuator setting of 70 dB. This value must be at least 40 dB below the level measured for the 1000 Hz input signal. For example, if the output of a TDH-49 earphone is 90 dB SPL, the system noise should be no greater than 50 dB SPL with the signal removed.

Cross talk is the presence of unwanted signal in the earphone opposite the signal earphone. A supplemental procedure for the evaluation of cross talk is discussed in Appendix B to the proposed standard. This procedure is performed using six otologically normal subjects, having hearing thresholds of 10 dB or less for test frequencies of 250 through 4000 Hz. The earphone to which the signal is delivered is disconnected, and subjects are asked to indicate the presence of a signal in the connected earphone. No signal should be audible at a 50-dB dial setting, with the tone switch in both the normally on and normally off positions.

An alternative method not discussed in the standard is an electroacoustic check for measurement of cross talk. This can be accomplished by measuring the output of the nonsignal earphone in an acoustic coupler, while using appropriate isolation of the signal generating earphone.

MASKER INTENSITY, MASKER ATTENUATOR INTERVAL, AND LINEARITY

The clinician may utilize either a speech spectrum or broad band noise for masking the speech test signal. Speech noise is defined as noise having equal energy per cycle from 250 through 1000 Hz, with a 12 dB per octave slope from 1000–4000 Hz. These characteristics must be met to within ± 5 dB. The broad band signal should produce an output to within ± 5 dB of that at 1000 Hz across the frequency range of 250–6000 Hz.

Manufacturers of audiometric equipment are required to supply calibration data showing the masking effect for each signal provided and the corresponding sound pressure level. If these specifications are not available, masking effectiveness may be determined by subjective calibration of the masking stimulus. This is accomplished by using six or more subjects with otologically normal ears and speech reception thresholds equal to or better than 10 dB HL. The subjects' unmasked threshold is measured and masking is introduced to the same ear in sufficient quantity to shift the SRT by 5 dB. The mean unmasked SRT is then subtracted from the mean masker dial reading necessary to produce the 5-dB shift. For example, if 20 dB of masking is required to shift the SRT by 5 dB, and the unmasked threshold is 10 dB, the level which represents zero dB effective masking is 10 dB (20 dB masking dial reading minus 10 dB SRT).

The masking level dial must be adjustable in steps of 5 dB or less, and may be calibrated either in effective masking or sound pressure level. Calibration tolerances for accuracy of these levels are essentially the same as those described in the intensity and attenuator interval and linearity sections above.

Sound Field Calibration

Calibration for soundfield auditory assessment is often approached with less rigor than earphone calibration, presumably because of the many problems involved with specification of signal parameters in this environment. However, the frequent use of this test setting by many audiologists necessitates a thorough working knowledge of instrumentation characteristics and the signal output. Due to the absence of national standards for such calibration, it becomes the responsibility of the audiologist to formulate an effective program based on his or her interpretation of the relevant literature.

Previous investigations have shown that variations in test room and equipment characteristics and test procedures alter soundfield thresholds measured. Dissimilarities in values obtained by several investigators (Breakley & Davis, 1949; Tillman et al., 1966; Dirks et al., 1972; and Tillman et al., 1973) while attempting to define the earphone–soundfield relationship for SRT in normal-hearing subjects may be resolved, at least in part, by attention to these variables. Specifically, loudspeaker placement and room absorption qualities have been shown to affect threshold measurements. While resultant variations in threshold data are predictable as to direction, the magnitude of the difference is not always forseeable, and may for certain conditions exceed 10 dB (Dirks et al., 1972).

Given the complex nature of the acoustic environment, the establishment of standard reference values for soundfield testing does not seem as appropriate as the formulation of a standardized procedure for such calibration. Such a procedure must not be compromised by the lack of uniformity among individual test settings or by variations in threshold sound pressure levels due to methodological differences in intensity determination. The utilization of a biological calibration procedure in conjunction with the more typical electroacoustic measurements allows simultaneous consideration of all aspects of the acoustic environment as well as accurate determination of normative threshold.

An approach to soundfield calibration for speech testing is considered below in two steps. A biological calibration procedure is performed only as an initial assessment technique. The electroacoustic calibration is used both for initial calibration and subsequent routine calibration checks, and seves to monitor the system for possible changes.

BIOLOGICAL CALIBRATION

Biological calibration for speech audiometry may be accomplished according to the following procedure. The SRT is determined both under earphones and in the soundfield for five to ten normal-hearing subjects, and the means computed in dial reading. Mean values for the earphone and soundfield SRT are then compared to obtain the correction factor for soundfield testing. For example, if the mean earphone SRT is 5 dB, and the mean soundfield threshold is 10 dB, a difference of 5 dB is noted. Therefore, 5 dB dial reading represents 0 dB HL for the soundfield SRT. This procedure should be followed for each loudspeaker and each placement in the field where testing is completed.

In an appendix to the proposed ANSI standard it is recommended that, if two loudspeakers are used, they are to be placed between 40° and 60° azimuth to either side of the subject, while if one loudspeaker is utilized, this is located 0° azimuth relative to the listener. The use of the biological procedure described above will effectively assess the influence of any loudspeaker placement on the threshold. The use of an adjustment factor in hearing level rather than sound pressure level obviates the need for exact measurement of SPL at the subject's eardrum, which is impractical in the clinical setting.

ELECTROACOUSTIC CALIBRATION PROCEDURE: INTENSITY

As suggested in Appendix A to the proposed ANSI standard, intensity of the speech signal should be calibrated by means of a masking noise, either speech or broad band noise, and measured using a "C" weighting on the sound level meter. The measurements are typically carried out with the field microphone of the sound level meter positioned at a point analagous to the center of the average subject's head. Presentation of the calibration stimulus at levels of at least 70 dB HL will assure that measurements are not contaminated by environmental noise. This procedure should be followed for each loudspeaker and for each input source used. When tape and disc recordings are employed for stimulus presentation, it may be necessary to utilize the 1000 Hz tone provided for earphone calibration for sound field assessment, if a noise source is not available for this purpose. Measurement of sound pressure levels at points adjacent to the center reference position will give an idea of the variability associated with the use of this stimulus. See the above section for recommendations concerning the signal source for calibration of the live-voice speech circuit. Although it is recognized in the proposed standard that soundfield intensity levels will depend upon the individual characteristics of the environment, it is suggested that for loudspeaker placements of 40°–60° azimuth, the typical standard reference sound pressure level is 13 dB.

The lack of constraint on the subject's movement in the soundfield test environment naturally allows for a great amount of variability in distance and orientation of the listener relative to the sound source. For this reason, it is advisable to conduct a more extensive sound survey in the test room than is described in the proposed standard. Using a speech spectrum or broad band noise stimulus, intensity level measurements made at various discrete locations within the test room will allow the clinician to determine the amount of variability that is incorporated in the test results as a function of subject movement. Should the differences measured exceed the tolerance limits for soundfield intensity calibration, a chart showing comparative intensity levels within the room may be constructed for use in reporting test data. It is suggested that, should the tolerance limits set for calibration exceed 5 dB, this fact be reported along with the test information. Intensity levels measured for one stimulus presentation can differ by as much as 15 dB between locations within the test environment (Tucci, Ruth, & Schoeny, 1978).

FREQUENCY RESPONSE

The frequency response of the loudspeaker is measured using narrow bands of noise or warbled tones, which are input through each source used for speech stimulus presentation in the soundfield. Specifications for the introduction of these sources are the same as used for earphone calibration. The intensity level used for measurement of frequency response is not given in the standard. It is suggested, however, that a soundfield output level of 90 dB SPL be used for this purpose. This value is high enough to eliminate interference of ambient noise and low enough to eliminate problems with acoustical feedback when testing the live-voice circuit. It is recommended in the proposed standard that the output levels measured at a given soundfield position at 250, 500, 750, 1000, 2000, 3000, and 4000 Hz not differ from that of 1000 Hz by more than ± 10 dB.

In order to realistically assess the interaction between the loudspeaker and a specific acoustic environment, it is important that the frequency response of the loudspeaker be measured in the setting in which it is to be used. If the measured response does not meet specified tolerance limits, steps may be taken to alter the environment in a manner which will allow these requirements to be met (Dirks et al., 1972; Dirks et al., 1976).

ATTENUATOR INTERVALS, LINEARITY, OVERALL DISTORTION, EQUIPMENT-GENERATED NOISE

Due to the addition of instrumentation used for sound field testing (i.e. booster amplifier and loudspeakers) that could serve as sources of intensity variation, distortion and equipment noise the calibration procedures as described in the earphone calibration section should be repeated for each loudspeaker.

Calibration for Bone Conduction

The value of speech audiometry by bone conduction was first demonstrated by Goetzinger and Proud (1955). The clinical application of this technique has not been widespread, however, primarily due to problems of signal calibration. At present, no standard exists for calibration of the bone vibrator for speech audiometry. The difference in thresholds for air- and bone-conducted spondees appears to depend upon the type of bone vibrator and particular audiometer used. For this reason, it is essential to implement a subjectively based calibration procedure.

Biological calibration is accomplished by testing five to ten normal-hearing subjects for SRT both under phones and with a bone-conducted presentation. The difference between the two presentation modes will then serve as a dial reading correction factor for bone-conducted speech tests. In addition, a subjective indication of the fidelity of the speech signal delivered through the bone vibrator may be ascertained by obtaining measures of speech discrimination as a function of intensity. Barry and Gaddis (1978) found that speech discrimination for normal-hearing subjects remained essentially unchanged for the stimulus presentation range from 20–70 dB above threshold, after which a sharp reduction in speech discrimination was observed. This was attributed to a substantial increase in overall distortion of the signal measured at higher presentation levels.

Physical calibration of the bone vibrator is accomplished by use of an artificial mastoid and associated analysis and display instrumentation. General procedures for measurement of fidelity, linearity, and distortion of the bone vibrator should be based on those previously given in the earphone calibration section. Attention should be given to the measurements of harmonic distortion, as this becomes critical at suprathreshold levels for the bone conduction transducer. The extent and frequency of the calibration procedures for bone-conducted speech stimuli will depend upon the amount of usage made of this method of speech presentation.

SUMMARY

Calibration is a responsibility of the audiologist that is as critical as other aspects of test administration and interpretation. A suggested plan for calibration in speech audiometry has been given, which is modeled on existing and proposed standards. Included in the present calibration protocol is a procedure for biological assessment, for use in situations in which standards are not provided, or in which physical measurements alone are not adequate. The attempt here has been to provide the clinician with a practical calibration format that involves sufficient rigor to assure adequate control and specification of the speech signal in all test situations. For a more general discussion of calibration procedures, including pure-tone and noise-signal quantification, the reader is referred to Wilber (1978).

REFERENCES

American National Standards Institute. Specifications for audiometers. ANSI S3.6-1969. New York: American National Standards Institute, Inc., 1970.

American National Standards Institute. Criteria for permissable ambient noise during audiometric testing. ANSI S3.1-1977. New York: American National Standards Institute, Inc., 1977.

Barry, J., & Gaddis, S. Physical and physiological constraints on the use of bone conduction in speech audiometry. *Journal of Speech and Hearing Disorders*, 1978, *43*, 220–226.

Bernaek, L. *Acoustic measurement*. New York: John Wiley and Sons, 1949.

Breakley, M., & Davis H. Comparisons of thresholds for speech: word and sentence tests; receiver versus field and monaural versus binaural listening. *Laryngoscope*, 1949, *59*, 236–250.

Burkhard, M., & Sachs, R. Anthropometric manikin for acoustic research. *Journal of the Acoustical Society of America*, 1975, *58*, 214–222.

Dirks, D., Morgan, D., & Wilson, R. Experimental audiology. In C. Smith and J. Vernon (Eds.), *Handbook of auditory and vestibular research methods*. Springfield, Ill.: Charles C. Thomas, 1976, pp. 498–547.

Dirks, D., Stream, R., & Wilson, R. Speech audiometry: earphone and soundfield. *Journal of Speech and Hearing Disorders*, 1972, *37*, 162–176.

Goetzinger, C., & Proud, G. Speech audiometry by bone conduction. *Archives of Otology*, 1955, *62*, 632–635.

Killion, M., & Studebaker, G. A-weighted equivalents of permissable ambient noise during audiometric testing. *Journal of the Acoustical Society of America*, 1978, *63*, 1633–1635.

Proposed American National Standard for Audiometers, May 1978.

Stream, R., & Dirks, D. Effect of loudspeaker position on differences between earphone and sound field thresholds. *Journal of Speech and Hearing Research*, 1974, *17*, 549–568.

Tillman, T., Johnson, R., & Olsen, W. Earphone versus sound-field threshold sound-pressure level for spondee words. *Journal of the Acoustical Society of America*, 1966, *39*, 125–133.

Tillman, T., Olsen, W., Killion, M., & Block, M. *MAP versus MAF for spondees: nothing's really missing*. Paper given before the American Speech and Hearing Association, Detroit, Michigan, 1973.

Tucci, D., Ruth, R., & Schoeny, Z. *Sound field calibration: a suggested procedure*. Paper given before the American Speech and Hearing Association, San Francisco, California, 1978.

Wilber, L. Calibration, pure tone, speech and noise signals. In J. Katz (Ed.), *Handbook of clinical audiology* (2nd ed.). Baltimore: Williams and Wilkins Co., 1978, pp. 81–97.

Zwislocki, J. An earlike coupler for earphone calbration. Syracuse University: Laboratory Sensory Communication, Report LSC-S-9, 1971.

Editors' Note: The first fifteen chapters in this book were written by the major contributors as a state of the art of speech-associated measurements in audiology. As the historical reviews in many parts of this book suggest, speech audiometry and the use of speech materials have had a colorful evolution. All fifteen chapters have reviewed where we have been and where we now are in the field of speech audiometry. The next and final chapter—on new frontiers and new horizons—gives our esteemed, established scholars an opportunity to share with our readership their thoughts and philosophy on the direction that future speech audiological approached will take.

We are indebted to those whose brief statements are quoted in the pages that follow and who willingly volunteered to gaze into their professional crystal balls and predict, suggest, as well as nudge the direction of speech audiology in the future.

A Series of Predictive Discussions
by a Group of Established
Scholars in Audiology

16

Speech Protocols: New Frontiers and New Horizons

John J. O'Neill, Ph.D.

"Audiologists have been making increasing use of variations of speech audiometry to assist in the location of sites of lesion in the auditory system, as they relate to involvement of the cochlea, auditory pathways, and the auditory cortex. Thus, attention is being directed to the various parts of the processing system with not too much attention being paid to the nature of the response in terms of the stimulus material itself (confusions, distortions or omissions). Interest in speech audiometry today is more frequently being directed toward models of speech perception with emphasis upon such areas as storage and recall, memory, attention, auditory experience, and linguistic ability.

"As a result of such interest, speech audiometry will be undergoing changes in terms of manipulation of stimulus materials and the development of 'base line' responses that can be related to responses obtained by a sample of persons with normal hearing and the major hearing disorders.

"With the advent of tape cassettes and the increasing availability and capability of computers, it is now becoming relatively simple to manipulate signals and store subject responses. At the same time, with increasing interest being paid to the linguistic aspects of stimulus materials, it would seem that new types of stimulus materials will be developed.

"Major changes that can be introduced involve changes in the temporal aspects of the stimulus or in the basic nature of the signal, i.e., filtering or compressing of signal, or masking with white noise or speech. What is needed at this stage is a detailed specification of task performance, i.e., what areas of speech perception does the examiner consider of importance in the evaluation. Before developing a test battery, there should be a specification of task performance.

"The following areas of testing interest (based upon a rather broad model of speech perception) can be evaluated through the use of the indicated types of speech audiometry.

1. Presentation of time-compressed materials with various pause times or various time sequences for the purpose of evaluating time-processing abilities.
2. Presentation of distorted materials (filtered, noise masked, competing messages, and time-interrupted materials) for the purpose of evaluating attentional factors.
3. Presentation of sentence materials (single and multiple) and sentences with selected, deleted words to test value of context-listening ability in terms of syntax and semantics and auditory memory; in essence, testing the intellectual activities associated with the perception of speech.

"The above tests will allow the examiner to relate the difficulties experienced by a listener to specific processes of speech perception (temporal processing, attention, memory, and previous auditory experience) as well as language comprehension.

"With the use of tape cassettes, a variety of stimulus materials can be easily presented, and with the use of computer programming, variations in the stimulus material can be easily presented in a controlled manner. Also, with the use of the computer it is possible to store responses to assist in the development of base line data or to store data to develop one's own clinic norms."

Moe Bergman, Ed.D.

"Present-day speech audiometry grew out of the 'articulation' tests in which telephone engineers used spoken-test material to evaluate various transmission systems. The use of similar tests to assess hearing began in earnest during World War II in the armed forces aural rehabilitation centers, where the Speech Reception Threshold and the 'discrimination score' were added to pure-tone audiometry in the diagnostic test battery.

"The current developmental thrust is for speech–hearing tests designed to expose central auditory system dysfunction. It is based upon the principle that higher level auditory functions involve perceptual behavior far more complex than can be revealed by the standard clinical tests. The result has been the introduction of such tests as the competing sentences, SSW, low-pass filtered speech, dichotic listening, and the interaural alternation of a message. Such tests are additions to the existing test battery for the medically oriented diagnosis of pathology. It is safe to predict that as they prove their value they will be refined and that new, even more sophisticated diagnostic speech–hearing tests will be added as behavioral measures to accompany the advancing technology of electrical response audiometry.

"I believe, however, that speech audiometry has even broader future applications, both inside and outside the medical and audiology clinics, to meet developing needs such as the following.

"We are now awakening to the realities of the inexorable changes in the makeup of our populations. The median age has been climbing steadily from young adulthood into the middle years. Whereas our present standards for communication systems (e.g., the telephone) and for acceptable noise interference are predicated primarily upon the performance of normally hearing young adults, who are in the prime period for speech perception, findings emerging from our studies and those of others show convincingly that when the listening conditions are less than optimal, listeners who have reached their middle years begin to suffer demonstrable deficits in speech perception compared with young adults.

"A second rapidly growing group of listeners with special needs is the result of the expanding migration of peoples from one culture and language to another. Much of this linguistic transplantation involves adults who are replacing the language they learned during their most plastic early years by one in which, our findings suggest, they will never completely overcome their deficits in the perception of noise-competed or distorted speech, regardless of their apparent fluency in their second-learned language.

"I believe, therefore, that we will be addressing our interests and skills, in the near future, to more sophisticated diagnostic speech–hearing tests, which stress the various parts of the complex auditory system selectively, and that a number of us will become deeply engaged in exploring the many aspects of speech perception as they affect different segments of our changing population. We will be looking more critically at the linguistics of the speech signal—that is, at its phonology, syntax, and semantics—as they affect its perception; at the acoustics of its transmission, and of the listening environment; and at the linguistics (language and dialect history), physiology (state of the auditory system) and psychology (vigilance, memory, cognitive abilities, etc.) of the listener. As specialists in auditory reception and perception, we will be concentrating heavily on that which is of prime importance in audition, the perception of speech."

Charles I. Berlin, Ph.D.

"While some may suggest that future developments in speech audiometry should include studies of connected speech, dichotic speech tasks, other filtered or low-redundancy messages, etc., I would like to suggest that the future in speech audiometry lies with the use of 'speech-like signals' (e.g., tone sweeps and glides) and synthetic speech in which the acoustic parameters of the signal can be meticulously controlled. Using these highly controlled acoustic stimuli, dichotic or monotic fusion studies, temporal integration studies, and basic principles pertaining to the acoustic building blocks of speech perception can be investigated. For example, I envision a predictive test of speech perception being based, in part, on a listener's ability to resolve brief tone glides. The technology necessary to perform such studies and generate such stimuli routinely is only now becoming available and promises to be part of the wave of the future.

"Other procedures will probably include broader, more linguistically oriented philosophies. Thus, stimuli will vary syntactical structure, morphology, or even pragmatics. Related to this, of course, will be speech perception tasks for younger children.

"We have few, if any, objective techniques for studying speech perception, at present. Electrophysiologic techniques which use the 'contingent negative variation' or some other late component-evoked potential may, in the future, enable us to get better insight into patients' central awareness of speech stimuli. At present, the extension of electrophysiology into speech research has been limited, and I suspect that this useful step is not long in coming."

David P. Goldstein, Ph.D.

"It is possible to sort out at least three different purposes for using speech stimuli in audiological testing. One is to evaluate the auditory system in order to make a statement about the site of lesion. The second is to evaluate the communication problem of the hearing-impaired individual. A third reason for the use of speech relates to the hearing aid selection process. I wish to confine my remarks about future trends and needs to this selection process.

"Audiology is entering into a new era in terms of hearing aid dispensing and managing the rehabilitation needs of the hearing impaired. It is appropriate at this time that we examine where we have been and where we need to go relative to the use of speech in the hearing aid selection process.

"Early speech stimuli were developed out of a need to test telephone communication systems and were borrowed by audiology for use in clinical evaluations. The percent correct intelligibility score, which originally reflected the 'articulation' capabilities of the electronic transmission system, now became a metric of the patient's discrimination ability. In other words, although the format did not change, the listener who was originally a part of the measurement system now became the focus of the measurement. Under this scheme the person is viewed as a transmission line—specify input, score output. In the case of the hearing aid evaluation, the listener was conceptually joined with the aid as a transmission system, while at the same time serving as a device to read out data used to make a decision about amplification.

"This format has persisted even as a wide variety of different speech simuli were introduced over the years. The approach represented the state of the art at the time and was logical in evaluating a passive transmission system such as a telephone. The human being, however, is not a passive transmission system, but can make insightful judgments about different qualitative dimensions of the acoustic signal being received and even dynamically adjust to signal qualities.

"One goal of a rehabilitation regimen which incorporates the hearing aid is to achieve user acceptance of the amplification system. This involves more than consideration of the percent correct discrimination score read out by a listener wearing various hearing aids. It also involves the person's auditory experiences and biases as well as his psychological status. An evaluation procedure must take cognizance of this fact.

"It may become necessary for audiology to grapple with the idea that although good speech perception ability is a necessary ingredient in communication, it is not necessarily a precise predictor of personal preference. An example of this fact can be found in whispered speech. This can be intelligible but not considered acceptable.

"What is needed is a formal procedure that either directly or indirectly probes the affective responses to acoustic properties unique to each hearing aid system. The approach must provide for quantification of response data, allow for statistical tests of significance underlying clinician decision processes, and satisfy the test of reliability and validity. It must also satisfy the constraints inherent in using a procedure in a clinical setting. Broadly speaking, quality judgment procedures fit into the discussed category. Available techniques, however, are relatively primitive, especially in so far as clinical utility is concerned.

"Past research efforts have stressed development of new and better speech stimuli. Future work may need to be focused at a more basic level. What is needed is a new approach which emphasizes precision in predicting user acceptance of a particular hearing aid system best suited to meet his [or her] needs."

Marion P. Downs, M.A.

"Standard speech reception tests have been greatly maligned in the last few years—and with just cause. No longer are we sanguine enough to believe that PB lists, sentence tests, rhyme tests, etc. differentiate between hearing aids or show fine differences between ears. The SSI tests have been a major breakthrough, and dichotic speech testing has given us new insights into speech processing. But whether there are any routine, clinical speech reception tests that are fine enough to make the distinctions that we need is questionable. At the heart of the problem is the awesome complexity of the speech reception process and its language substrate. For too long we audiologists have considered speech reception only as a series of acoustic events that impinge upon the ear and are isomorphically spewed out by the listener. We have ignored the intermediary processing that is accomplished by the brain and how that processing differs between individuals. What we must consider is the fact that people develop different strategies for understanding the language that speech transmits, and we can perhaps never eliminate those strategies from participation in the speech reception process.

"However, the standard tests do discriminate gross differences in the way people hear speech. These gross differences can be of infinite value to medical diagnosis and in understanding individuals' hearing needs in the clinical situation. For example, their very grossness makes for more reliable diagnosis of such entities as Meniere's disease, acoustic tumors, hearing loss due to syphillis, and phonemic regression. The deviations in such cases are usually dramatically larger, and consequently they will pinpoint the diagnosis unequivocally. The clinician or surgeon is thus given added confidence in his decision regarding medical or surgical management. And where large deviations emerge in presbycusis cases, they highlight the need for careful hearing aid fitting and for a strong aural rehabilitation program.

"So, in our zeal to develop finer speech reception tests, let us not discard the standard traditional procedures that still serve us well in many situations. Our attitude toward them should be that they screen out those individuals who require more detailed diagnosis, much as any screening test identifies children or people at risk for a problem. Viewed in this light, standard speech reception tests are as fine a tool as we have in our armamentarium."

Phillip A. Yantis, Ph.D.

"The perception of speech stimuli as meaningful information is fundamental to normal interhuman communication. The audiologist's greatest service to the hearing impaired is to enhance this critically important skill. We therefore must place a high priority on the development and use of techniques yielding valid, reliable information about the processing of speech. Although input through the auditory channel is of obvious interest, we must continue to focus on the potential of visual and tactile stimulation as well.

"This book amply demonstrates that there has been no paucity in the creation of word and sentence lists available to the audiologist for prognostic, rehabilitative, or diagnostic purposes. Even so, relatively little of this material is being utilized in clinical practice. The methods and techniques by which these stimuli are applied remain quite variable in clinical practice. Although many avenues of future research and development in this area can be specified, three appear to me to be of primary importance.

"First, we must continue to define those methods of lowering speech redundancy (time–frequency–intensity distortion and S/N variations) having the highest sensitivity potential in the evaluation of differential auditory function. Recorded stimuli representing the many available approaches must be presented to single subjects having well-defined sensorineural pathology so that comparative data can be analyzed. Such research necessitates the utilization of patient populations in large medical centers having highly structured diagnostic services. Comparative data of this type will continue to be needed by the clinician as the number of techniques having diagnostic potential enlarges.

"Secondly, standards must be developed which define certain of the conditions under which speech intelligibility is assessed. Evidence is now ample to show that even though similar lists of words are used, test difficulty can vary significantly with changes in the acoustic characteristics uttered by various talkers, with variations in carrier phrases, with differences in methods used for lowering redundancy, and with variations in intensity level. Lists of sounds, words, or sentences are *not* tests of speech intelligibility or discrimination. Only recorded versions of such lists, presented under similiar acoustic conditions, meet sufficient tests of equivalency to be called standard stimuli. Guidelines promoting consisiency in test administration, carefully defined in ANSI standards for pure-tone and speech sensitivity measures, are still lacking for speech tests conducted at supra-threshold levels. It is time to close this gap.

"A third major need relates to the continued lack of materials and techniques having satisfactory predictive value in the assessment of social efficiency. A reliable test having specific relevance to the day-by-day communicative capacity of a person would have numerous applications. Such a metric might finally allow us to abandon our dependence on tonal sensitivity as the primary means of assessing handicap and disability. Certainly, the rehabilitative potential of speech audiometry would be significantly improved.

"This brief synopsis by no means exhausts the many lucrative paths of investigation that should be pursued in assessing the auditory processing of speech. Serious questions remain regarding the most desirable degradation effects of background noise on primary acoustic signals, and how these conditions should vary depending on the clinician's goal. Means by which the potential effects of peripheral auditory dysfunction can be reduced or eliminated in evaluating the central auditory nervous system must continue to be explored. There are many others. The complex nature of the acoustic stimulus we call 'speech,' coupled with the extremely variable status of linguistic information in storage, often lead to unique difficulties in reseach design, most of which do not occur when tonal stimuli are being processed. Although challenging in conception, the outcome of such investigations will continue to have a direct impact on audiologic practice."

David M. Lipscomb, Ph.D.

"Speech audiometry has many applications, as has been pointed out in this book. It is my feeling that the greatest use to which one might put speech audiometry is in the assessment of cochlear reserve. With few exceptions, impairments of the external and middle ear are problems of amplitude rather that of perception. Since the reception and perception of speech stimuli by persons with classical conductive hearing impairments are routinely unimpaired, speech testing serves a less important role and the response to pure tones is of primary importance.

"I shall concentrate on the value of speech audiometry in increasing our feel for the impact of cochlear pathologies. One premise for my desire to base heavy weighting on the speech test for cochlear pathologies is that recent evidence has accumulated in which it is becoming clear that the pure-tone hearing test is inadequate as an index of cochlear reserve, i.e. the degree to which the hair cell populations are impaired or intact (Bredberg & Hunter-Duvar, 1975; Lipscomb, 1975a; Lipscomb, 1975b; Lipscomb, Axelsson, Vertes, Roettger, & Carroll, 1977). In view of this insight, it is becoming increasingly important that better use be made of testing materials which put the inner ear to the test so that various degrees of pathological development will yield differential response results. We must return to the concept that the purpose of audiometric evaluations is first and foremost the *testing* of auditory function. By definition, to 'test' means to put the ear to the test. Using pure tones, the simplest signal the ear is ever asked to handle does not always *test* the ear. Speech stimuli presented live voice via very expensive high fidelity equipment by a well-trained, highly intelligible speaker is not universally a *test* of auditory capabilities. Speech-in-noise, filtered speech, difficult speech, competing signals, etc., are approaches which have offered some benefits in the past. I look for additional developments in this direction for the future so that we can test for cochlear reserve more effectively.

"A second hope I have for the future of speech audiometry bears on the resurrection of using some form of articulation function testing. Earlier in this book, the articulation function was discussed as a means whereby one can observe changes in speech intelligibility as a function of stimulus amplitude. Because articulation functions are time consuming and place rather severe demands on the stamina of patients, their use in routine clinical audiometric activities have been largely discontinued. However, the information one can glean from a completed articulation function makes it possible that we can have given away too much clinical utility in the name of clinical expediency. Of course, it would be nice if something akin to the articulation function can be obtained more rapidly and with less effort by the patient. This appears to be another fruitful avenue of investigation for our field. If the longer, more rigorous testing for articulation function is the best avenue we have for evaluating one's cochlear reserve, then, it behooves us to remember to use that approach when it is essential that we discover the true limits of hearing for our patients."

REFERENCES

Bredberg, G., & Hunter-Duvar, I. Behavioral tests of hearing and inner ear damage. In W. D. Keidel & W. D. Neff (Eds.), *Handbook of sensory physiology*. Vol. V: *Auditory system: physiology (CNS), behavioral studies, psychoacoustics*. Berlin: Springer-Verlag, 1975, pp. 261–306.

Lipscomb, D. M. What is the audiogram really telling us? Part I: Audiometrics versus cochlear damage. *Maico Audiological Library Series,* 1975a, *Vol. 13,* Report 5.

Lipscomb, D. M. What is the audiogram really telling us? Part II: Sensorineural hearing losses. *Maico Audiological Library Series,* 1975b, *Vol. 13,* Report 6.

Lipscomb, D. M., Axelsson, A., Vertes, D., Roettger, R., & Carroll, J. The effect of high level sound on hearing sensitivity, cochlear sensorineuroepithelium and vasculature of the chinchilla. *Acta Otolaryngologica,* 1977, *84,* 44–56.

Victor P. Garwood, Ph.D.

"The most extensive use of speech audiometry today is for hearing aid evaluation procedures. A growing dissatisfaction with speech testing suggests that speech lacks precision, is not measurable, and involves variables that are confounding. As a result, noise bands as stimuli are in limited use for those cases able to respond to threshold and suprathreshold measurements. A recent pilot study of 'successful' hearing aid users showed, however, that 80 percent of the subjects were unsuccessful in meeting even minimal criteria set up by the experimenter's noise band hypothesis (Goldberg & Sandlin, 1978). This finding indicated to me that if the criterion for fitting is usable hearing in everyday life, noise bands will never be a procedure of choice, despite its claimed objectivity.

"The problem, as I see it, lies in the many unknown parameters of the human speech stimulus. The use of 'synthetic' sentences seems to be of significance as a language, rather than a speech variable. By slightly changing the focus, using synthesized speech might be a more plausible goal for research. Early efforts by Lawrence (1955) with synthesized speech demonstrated a method by which the relative parameters of time, pitch, intensity, and quality might be systematically changed. He demonstrated that manually drawn variations of his own spectrographic recording yielded strikingly different speech patterns by systematically changing the format structure, speed, and buzz and hiss controls. The reproduction of this sample was readily discernible as being significantly different than his own characteristic speech. Alas, all recordings had a British accent!

"The technique does, however, point the way toward developing speech materials that can be controlled. With the tremendous increase in sophistication of computer sciences, it seems but a small step to utilize this information to generate stimulus materials that would lead to the development of microamplification circuits that in turn could be sensitive to the nuances of the parameters of phoneme production, prosody, inflectional patterns, and other cogent parameters of speech.

"Although multifiltered devices are now on the market, they have been designed on the basis of acoustic rather than linguistic models. Given that such devices might be more bulky than those designed today to be inconspicuous, if the signal were linguistically accurate, the fetish of a 'hidden' hearing aid might be overcome. Circuits can be designed to effectively separate input from output at early level and from a body worn 'black box' if necessary.

"Current research on extended high-frequency hearing aid circuits for certain types of profound hearing loss also suggests that these neglected frequencies also may supply important cues for speech comprehension.

"As a final comment, may I add my name to a number of audiologists who favor the elimination of the use of hearing level (HL) as a reference and that we return to the use of sound pressure level. The current level of sophistication even now denies the time-consuming task of converting this artificial portrayal of the auditory response. Obviously, a practical use of this level will demand further study of more accurate calibration methods to establish reliable threshold, comfort, discomfort and discrimination reference points."

REFERENCES

Goldberg, H., & Sandlin, R. E. Minimal standards for hearing aid performance. *Board of Medical Quality Assurance, State of California,* August, 1978.

Lawrence, W. The use of synthetic speech as an aid to the study of speech apprehension—a lecture demonstration. *Signals Research and Development Establishment, Christ Church, England, 1955.*

James T. Yates, Ph.D.

"What does the future hold for speech audiometry? For the short-term answer, we can probably look to the present. As a profession, we have shown remarkable resistence to change in the face of good and compelling reasons to do so.

"The Martin and Forbis (1978) study of the status of audiometric practice showed that the majority of all audiologists who responded use speech material that were developed years ago. For Speech Reception Threshold testing, 82.9 percent use either the CID-W-1 or W-2 lists and an additional 5.1 percent use the Harvard Test no. 9. Most of those who use the latter present live voice and not the recorded versions. So, 88 percent of the practicing audiologists sampled use materials developed no later than 1952 (Hirsh et al., 1952).

"For discrimination testing, 70.7 percent use the CID W-22, and 12 percent use the CNC tests in one form or another, with most preferring the Tillman and Carhart (1966) version. If we are to accept the Martin and Forbis study as typical of contemporary practice, most audiologists use ST and discrimination materials that are decades old, over 30 years (old) in the case of the W-1, W-2, and W-22 word lists. Moreover, the materials were developed originally for purposes other than the evaluation of human hearing.

"The discrimination test word lists were subject to immediate and continuing criticism (see, for example, Hirsh et al., 1952; Silverman & Hirsh; Lehiste & Peterson, 1959; Newby, 1972). Consensus is that, among other things, single words simply are not analogous to real life communication situations.

"Recently, the standard materials and procedures for Spondee Threshold testing has been 'endorsed' by the ASHA, which adopted 'Revisions of the Central Institute for the Deaf W-1 Auditory Tests' in the

ASHA 'Guidelines for Determining the Threshold Level for Speech' ASHA, 1979, *21*, 356). Although guidelines are not mandates, those of us who believe in standardization will find it difficult to resist adopting ASHA's recommendation. No doubt when a guideline for determining discrimination ability appears, it will specify (recommend?) the CID W-22s used by 70.7 percent of the respondents to the Martin and Forbis study.

"Although I normally am a supporter of guidelines, it is too early in our profession's development to engage in 'hardening of the categories.' I firmly endorse guidelines as a means of illustrating accepted procedures or supporting minimum standards of accuracy and performance, but they have, as their opponents argue, a tendency to become policy. They represent de facto acceptance of the present methods when a large segment of the professional population agrees that these measures (at least the discrimination tests) are in dire need of the attention of qualified researchers.

"Another circumstance that mitigates against rapid and/or startling progress in this field is the fact that our profession is in the midst of a vast expansion of its technological base. New techniques and innovations are being developed and adapted that are capturing the attention of the clinician-researchers. With BERA, ECOG, implants, Biofeedback, etc., there is no glamour in the mundane procedures. Worse, there is no sense of urgency to replace or refine existing techniques. It is like Mark Twain's supposed comment about the weather: everyone complains about speech audiometry, but nobody does anything about it. Although a number of new tests have appeared over the years, none has gained any measure of acceptance. The research that is being reported now seemingly is directed toward detection of dysfunction deep within the CNS.

"In the future, we will see a re-emergence of research and resulting tests in response to broad empahsis on the restoration process.

"The present word discrimination tests probably are adequate to demonstrate most types of gross disturbances in auditory function. However, for finer judgments, such as attempting to demonstrate everyday communication function, for demonstrating differences in hearing aid performance, and for diagnostic-evaluative uses, they are clearly inadequate. The use of word lists simply does not equate to everyday auditory tasks. In fact, word discrimination tests may be no more predictive of functional ability than are judgments based upon evaluation of the pure-tone audiogram by an experienced clinician.

"The problems with the tests cannot be alleviated by modification of existing materials. First, we must abandon the communication testing model of the past and redefine both the approach and the mechanism for evaluating the response.

"Although a segment of the profession will cling tenuously to the

ST–PB approach, an increasingly large percentage will move to a bilevel system, retaining the PB concept as a screening or identification tool. SRT (ST) tests for adults won't change much because there will not be a great perceived need.

"For children, we may see an approach utilizing a series of short tests to evaluate simple discrimination and figure ground perception, closure, attention span, sequencing, and other important features of auditory perception. The long needed prescriptive diagnostic materials will appear. For smaller children, we may see the use of tests that stress phonemic perception and discrimination. The new awareness of hearing aid evaluation procedures for children should result in refined techniques for assessing aided performance.

"The term Speech Discrimination Testing should give way to a new title that recognizes the complex nature of the auditory system and of its evaluation. Speech stimuli will still be the choice for the text materials but series of subtests using phrases, sentences, pivot phrases, etc., will allow the tester to apply item analysis to the patient's performance to assess the contributions of numerous variables to the 'score'. A composite score and subtest scores will reflect overall function and individual skills functions. Subtests probably will be limited in scope initially, but eventually will apply to bilingual/bicultural and other special populations.

"Advances in speech test materials will be accompanied by greater sophistication of instrumentation. Multiple-channel instruments will allow more realistic recreation of real environments in controlled conditions. The ability to control phase, for example, would allow application of MLD concepts to speech audiometry. Computer-controlled AGC circuitry could make use of recorded speech practical as a competing stimulus. Additional circuitry or speech tests to demonstrate binaural fusion may become commonplace in hearing aid evaluation, especially in binaural fittings.

"New tests and materials may result from a massive coordinated effort among research laboratories and foundations, philanthropic organizations, and possibly government support. There is little likelihood of private enterprise developing such materials because there is little incentive to do so. It is more probable that a national center will be developed that will generate research such as this on a wide scale."

REFERENCES

ASHA Committee on Audiometric Evaluation, Guidelines for determining the threshold level for speech. *ASHA,* 1979, *21,* 353–356.

Hirsh, I. J., Davis, H., Silverman, S. R., Reynolds, E. G., et al., Development of materials for speech audiometry. *Journal of Speech and Hearing Disorders,* 1952, *17,* 321–337.

Lehiste, I., & Peterson, G. Linguistic considerations in the study of speech intelligibility, *Journal of the Acoustical Society of America,* 1959, *31,* 280–286.

Martin, F. & Forbis, N. The present status of audiometric practice: a follow-up study, *ASHA,* 1978, *20,* 531–533.

Newby, H. A. *Audiology* (3rd ed.). New York: Appleton-Century-Crofts, 1972, p. 127.

Silverman, S. R., & Hirsh, I. J. Problems related to the use of speech in clinical audiometry. *Annals of Otology, Rhinology, and Laryngology,* 1955, *64,* 1234–1244.

Tillman, T. W., & Carhart, R. An expanded test for speech discrimination utilizing CNC monosyllabic words. Northwestern University Test Number 6, Technical Report, SAM-TR-66-55. Brooks Air Force BAse, Texas: USAF School of Aerospace Medicine, Aerospace Medical Division (AFSC), 1966.

Index

Page numbers in *italics* indicate illustrations.

a
b
c
d
e
f
g
0 h
1 i
8 2 j